Orthopaedic Knowledge Update
Pediatrics

American Academy of Orthopaedic Surgeons

Orthopaedic Knowledge Update
Pediatrics

Edited by
B. Stephens Richards, MD

Developed by the
**Pediatric Orthopaedic Society
of North America**

Published by the
American Academy of Orthopaedic Surgeons
6300 North River Road   Rosemont, IL 60018

Orthopaedic Knowledge Update: Pediatrics

American Academy of Orthopaedic Surgeons

The material presented in *Orthopaedic Knowledge Update: Pediatrics* has been made available by the American Academy of Orthopaedic Surgeons for educational purposes only. This material is not intended to present the only, or necessarily best, methods or procedures for the medical situations discussed, but rather is intended to represent an approach, view, statement, or opinion of the author(s) or producer(s), which may be helpful to others who face similar situations.

Some drugs and medical devices demonstrated in Academy courses or described in Academy print or electronic publications have Food and Drug Administration (FDA) clearance for use for specific purposes or for use only in restricted settings. The FDA has stated that it is the responsibility of the physician to determine the FDA status of each drug or device he or she wishes to use in clinical practice, and to use the products with appropriate patient consent and in compliance with applicable law.

Furthermore, any statements about commercial products are solely the opinion(s) of the author(s) and do not represent an Academy endorsement or evaluation of these products. These statements may not be used in advertising or for any commercial purpose.

The material contained in this volume was submitted as previously unpublished material, except in the instances in which credit has been given to the source from which some of the illustrative material was derived.

First Edition
Copyright © 1996 by the
American Academy of Orthopaedic Surgeons

ISBN 0-89203-159-X

Acknowledgments

Contributors

Michael D. Aiona, MD
Shriners Hospital for Crippled Children,
  Portland Unit
Portland, Oregon

Stephen A. Albanese, MD
Associate Professor, Orthopedic Surgery
SUNY Health Science Center at Syracuse
Department of Orthopedic Surgery
Syracuse, New York

George S. Bassett, MD
Chief, Pediatric Orthopaedic Surgery
Washington University School of Medicine
St. Louis Children's Hospital
St. Louis, Missouri

J. Sybil Biermann, MD
Assistant Professor
Orthopaedic Surgery
University of Michigan Medical School
Ann Arbor, Michigan

Brian Black, MD
Medical Director
Children's Orthopedic and Scoliosis Center
Milwaukee, Wisconsin

John S. Blanco, MD
Associate Professor of Orthopaedic Surgery and
  Pediatrics
University of Virginia Health Sciences Center
Charlottesville, Virginia

R. Dale Blasier, MD, FRCS(C)
Associate Professor of Orthopaedic Surgery
Division of Pediatric Orthopaedics
Arkansas Children's Hospital
University of Arkansas for Medical Sciences
Little Rock, Arkansas

Steven L. Buckley, MD
Assistant Professor
Department of Orthopaedic Surgery
Emory University School of Medicine
Atlanta, Georgia

Alvin H. Crawford, MD, FACS
Professor of Pediatrics and Orthopaedics
Children's Hospital Medical Center
Cincinnati, Ohio

Richard S. Davidson, MD
Associate Professor
Children's Hospital of Philadelphia
Philadelphia, Pennsylvania

Peter A. DeLuca, MD
Pediatric Orthopaedic Surgery
Connecticut Orthopaedic Specialists
New Haven, Connecticut

Donald Diverio, DO
The Orthopedic Center, PA
Cedar Knolls, New Jersey

David Gray, MD
Scottish Rite Children's Medical Center
Atlanta, Georgia

John J. Grayhack, MD, MS
Assistant Professor of Orthopedic Surgery
The Children's Memorial Medical Center
Northwestern University Medical School
Chicago, Illinois

Jan S. Grudziak, MD
Visiting Instructor
University of Pittsburgh Medical Center
Department of Orthopaedic Surgery
Pittsburgh, Pennsylvania

Lori Karol, MD
Assistant Professor, Department of Orthopaedic Surgery
University of Texas-Southwestern
Texas Scottish Rite Hospital for Children
Dallas, Texas

Steven E. Koop, MD
Gillette Children's Hospital
St. Paul, Minnesota

Randall T. Loder, MD
Associate Professor, Section of Orthopaedic Surgery
University of Michigan
Ann Arbor, Michigan

Shobha Malviya, MD
Assistant Professor of Anesthesiology
The University of Michigan Medical Center
Ann Arbor, Michigan

Jack K. Mayfield, MD, MS
Adjunct Professor
Department of Biochemical and Materials Engineering
Arizona State University
Phoenix, Arizona

Gregory A. Mencio, MD
Assistant Professor
Department of Orthopaedics
Vanderbilt University Medical Center
Nashville, Tennessee

Sandra Merkel, RN
Clinical Nurse Specialist
University of Michigan Medical Center
Ann Arbor, Michigan

Vincent S. Mosca, MD
Associate Professor and Chief of Pediatric Orthopedics
University of Washington School of Medicine
Seattle, Washington

B. Stephens Richards, MD
Associate Professor, Department of Orthopaedic Surgery
University of Texas-Southwestern
Texas Scottish Rite Hospital for Children
Dallas, Texas

William J. Shaughnessy, MD
Associate Professor of Orthopaedics
Mayo Medical School
Rochester, Minnesota

James E. Shook, MD
Assistant Professor of Orthopedic Surgery
Loma Linda University School of Medicine
Loma Linda, California

Kit M. Song, MD
Assistant Professor of Orthopedics
University of Washington School of Medicine
Seattle, Washington

Paul D. Sponseller, MD
Associate Professor and Head, Pediatric Orthopaedics
Johns Hopkins University
Baltimore, Maryland

Carl Stanitski, MD
Chief, Orthopaedic Surgery
Children's Hospital of Michigan
Detroit, Michigan

Deborah Stanitski, MD
Associate Chief of Orthopaedic Surgery
Children's Hospital of Michigan
Detroit, Michigan

John G. Thometz, MD
Associate Professor
Department of Orthopaedic Surgery
Medical College of Wisconsin
Milwaukee, Wisconsin

J. David Thompson, MD
Assistant Professor
Medical University of South Carolina
Charleston, South Carolina

Laura L. Tosi, MD
Assistant Professor of Orthopaedics and Pediatrics
George Washington University
Washington, District of Columbia

W. Timothy Ward, MD
Associate Professor
University of Pittsburgh Medical Center
Department of Orthopaedic Surgery
Pittsburgh, Pennsylvania

Peter M. Waters, MD
Clinical Director, Hand Surgery Clinic
Children's Hospital
Boston, Massachusetts

Table of Contents

Preface

This *Orthopaedic Knowledge Update: Pediatrics* edition, intended for the general orthopaedist rather than the subspecialist, presents current information on pediatric-related conditions that often are seen in practice. The update is organized into four areas: general issues, spinal disorders, lower extremity abnormalities, and trauma. New concepts that have been introduced in the recent literature are incorporated into this review and provide the reader with up-to-date classifications, terminology, and approaches to treatment. Annotated bibliographies, with emphasis on recent articles, accompany each chapter.

This book is the result of the hard work and organiza-tion provided by the section editors, George S. Bassett, MD, Randall T. Loder, MD, Paul D. Sponseller, MD, Deborah Stanitski, MD, and W. Timothy Ward, MD; the many individual contributors; and the editors at the American Academy of Orthopaedic Surgeons, particularly Jane Baque and Lisa Moore. I thank them all—each deserves a large amount of credit.

We hope that the reader will find this a useful source of information for pediatric-related conditions that are seen so often today.

B. STEPHENS RICHARDS, MD
EDITOR

I

General Pediatric Orthopaedics

Randall T. Loder, MD
Section Editor

1

The Limping Child

Introduction

The limping child may present a significant challenge to the orthopaedist. In order to arrive at the correct diagnosis, the clinician must approach each patient in an organized fashion. This chapter reviews the different types of childhood limps and describes many of the conditions that may be responsible. Most problems that can lead to a limp in childhood (ie, developmental dysplasia of the hip, Legg-Calvé-Perthes disease [LCPD], or slipped capital femoral epiphysis [SCFE]) will be discussed in depth in other chapters and, therefore, will be mentioned only briefly here. Injuries that could cause a limp, which are obvious to both the parent and clinician, will not be reviewed.

In general, disorders that cause limping vary from age group to age group. Therefore, three different age groups will be examined relative to the disorders leading to gait disturbances. The three groups are toddlers (aged 1 to 3 years), children (4 to 10 years), and adolescents (11 to 15 years). This age breakdown should enable the clinician to organize a more effective approach to this problem.

A thorough history taken by the clinician is important in evaluating the limping child. The history may allow for an early diagnosis, perhaps even before the physical examination is performed. The history helps provide guidance for the proper workup, which may include a variety of laboratory studies, radiographs, and, less frequently, ultrasound studies, bone scan, computed tomography (CT), or magnetic resonance imaging (MRI).

Gait Disturbances in Children

The walking pattern of the young toddler has not matured to the level of the adult, a fact that must be taken into consideration when evaluating their gait. For better balance, toddlers walk with a wide-based gait, increased flexion of the hips and knees, and the arms held out to the side with elbows extended. Their movements appear uncoordinated and rapid. During their gait cycle, an increased amount of time is spent in double limb stance, again, to maintain balance. Because neuromuscular development is immature, a toddler cannot achieve an increase in speed by increasing the step length, but instead, must do so by an increase in cadence. As the toddler matures, the movements become smoother, reciprocal arm swing appears, and step length and walking velocity increase. Velocity increases to a stable pattern by the age of 5, and an adult pattern of gait is achieved by the age of 7.

Children most often limp to achieve relief from a painful extremity. Sometimes, however, they will limp for reasons other than pain. This is particularly true in toddlers, in whom limping may be the result of painless disorders such as developmental dislocation of the hip (DDH), limb length discrepancies, or mild static encephalopathies, to name a few. The orthopaedist may find himself the first to make the diagnosis of one of these.

Antalgic Gait

In general, the most common type of limp will be antalgic or pain related. The child takes quick soft steps on the painful extremity in an effort to shorten the amount of time spent in stance phase. The normal extremity comes forward more quickly to bear the weight and, thus, the normal leg has a longer stance phase. Painful abnormalities anywhere in the lower extremity can lead to this pattern. What could also be termed an antalgic gait in another form is seen in children with painful spinal disorders such as diskitis or osteomyelitis. These children walk slowly, or may refuse to walk at all, in an effort to avoid jarring of the back.

Trendelenburg Gait

A Trendelenburg gait results from functionally weakened abductor muscles and is commonly seen in the child with DDH. With a dislocated hip, the abductor muscles are at a mechanical disadvantage and are effectively weakened, which makes it difficult for them to support the child's body weight. As a result, the pelvis tilts away from the affected hip. In an effort to minimize this imbalance during the stance phase of gait, children lean over the affected hip. After the gait cycle has been observed several times, the presence of a characteristic Trendelenburg gait pattern will be evident. In contrast to the antalgic gait pattern, the amount of time spent in stance phase on the affected extremity may not be decreased in someone with a Trendelenburg gait, because pain is not present.

Short Limb Gait

In the short limb gait, the child walks on the toes on the affected side throughout the gait cycle. This is done in an effort to maintain a level pelvis. If the discrepancy between limb lengths is large, the longer extremity may remain flexed at the hip and knee during stance phase.

Spastic Gait

A spastic gait, seen in cerebral palsy, reflects hypertonicity and an imbalance between muscle groups. Sustained activity of the gastrocnemius-soleus muscles may lead to ankle equinus and toe walking. Spastic hamstring muscles limit knee extension and may lead to crouching at the knee and a shortened stride length. Spastic quadriceps muscles may lead to a stiff extended knee gait. The clinical presentation may be extremely subtle. For example, in a child with mild hemiplegia, slight ankle equinus forces the knee to hyperextend during the stance phase of gait so that the foot can be placed flat to the ground. This hyperextension of the knee may be the only abnormality noted during gait. Usually, however, the spasticity is more evident (ankle equinus and knee flexion), which makes the diagnosis easier. Often, when the child is asked to run, the lower extremity spasticity and subtle upper extremity posturing (elbow flexion, forearm pronation, wrist flexion, and clenched fist) become more evident, which also helps in making the diagnosis. These patterns can be very subtle and a number of consultations may have been obtained before the proper diagnosis is made.

Proximal Muscle Weakness Gait

Limping from proximal muscle weakness may present in the older toddler or in the early childhood period. A prime example would be a young boy with muscular dystrophy. Because the hip extensor muscles are weak, the child may have a lordotic gait to maintain hip extension. A positive Gower's sign, in which the child "climbs up on himself" by placing hands first on knees, then on thighs, and finally on hips, also reflects the proximal muscle weakness.

Additional abnormal gait patterns exist, but the general orthopaedist who is familiar with those described above should be able to categorize accurately many of the limps that occur in childhood and should be able to proceed down the correct diagnostic pathway.

The Limping Toddler (Ages 1 to 3 Years)

Of the three age groups mentioned, toddlers probably offer the most difficulties for the orthopaedist who must accurately diagnose a limp. A reliable history may be difficult to obtain because of the toddlers' inability or refusal to communicate. If they do talk, their description of the problem may not be accurate. Furthermore, if the history is taken from their parents, the description of the problem still may not be accurate. Minor events that can lead to a limp, such as a splinter in the foot or a toddler's fracture of the tibia, may have been overlooked.

The physical examination should be complete and undertaken with the child gowned and barefoot. Because toddlers are frequently apprehensive, the least threatening portions of the examination are best done first. Check their gait, allowing them to walk freely with their parents. Observing the child's gait can help the orthopaedist localize an abnormality, which might be anywhere from the spine down to the foot. Lack of spine motion or limitation of joint range of motion is usually quickly evident. Tenderness to palpation, warmth, redness, and swelling of an extremity are all helpful in narrowing the differential diagnosis.

Infection Versus Noninfection

Transient synovitis and septic arthritis must often be differentiated from one another. Although both conditions produce a limp in the toddler because of pain, patients who have the latter condition are usually more irritable and frequently refuse to walk. Transient synovitis—probably the most common cause of lower extremity joint pain—generally has a favorable outcome. Septic arthritis, on the other hand, has the potential for significant complications.

Septic Arthritis

Septic arthritis usually presents with a rapid onset of joint pain, usually progresses to a febrile systemic illness, and leads to the toddler's refusal to use the extremity. There may be a history of mild trauma to the extremity or simultaneous illness or infection. On examination, the joint is held immobile, may be swollen and tender to palpation, and weightbearing is painful. Range of motion to the affected joint causes obvious pain to the child. Radiographs obtained at the time of the onset of symptoms may be unremarkable except for soft-tissue swelling. Radiographic changes in the bone caused by infection are visible after a period of 7 to 10 days and, if seen, signify a prolonged active process. The white blood cell (WBC) count, C-reactive protein, and erythrocyte sedimentation rate (ESR) are usually elevated. Blood cultures may also be helpful in up to 50% of patients with septic arthritis. Bone scans are not necessary if the joint or periarticular region is identified. If, however, the clinician is unable to localize the lesion or make the diagnosis following the above described evaluation, then acute triphase scintigraphy has been shown to be very effective and sensitive in localizing the abnormality. Aspiration of the joint is necessary to confirm the diagnosis and identify the bacterial organism. Analysis of the joint aspirate generally reveals a WBC count between 80,000 and 200,000, with more than 75% polymorphs. Gram stains are helpful in the preliminary antibiotic selection. Though *Staphylococcus aureus* is the most common organism responsible for septic arthritis, *Haemophilus influenzae* and Group B streptococci must be considered in the toddler age group.

Transient Synovitis

Transient (toxic) synovitis also presents as an acute onset of joint pain, limp, and restricted joint range of motion in the older toddler. The most common age range for transient synovitis is between 3 and 8 years, and so it is less common in the toddler than in the older child. In contrast to septic arthritis, children with transient synovitis usually do not have fever and systemic illness. The clinical symptoms generally show a gradual and complete resolution over several days to weeks, usually averaging 10 days.

However, it is during the acute phase that the clinician must astutely differentiate between septic arthritis and transient synovitis in a timely fashion. The findings during physical examination may be similar for both of these entities, but usually children with septic joints are more irritable. As mentioned, it is uncommon for the temperature to be greater than 38°C in transient synovitis. Laboratory values (ESR, C-reactive protein, and WBC count) usually are within the range of normal. Radiographs are normal. Ultrasound of the irritable hip demonstrates the effusion associated with transient synovitis. Joint aspiration should be done only to assist in the diagnosis, because routine aspiration has not been shown to have therapeutic value. The aspirate WBC count is usually between 5,000 and 15,000, with fewer than 25% polymorphs. The goal of treatment, to hasten the recovery of the underlying inflammatory synovitis, can be accomplished by many different modalities, including activity restriction, bed rest, nonweightbearing, and oral nonsteroidal anti-inflammatory medication.

Diskitis

The inclusion of diskitis in this chapter on the limping child is important because toddlers may present to the clinician with difficulty walking, or they may have progressed to the point where they refuse to walk. During the evaluation, if the toddler is asked to pick up an object from the floor, the child will either refuse or will bend only at the hips while holding the lower back straight to avoid motion of the spine. Toddlers may not appear ill, but in over 80% of the cases the sedimentation rate will be elevated. Blood cultures may be positive and, if so, usually reveal *S aureus.* Needle biopsy and open biopsy can confirm this but because the organism is commonly *S aureus,* biopsy is currently not recommended. Early radiographs may be normal. Over the course of several days to weeks, disk space narrowing and vertebral end plate irregularities may become apparent. A bone scan is helpful in confirming the preliminary diagnosis and assists in localizing the infection. The treatment of choice, systemic antibiotics, has been shown to lead to a more rapid resolution of symptoms than oral antibiotics alone or no antibiotics at all. Bed rest is usually the only form of immobilization required, if needed, although casts are also occasionally used. Infectious spondylitis, a newer term, represents the convergence of diskitis and vertebral osteomyelitis—two conditions previously thought of as separate disorders. Through the use of MRI, the two have been shown to represent similar infectious processes.

Toddler's Fracture

A torsion type of injury to the foot may produce a spiral fracture of the tibia without a fibular fracture. There may be no history of recognized trauma yet the child presents with a limp or refuses to bear weight. Radiographs may demonstrate a spiral fracture or may be unremarkable.

Follow-up radiographs 1 to 2 weeks later likely will reveal subperiosteal new bone formation, either slight or abundant. Short-term immobilization is all that is necessary.

Neurologic Disorder

If the toddler's gait has always been abnormal, and if the beginning of ambulation was delayed, an underlying neurologic disorder should be sought as the cause of a limp. Most toddlers begin to walk when they are approximately 12 months old, but the normal range extends up to 18 months. Beyond this, the toddler would certainly be considered delayed. A thorough prenatal, perinatal, and postnatal history is needed and, once obtained, may provide an explanation for the limp. The clinician must ask if there was a history of prematurity, difficulty with pregnancy or delivery, low birth weight, ventilator requirements, infections, or failure to thrive.

Cerebral Palsy

The most common neurologic disorder that leads to limping in the toddler is mild cerebral palsy. The limping, caused by muscle spasticity, varies in its severity. If severe, the diagnosis has usually been made prior to the initial visit to the orthopaedist, and these children do not pose a diagnostic challenge. Rather, the difficulty that the orthopaedist faces is in the child whose muscle imbalance is minor and who presents with a mild limp. A thorough examination will help to differentiate the problem. Limited range of motion of the knee and ankle, hyperreflexia, and clonus provide confirmation. Radiographs are usually normal, and other tests are not needed. The general orthopaedist may be the first doctor to introduce this diagnosis to young parents and, in doing so, may find himself trying to explain a general condition that is better addressed by the pediatric specialist.

Muscular Dystrophy

This uncommon problem leads to a gait disturbance in children between 2 and 5 years of age. The toddler, a male, may have a history of delayed ambulation and now presents because of stumbling, falling, and difficulty climbing stairs. The examination may demonstrate toe walking, but proximal muscle weakness and a positive Gower's sign are also evident. Calf pseudohypertrophy may be present. Measurement of the serum creatine phosphokinase (CPK) levels will aid in making the diagnosis.

Congenital/Developmental Disorders

Developmental Dislocation of the Hip Developmental dislocation of the hip, previously termed congenital dislocation of the hip, causes a painless limp in toddlers. Onset of ambulation may be mildly delayed. Examination of the toddler's gait may demonstrate a limp, a short leg, one-sided toe walking, or, if bilateral, a swayback appearance accompanied by a waddle. The abductor lurch to the affected side (Trendelenburg gait) is readily evident. If the toddler is cooperative during the examination, the pelvis drops to the opposite side when standing on the affected extremity and the trunk will lean over the dislocated hip (Trendelenburg sign). On supine examination, the toddler's hip has a limited amount of abduction when compared to the normal side and may have a mild flexion contracture. By the age of 1 year (when the toddler presents walking), a standing radiograph of the pelvis easily confirms the diagnosis. Ultrasound evaluations, MRI, or CT provide no additional useful information.

Coxa Vara Congenital or developmental coxa vara may present with a clinical picture similar to that of DDH in the toddler, but it is much less common. If unilateral, this painless condition may have an abductor lurch secondary to functional weakness of the abductor muscles. If bilateral, a waddling gait pattern may be evident. When examined in the supine position, hip abduction is limited. But, in contrast to the toddler with dislocation of the hip, hip rotation is also limited. Again, the diagnosis is easily made radiographically. The femoral neck-shaft angle is decreased and the physis has a vertical orientation.

Pauciarticular Juvenile Arthritis

The toddler with pauciarticular onset arthritis, the most common subgroup of juvenile arthritis, usually presents around the age of 2 years with a mildly painful limp. Girls are affected four times more often than boys. Symptoms develop slowly and are accompanied by mild swelling, warmth, and restriction of joint range of motion. The subtalar joint, ankle, or knee are commonly involved in the lower extremity. Laboratory evaluation, including ESR, WBC count, and rheumatoid factor, may be unremarkable. The antinuclear antibody (ANA) may also be negative in 50% of the toddlers. This may change over time and therefore should be repeated, if needed, at a later period in the child who is suspected of having this disorder. By that time, if swelling has been persistent, referral to a children's rheumatologist should have already been made. The vast majority of children with pauciarticular arthritis will do well with no orthopaedic intervention and will return to normal function.

Neoplasms

Bone tumors are uncommon and, therefore, are rarely responsible for a toddler's limp. If present, plain radiographs may often identify the abnormality. In the recent literature, however, two neoplasms have been emphasized, both of which may be unremarkable on initial radiographic evaluation. Leukemia and osteoid osteoma have again been shown to be responsible for painful limps in toddlers.

Leukemia Acute leukemia, the most common neoplasm in children under 16 years, has a peak incidence between 2 and 5 years of age. Musculoskeletal complaints are a presenting feature in 20% of children with this disorder.

Bone pain in the lower extremities may be described as discomfort in an adjacent joint. Generalized symptoms should be recognized, and these include lethargy, pallor, bruising, fever, and bleeding. In addition to the joint symptoms and bone pain, appreciation of skin bruising and hepatosplenomegaly are helpful in making the diagnosis. With the exception of bruising, bleeding, and hepatosplenomegaly, the clinical picture may be similar to that of septic arthritis, osteomyelitis, cellulitis, or arthritis. Therefore, leukemia should always be included in the differential diagnosis of these other disorders. Laboratory evaluation may reveal elevated ESRs and peripheral leukocyte counts. Radiographically, lucent metaphyseal bands may be one of the earliest findings. Bone scans may be normal and therefore contribute little information. If, after a thorough general evaluation, the suspicion of leukemia persists, then referral to the pediatric hematologist is warranted for bone marrow evaluation.

Osteoid Osteoma Osteoid osteomas are uncommon in children younger than 5 years of age. This diagnosis is especially difficult to make in toddlers who are just learning to walk. Although pain is the most frequent clinical manifestation, limping is common. If radiographs are negative, bone scans provide considerable guidance in identifying the lesion.

The Limping Child (Ages 4 to 10 Years)

Older children can communicate better than toddlers, usually are more cooperative during examination, and have mature gait patterns, all of which assist the clinician in the evaluation of the problem. Complaints by children in this age group should be taken seriously, because these children usually are more interested in play than they are in secondary gains. Periodically parents describe a situation in which their child complains of aching in the legs, generally in the evening before bedtime. This pain responds to a rubdown and infrequently requires medication. Prior to reassuring the parents that this represents benign "growing pains," an evaluation of the child should be completed in order to avoid missing an underlying disorder. All of the disorders presented in the section on the toddler must be kept in mind when evaluating an older limping child.

Transient Synovitis

Transient synovitis is seen most commonly in the 3- to 8-year age group and probably is responsible for the majority of limping due to an irritable joint. Its proper evaluation has been discussed and, again, it must be properly differentiated from a septic process. Two other disorders responsible for irritable joints in this age group include LCPD and discoid menisci.

Legg-Calvé-Perthes Disease

LCPD is most common in children aged 4 to 8 years, although older children may also be affected. For reasons unknown, boys are involved four to five times more frequently than girls. The children present with limping, but complaints of hip pain are infrequent. If pain is present, it may be described in the hip, groin, thigh, or knee and is usually increased following activity. Observing the child's gait demonstrates an antalgic limp with less time spent on the affected extremity. The physical examination quickly localizes the problem to the hip, because rotation, particularly internal rotation, is limited and causes discomfort to the child. The earliest radiographic appearance in this disorder is seen on the lateral projection of the hip and appears as a subchondral lucency (crescent sign). This crescent sign precedes the collapse and fragmentation of the femoral epiphysis seen in later radiographs. If the child presents very early in the course of the disorder, radiographic changes may not yet be apparent. In this instance, bone scintigraphy or MRI may prove diagnostic. Once diagnosed, the clinician must decide on what type of treatment to initiate. Much debate continues regarding the most effective treatment. This will be discussed later in the chapter on LCPD.

Discoid Meniscus

A discoid meniscus is a rare cause of limping in the child. It usually presents as knee pain, periodic knee swelling, lack of full knee extension, or a clicking sensation. Although a common age range for presentation has been described as 8 to 12 years, this disorder may also present in the young child between the ages of 3 and 8. Parents and patients both usually deny a history of trauma and the child's symptoms are magnified with increased activity. Tenderness may be noted on the lateral joint line. Radiographs may be normal or, infrequently, may demonstrate widening of the lateral joint space with flattening of the lateral femoral condyle. An MRI will confirm the diagnosis.

Limb-Length Discrepancy

A progressive limb-length discrepancy (LLD) may become evident in this age range. The child may toe walk on the short extremity in an effort to achieve a level pelvis and smooth gait pattern. Clinically, this discrepancy can best be measured by having the child stand on blocks until the pelvis is leveled. Radiographically, a standing film (long cassette) of both entire lower extremities is needed to determine which region of the limb is responsible for the discrepancy. Subtle findings on this radiograph may provide the diagnosis. Examples include a mild fibular hemimelia, a physeal abnormality following a remote infection, or a congenitally short femur.

The Limping Adolescent (Ages 11 To 15 Years)

The adolescent with a limp usually can provide an accurate history of the problem. However, the symptoms that are described may be minimized if, for example, the patient wants a quick return to sports. Likewise, the symptoms may be overemphasized if the patient wishes to avoid physical activities such as gym class. Over the course of the evaluation, the clinician can usually gain an accurate assessment of the patient's real symptoms. As mentioned earlier, many of the same disorders already presented must be taken into consideration when evaluating the adolescent who is limping. In addition, several other disorders that are more common in the adolescent age group should be included. These include slipped capital femoral epiphysis, hip dysplasia, chondrolysis, overuse syndromes, osteochondritis dissecans, and tarsal coalitions.

Slipped Capital Femoral Epiphysis

SCFE is believed to be the most common hip disorder occurring in adolescence. Clinically, boys present around the age of 14 years and girls around age 12 years. Most often the adolescents, who generally are overweight, describe a mild but constant pain in the hip, groin, thigh, or knee. The duration of symptoms is usually several months (chronic stable slip). On examination, an antalgic limp accompanies the pain. Range of motion of the hip is limited in internal rotation and abduction. As the lower extremity is flexed at the hip, it often assumes an externally rotated appearance. (Less frequently, the adolescent may present with acute excessive pain and actually is unable to walk at all. This acute unstable slip is much like an acute fracture. With it comes a worse prognosis because of an increased incidence of osteonecrosis.) Radiographs are mandatory, particularly the lateral projection, to confirm the diagnosis. Other imaging tests are not necessary.

Hip Dysplasia

Hip dysplasia may first become clinically apparent in the adolescent age group as a source of hip pain and limp. Prior to this, the patient may have been unaware of any hip disorder. Complaints of an aching discomfort after prolonged activity are common. The physical examination may be normal or may demonstrate mild limitation in hip range of motion. The diagnosis is made with standing radiographs of the pelvis.

Chondrolysis

Chondrolysis of the hip is an uncommon disorder. Although its occurrence is most often associated with SCFE (in which an incidence of up to 8% is reported), its etiology remains unknown. Proposed theories have included nutritional abnormalities, ischemia, mechanical injury, and abnormal intracapsular pressures. Females are affected five times more frequently than males and the age of presentation is in the 12- to 14-year age group. As with a stable slipped capital femoral epiphysis or hip dysplasia, the complaint commonly is insidious aching in the hip or groin. In addition to a limp, the examination demonstrates a stiff hip with limited range of motion in all directions. Laboratory investigation is usually normal. Chondrolysis is diagnosed from hip radiographs, which demonstrate osteopenia from disuse in the hip region, classic joint space narrowing as compared to the normal side (greater than 2 mm difference), and subchondral lucencies. Bone scans demonstrate increased uptake on both sides of the joint but have not been shown beneficial in guiding treatment.

Treatment of idiopathic chondrolysis is aimed at resolving the synovitis, improving and maintaining joint range of motion, and providing a lengthy period of weight relief to the involved joint. Beginning with nonsteroidal anti-inflammatory medication, traction, and aggressive physical therapy, the treatment program may progress to soft-tissue releases in an effort to address contractures. Beneficial results from subtotal capsulectomy and muscle releases (followed by physical therapy) have been reported, but the role of this aggressive management must be better defined in future larger studies.

Overuse Syndromes

As adolescents become more active in organized sports, overuse injuries occur with increasing frequency. Although these overuse syndromes typically present with pain, they can on rare occasion also present as a limp. The knee is the most common site for this. Patellar tendonitis or apophysitis of the tibial tubercle (Osgood-Schlatter disease) cause persistent pain. Point tenderness to palpation is helpful in confirming these disorders. For those with apophysitis, radiographs may demonstrate apparent fragmentation of the tibial tubercle. Rest, ice, and anti-inflammatory medicines are needed in the acute stage. For the long term, consideration must be given to altering the activities or changing the training regimen.

Stress fractures are seen in patients whose activities lead to repetitive loading of the lower extremities. The tibia and fibula are most susceptible. Radiographs may demonstrate the subtle sclerotic line or periosteal reaction, or they may be normal. If suspicion of a stress fracture is high, a bone scan is very useful in confirming the diagnosis. Again, rest is needed in the acute phase and an alteration of training or equipment may be necessary for the long term.

Osteochondritis Dissecans

Osteochondritis dissecans is most common in the adolescent age group, and typically presents with pain, but it also can, on rare occasion, present with a limp. The knee is affected most, but the hip and ankle can also be involved. Radiographically, the "tunnel" view of the knee allows the viewer to appreciate the defect in its classic location on the lateral side of the medial femoral condyle.

Tarsal Coalitions

Tarsal coalitions become clinically evident in this age group as the cartilaginous coalitions begin to ossify. Contracture of the peroneal muscles is common and leads to a stiff everted flatfoot. Calcaneonavicular coalitions can readily be identified on the oblique radiographs of the feet. If a talocalcaneal coalition is suspected, a radiograph of the subtalar joint (Harris view) may be helpful in revealing the abnormality. More often, though, a CT scan of the hindfoot is necessary to confirm the diagnosis of a subtalar coalition.

Annotated Bibliography

Aronson J, Garvin K, Seibert J, et al: Efficiency of the bone scan for occult limping toddlers. *J Pediatr Orthop* 1992;12:38–44.

Fifty consecutive occult limping toddlers (8 to 48 months of age) were prospectively evaluated by triphase bone scan. Only patients with a limp that could not be diagnosed by an orthopaedist were included. The bone scan proved valuable in localizing the abnormality in 27 patients. It was highly sensitive, specific, efficient, predictive, and was superior to other screening tests (WBC, ESR, temperature, plain radiographs).

Blatt SD, Rosenthal BM, Barnhart DC: Diagnostic utility of lower extremity radiographs of young children with gait disturbance. *Pediatrics* 1991;87:138–140.

Eighty-four well-appearing children (1 to 5 years of age) were evaluated as outpatients whose predominant complaint was a limp. Physical examinations were unremarkable. Lower extremity radiographs were obtained in all. These yielded no diagnostically important information. All but one patient had spontaneous resolution of symptoms. In this setting, the authors recommend deferring radiographic evaluation, assuming that timely follow-up is assured.

Choban S, Killian JT: Evaluation of acute gait abnormalities in preschool children. *J Pediatr Orthop* 1990;10:74–78.

This is a retrospective evaluation of 60 children (under age 5 years) hospitalized for evaluation of limp. The most common final diagnosis was transient synovitis (24 patients). Only one of 22 patients with a normal CBC, ESR, and temperature had an infection. Of the 14 patients with infection, only one had a normal CBC, ESR, and temperature. Radiographs were diagnostic in only four cases (osteomyelitis in two, LCPD in one, and diskitis in one). Aspiration identified nine of 13 infections. Eighteen of 35 bone scans were helpful in arriving at the definitive diagnosis. The authors advocate a liberal use of diagnostic aspiration. If aspiration proves negative, and the temperature, WBC count, or ESR is elevated, then a bone scan should be obtained to rule out osteomyelitis.

Kaweblum M, Lehman WB, Bash J, et al: Osteoid osteoma under the age of five years: The difficulty of diagnosis. *Clin Orthop* 1993;296:218–224.

Seven patients were included in this study, most of whom were initially diagnosed incorrectly. The time between the onset of symptoms and the diagnosis varied from three months to five years. Limping was the second most frequent finding (behind pain) and was always present when the lower extremity was affected. Bone scans were very sensitive.

Kaweblum M, Lehman WB, Bash J, et al: Diagnosis of osteoid osteoma in the child. *Orthop Rev* 1993;22:1305–1313.

In addition to the information provided by the previous article, the English literature regarding osteoid osteomas in children under age 5 years (52 cases) is reviewed.

MacEwen GD, Dehne R: The limping child. *Pediatr Rev* 1991;12:268–274.

The differential diagnosis of a painful limp is presented as it relates to the hip (septic arthritis, transient synovitis, LCPD, SCFE), knee (septic arthritis, juvenile arthritis, tumor, overuse injuries), and spine.

Mubarak SJ: Osteochondrosis of the lateral cuneiform: Another cause of a limp in a child. A case report. *J Bone Joint Surg* 1992;74A:285–289.

A 2.5-year-old male presented with a 2-month history of painful limp. Sclerosis of the lateral cuneiform was evident radiographically and bone scan was normal. Without treatment, symptoms resolved and radiographs returned to normal within 6 months. This appears similar to osteochondroses involving the medial cuneiform, intermediate cuneiform, and tarsal navicular.

Phillips WA: The child with a limp. *Orthop Clin North Am* 1987;18:489–501.

The normal gait pattern of a child is reviewed and the different types of limps are explained. The differential diagnosis of limping is presented by age groups: toddlers (1 to 3 years), children (4 to 10 years), and adolescents (11 to 16 years). Trauma, as a cause of limp, is excluded in this article.

Royle SG: Investigation of the irritable hip. *J Pediatr Orthop* 1992;12:396–397.

Sixty-two children (age 2 to 12 years) with irritable hips were evaluated with conventional radiography, ultrasound scanning, and bone scan. The patients were afebrile, had normal WBC counts and ESRs, and low suspicion of sepsis, but had failed to improve with 2 days bed rest. All patients with demonstrable effusions were aspirated. One patient subsequently developed Perthes disease; the others had an uneventful outcome. The author recommended that radiographs and ultrasound be routinely performed. Bone scan should be reserved for those with positive findings on ultrasound, as an abnormal bone scan was unusual when the ultrasound was normal.

Stahl JA, Schoenecker PL, Gilula LA: A 2 1/2-year-old male with limping on the left lower extremity: Acute lymphocytic leukemia. *Orthop Rev* 1993;22:631–636.

A case report of a toddler with acute lymphocytic leukemia is presented. The radiographic findings of a young child with leukemia, general information of leukemia, and a differential diagnosis are discussed.

Terjesen T, Osthus P: Ultrasound in the diagnosis and follow-up of transient synovitis of the hip. *J Pediatr Orthop* 1991;11:608–613.

Fifty-nine patients (age 2 to 15 years) with acute synovitis of the hip were evaluated using ultrasound. The diagnostic criteria for effusion was an ultrasound difference of 2 mm (between sides) in the distance between the anterior joint capsule and the femoral neck. All but one patient (who later developed LCPD) had a final diagnosis of transient synovitis. Ultrasound was recommended as the main imaging technique (instead of radiographs) for those suspected of having transient synovitis. Radiographs should be used in those suspected of having LCPD. No mention was made in the article about differentiating between septic arthritis and transient synovitis.

Ring D, Johnston CE II, Wenger DR: Pyogenic infectious spondylitis in children: The convergence of discitis and vertebral osteomyelitis. *J Pediatr Orthop* 1995;15:652–660.

Forty-seven patients with pyogenic infectious spondylitis (diskitis) were reviewed to determine the spectrum of disease. MRIs were obtained in nine patients and were found to be identical to MRI findings in adult vertebral osteomyelitis. This provides strong evidence for an infectious process in diskitis. The investigation confirmed the usually benign course of spine infections in children but also emphasized the potential for serious sequelae. Symptoms were resolved more rapidly with intravenous antibiotics than they were with oral antibiotics or no antibiotics.

2

Evaluation of Back Pain

Traditional teaching has been that back pain in young children is usually attributable to true pathology. In a 1985 study, a definite diagnosis was found in 84 of 100 children who presented with complaints of back pain. However, it is also known that many older children and adolescents have back pain that mimics that of the adult population, and not that of the very young child. In this era of cost containment, a complete diagnostic evaluation for back pain, including radiographs, blood tests, and special scans is very expensive. Clearly not all of these children need to receive a full evaluation complete with radiographs, bone scan, computed tomography (CT), magnetic resonance imaging (MRI), and blood tests. The task of the orthopaedic surgeon is to decide which children require treatment for underlying pathology leading to their back pain, and to differentiate them from those who simply can be observed.

The changing patterns in diagnosis of children with back pain was studied in 1995 by a group from Toronto. An analysis of 226 consecutive single photon emission computed tomography (SPECT) scans in children with a primary complaint of back pain resulted in no diagnosis in 78%, spondylolysis in 7%, tumor in 5%, and other diagnoses in 10%. Thus, a definitive diagnosis could be made in only 22% of children. The factors that were associated with positive diagnoses were the nature of the pain (constant versus intermittent), radicular pain, male gender, and shorter duration of symptoms. Plain radiographs were the best screening test.

If the child is very young, or if an older child or adolescent fits these criteria, the possibility of a distinct diagnosis responsible for the back pain exists, and appropriate concern should be given. The remainder of this chapter discusses the approach to a child or adolescent in whom the likelihood of true pathology exists as a cause of back pain.

History

As always, the initial screen for pathology is a comprehensive history and physical examination. The location, intensity, and duration of pain must be determined. A history of trauma must be pursued. Mild pain of short duration after athletic trauma is most likely due to muscle strain. The presence or absence of night pain must be established, as night pain has been linked to tumors, particularly in young children. Fever, chills, or weight loss indicate a malignant or infectious etiology. Radiation of pain down the legs or into the buttocks is suggestive of a herniated nucleus pulposus or fractured apophysis. The examiner must ask about numbness, weakness, or bowel or bladder

changes. The association of pain with activity is important to recognize. Pain secondary to spinal tumors does not vary with activity, but is constant and progressive.

The age of the patient is helpful in directing the diagnostic workup. Children 4 years of age or younger who complain of back pain must be thoroughly evaluated, because this group of patients is most likely to have either a tumor or an infection requiring prompt treatment. Adolescents are more likely to develop spondylolysis or Scheuermann's kyphosis than infection or tumor.

The physician should inquire about athletic activities, the position played, and the level of participation of the child. Certain sports, such as gymnastics, ballet, football, and rowing, place shear forces across the lumbar spine, and predispose participants to spondylolysis and spondylolisthesis. Overuse injuries of the lumbar spine have become more common recently due to the intense training regimens currently in favor with coaches and parents.

Physical Examination

A careful physical examination must be performed with the child unclothed. Spinal examination must include palpation and inspection, particularly looking for midline defects such as hemangiomas, sinuses, or hair patches. The presence of scoliosis can be detected with forward bending, and trunk decompensation can be helpful in detecting underlying pathology. Flexibility must be evaluated. Reversal of the normal lumbar lordosis should occur with forward bending. Stiffness is a sign of underlying pathology. Hyperextension of the spine performed while standing on one leg can elicit symptoms in patients with pars interarticularis lesions. Lastly, hamstring tightness, elicited by a diminished straight leg raise and inability to touch the floor with the fingers, should be tested.

A meticulous neurologic examination is paramount to making the diagnosis of spinal cord pathology. Strength, sensation, and reflexes should all be evaluated. Asymmetry of the examination must be recognized. The presence of clonus or an abnormal Babinski reflex may indicate a central abnormality. The abdominal reflex should be tested by stroking the skin in each of the four quadrants of the umbilicus and observing movement of the umbilicus toward the quadrant stroked. Asymmetry of the abdominal reflex may lead to a diagnosis of syringomyelia.

As mentioned, the skin must be examined for cutaneous lesions linked with spinal abnormalities, particularly midline defects or café-au-lait spots. Lastly, a general physical examination is necessary to rule out nonorthopaedic etiologies of back pain, such as pneumonia with chest wall pain or a urinary tract infection leading to lumbar pain.

Radiographic Examination

The first branch of the decision tree is now reached—who should have standard radiographs performed? All children 4 years of age or younger should be studied on presentation. Children complaining of pain that has been present for 2 months or longer should be radiographed, as should children complaining of pain that wakes them from sleep or who have associated constitutional symptoms. Only older children with activity-related pain of short duration, normal neurologic evaluation, and normal general physical examinations may be observed without further diagnostic workup for a period of approximately 1 month.

Plain radiography is the most helpful imaging modality in children with back pain. Meticulous scrutiny must be done, looking for vertebral scalloping, disk space narrowing, alignment, and lytic or blastic lesions. Posteroanterior and lateral views of the spine without shielding are usually adequate. In the adolescent in whom spondylolysis or spondylolisthesis is suspected, oblique radiographs and a spot lateral of the lumbosacral junction may also be useful. The pelvis must be adequately visualized on radiographs, because pelvic lesions can present as back pain. Questionable lesions seen on plain radiographs may be seen more clearly with a coned-down spot radiograph, which yields superior bony detail.

Plain radiographs may reveal scoliosis in the patient with back pain. Although the radiographic appearance may lead the physician and family to attribute the pain to the deformity seen, scoliosis generally does not cause back pain. The presence of scoliosis in a patient with back pain should lead to further investigation into what has produced the pain, as well as the scoliosis. Occasionally, careful examination of the apex of the curvature on the convex side may reveal a bony lesion, with the spine deviating away from the irritating process. Scoliotic curves with left-sided apices are unusual, and are often associated with neurologic abnormalities.

In those children with normal plain radiographs and normal neurologic examinations, the next imaging modality recommended is the triphasic technetium bone scan. The bone scan is very sensitive in the detection of bony processes such as infection, malignant and benign tumors, and fractures, yet is not specific in its identification of a precise diagnosis. Pinhole collimation can be helpful in localizing increased uptake more accurately. A new imaging technique, SPECT, has been found to be superior to the standard technetium bone scan in detecting spondylolysis and for localizing lesions within the spine more precisely.

If the neurologic examination is abnormal, imaging of the neural axis should be performed. Although at one time the CT myelogram was the gold standard for spinal cord imaging, now MRI is performed more frequently. Tumors, syrinxes, and herniated disks are all seen clearly on MRI.

Bony lesions, such as tumors and fractures, can also be seen on MRI, but surrounding edema may obscure the exact location or extent of the process. When a bony lesion is seen on plain radiographs or bone scan, CT is usually more helpful than MRI in further clarifying the abnormality.

Laboratory Evaluation

Laboratory evaluation should be performed without hesitation on children with constitutional symptoms, on young children, and on those patients who complain of night pain. Initial screening consists of a complete blood count with differential and sedimentation rate. The C-reactive protein has recently gained favor as a measure of an acute phase reactant, but its role in the evaluation of back pain has not been specifically addressed.

Causes of Back Pain

Infectious Etiologies

Infection is the most common cause of back pain in the very young child. Diskitis typically affects children who are 1 to 5 years of age. The child may complain of pain in the back or abdomen, may refuse to walk, or present with a limp. Clinically, there is a limited range of spinal motion, and, commonly, tenderness to palpation. Often, these children will not bend to retrieve a toy from the floor, but rather will squat down with a straight spine. Fewer than half will be febrile, but often the children appear sick.

Radiographic changes lag behind clinical findings. Early on, the only radiographic sign may be subtle narrowing of the affected disk space. Increased activity on bone scan will localize the diskitis when plain radiographs are equivocal (Fig. 1). Later, end plate erosions can be seen at the adjacent vertebra. Recently, the use of MRI has been advocated for the evaluation of diskitis, and it has been helpful in identifying associated abscesses that required surgical drainage. Diskitis in older children has been confused with herniation of the intervertebral disk on MRI scan.

Controversy exists as to whether or not diskitis is a bacterial infection that requires antibiotics. Most feel it is, and *Staphylococcus aureus* has been most frequently isolated when positive cultures are obtained. Cultures of the disk space are positive only 60% of the time, however.

Treatment, as implied above, is controversial. Intravenous antibiotics are advised by most authors, with coverage for *Staphylococcus*. Some physicians advocate bed rest, casting, or bracing for children with diskitis. Routine biopsy and debridement is not necessary, and surgery should be reserved for children whose condition does not improve after several days of rest and antibiotics, or who demonstrate an abscess on imaging studies.

It can be difficult to distinguish between diskitis and osteomyelitis in children. Most clinicians feel that osteomyelitis is a continuation of diskitis, which results in greater

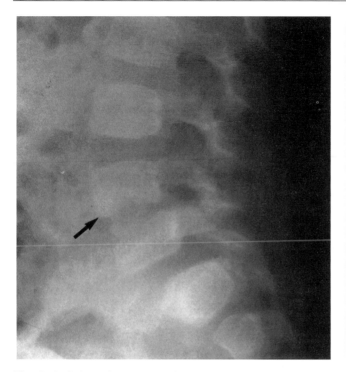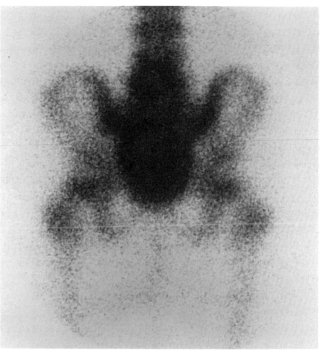

Fig. 1   Left, Lateral radiograph of a 2-year, 5-month-old female with diskitis at the L4-5 disk space, taken 9 days after the diagnosis was made. Note the end plate irregularities and disk space narrowing (arrow). **Right,** Bone scan reveals increased uptake.

vertebral bony changes. *S aureus* again is the most common organism in otherwise healthy children. Tuberculosis is gaining in prevalence once again, and should be suspected in particular in children from third world countries. Spinal tuberculosis is more likely to produce significant radiographic deformity, such as kyphoscoliosis, and soft tissue abscesses.

Developmental Etiologies

Scheuermann's Disorder   Scheuermann's kyphosis is the most common cause of thoracic back pain in adolescents. Males are affected more often than females, and the peak incidence is in adolescents 14 to 17 years of age. The teens localize their pain to the midscapular region, usually in the middle of their kyphosis. The pain is not associated with burning, tingling, or numbness, and is described as aching in nature. Constitutional symptoms are absent. Often, poor posture is the presenting complaint, with pain being present but not severe.

Physical examination reveals increased thoracic kyphosis, which is not flexible. Normal thoracic kyphosis ranges between 20° and 45°. Compensatory lumbar hyperlordosis is notable. Hamstring tightness may be present. Neurologic examination should be normal.

Radiographic diagnosis is classically made by the presence of more than 5° of anterior wedging at three contiguous vertebrae. End plate irregularities or sclerosis, and

Schmorl's nodes, may be present. Thoracic kyphosis is increased (Fig. 2).

Treatment is predominantly nonsurgical. Brace treatment can improve the kyphosis during the time of spinal growth. The most effective brace is the Milwaukee brace. It applies a three-point mold, anteriorly on the pubis and sternum and posteriorly at the apex of deformity. Lower profile braces have not been shown to be effective in this condition. Prerequisites for brace treatment include sufficient remaining spinal growth and flexibility of the kyphosis seen on stress radiographs. If the kyphosis is rigid, serial casting may improve the deformity. Exercises to stretch the hamstrings and lumbodorsal fascia and to strengthen the abdominal musculature may improve symptoms of pain but will not change the deformity. Surgical correction via spinal fusion is controversial. Currently accepted indications include deformity greater than 70°, progressive deformity, pain, and genuine concern regarding appearance. If surgery is performed, successful fusion is more likely with combined anterior and posterior approaches, although good results have recently been reported with a posterior only procedure.

A separate entity causing low back pain in adolescence is lumbar Scheuermann's disease. The peak age of incidence is in older adolescents, between 15 and 17 years of age. Males are affected twice as often as females. Radiographically, end plate irregularities, disk space changes, and, occasionally, wedging of the vertebrae are seen, with

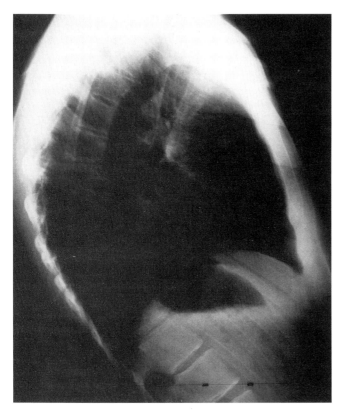

Fig. 2 Lateral radiograph of a 17-year-old female with progressive thoracic kyphosis secondary to the Scheuermann's kyphosis. Anterior wedging of the vertebral bodies is present.

the lesions most often at the thoracolumbar junction. The etiology is felt to be overuse, with microfractures of the vertebral endplates producing pain. Bracing can be helpful in relieving symptoms.

Spondylolysis and Spondylolisthesis Spondylolysis and spondylolisthesis are the most common causes of identifiable lumbar back pain in adolescents. Those most likely to be affected are gymnasts, divers, dancers, and football linemen. Impact on the hyperextended spine may lead to a stress fracture of the pars interarticularis, with resultant pain and/or listhesis. The most common time of onset is during the adolescent growth spurt. Presenting symptoms are lower back and buttock pain, possibly with radiation into the legs. The pain is associated with activity and improves with rest. It is exacerbated by twisting and hyperextension of the lumbar spine. Changes in posture may be noted, particularly flattening of the lumbar lordosis. A shuffling gait may be present.

The classic radiographic finding of a spondylolysis is a lytic area in the pars interarticularis. Associated spondylolisthesis may also be seen. Bone scintigraphy can be

helpful in identifying an occult pars fracture, and SPECT imaging has recently been shown to offer superior visualization of occult pars fractures and prefractures.

Traumatic Etiologies

A herniated intervertebral disk is seen occasionally in children and adolescents. Back pain with radiation into the legs is the most frequent complaint. Often, a history of trauma will be given. Mobility of the spine is compromised, and the patient may list on forward bending. A positive straight leg raise (Lasègue's sign) is almost always present. However, neurologic findings, such as absent reflexes, numbness, and weakness, are less common in children than they are in adults.

Plain radiographs are usually normal, but on occasion scoliosis is present. MRI will reveal the disk herniation, and this examination is gaining favor over CT myelography (Fig. 3). Caution is needed when interpreting disk degeneration using MRI, because its presence has been documented in asymptomatic adolescents. The findings on MRI must be correlated with the symptoms and physical examination of the patient. CT is helpful in determining the presence of congenital lumbar spinal stenosis, which is associated with herniated nucleus pulposus in young patients.

Initial treatment is conservative. Activity should be restricted and anti-inflammatory medications prescribed. A recent study of adolescents with herniated disks showed

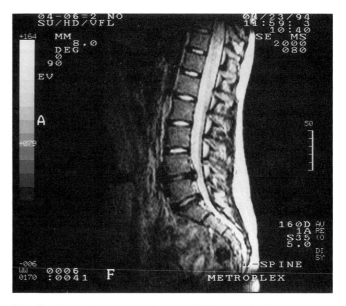

Fig. 3 Magnetic resonance imaging (MRI) scan of a 14-year-old female with complaints of back pain radiating into the legs, and numbness of the lateral leg. Herniation of the L4-5 and L5-S1 disks is present. Correlation of MRI and physical examination findings is paramount.

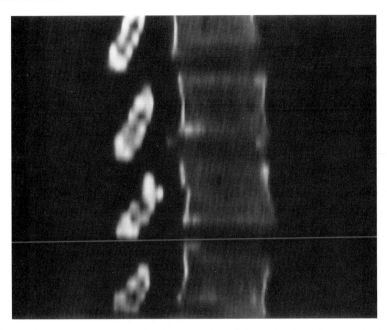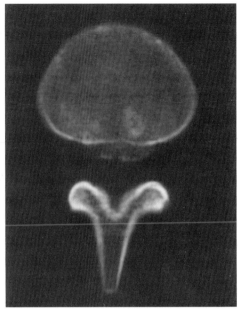

Fig. 4 Computed tomograms showing protrusion of the avulsed vertebra apophysis (posteriorly into the spinal canal) on the sagittal reconstruction (**left**) and transverse projection (**right**).

that adolescents who did not respond to an initial trial of conservative treatment improved after surgical diskectomy. Less favorable results were seen when surgery was not performed.

An entity specific to adolescence is the slipped vertebral apophysis. Male weightlifters are most commonly affected. The mechanism of injury is rapid flexion with axial compression. Symptoms mimic a herniated nucleus pulposus, but the onset of pain is always acute. Radiographs reveal a small fleck of bone representing the avulsed vertebral apophysis adjacent to the vertebral body. The most common location is the posterior inferior apophysis of the fourth lumbar vertebra. As this bony fragment may be difficult to see on plain radiographs, CT scan can be helpful (Fig. 4). Surgical management is always necessary, and the fragment of bone must be removed.

A relatively common cause of back pain in the teen athlete is muscle strain. The duration of symptoms is helpful in making the diagnosis, neurologic examination will be normal, and the pain should not radiate. Modification of activity, anti-inflammatory medication, and the application of heat or ice is advocated. Resumption of athletics can be allowed when the pain is resolved, but special attention to training techniques is necessary to prevent recurrence. Muscle strains resolve quickly. If the pain is persistent, radiographic evaluation, to look for spondylolysis and other etiologies, is indicated.

Obviously, spine fractures produce back pain. If the energy of injury or magnitude of pain is severe enough that

a fracture could have occurred, radiographs should be obtained at once.

Inflammatory Etiologies

Juvenile rheumatoid arthritis may produce back pain. Usually the patient will complain of pain or stiffness in other joints as well. Although the neck is more commonly involved than the thoracic or lumbar spines, and cervical instability in rheumatoid arthritis is well recognized, a thorough investigation for other causes of pain (ie, infection, tumor, or fracture) should be carried out when a child with rheumatoid arthritis complains of discomfort in the neck or back.

Ankylosing spondylitis may become evident during adolescence. Males are more frequently affected than females. The physical examination will reveal stiffness of the spine, with inability to reverse lumbar lordosis on forward bending. Abnormal kyphosis can be present, and chest excursion with deep inspiration can be limited. Sclerosis, narrowing, blurring, or fusion of the sacroiliac joints is seen on radiographs. A positive HLA-B27 blood test is linked with ankylosing spondylitis.

Neoplastic Etiologies

Eosinophilic Granuloma Children with eosinophilic granuloma (histiocytosis X) who present with back pain are usually younger than 10 years of age. Pain is localized over the involved vertebrae, and neurologic signs are uncommon. The skeletal lesions may occur singularly or as part of a systemic disease, such as Hand-Schüller-Christian disease or Letterer-Siwe disease. The spine is involved in 10% to 15% of children with histiocytosis X.

Radiographs may reveal a lytic lesion within the vertebral body. With larger lesions, collapse of the vertebral body results in vertebra plana, or the coin-on-end appearance (Fig. 5). More extensive collapse is generally seen in younger children. Differential diagnosis should always include infection. Resolution of skeletal lesions and back pain may occur without active treatment, and, therefore, the need for surgical or radiation treatment remains controversial. Surgical biopsy may be needed for diagnosis of the uncharacteristic lesion. The pain can be treated by bed rest or by immobilization in an orthosis or cast. Irradiation is used by some for children with neurologic deficits. Occasionally, surgical debridement and fusion is indicated in patients with severe neurologic compromise.

Osteoid Osteoma and Osteoblastoma   Osteoid osteomas usually involve the posterior elements of the spine. Patients complain of back pain, particularly at night, and find relief with nonsteroidal medications. The peak ages of incidence range between 6 and 17 years. Physical examination may reveal decreased spinal mobility or mild scoliosis with a list.

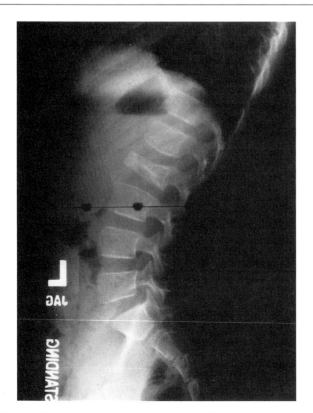

Fig. 5 Seven-year-old female with eosinophilic granuloma and coin-on-end appearance of the second lumbar vertebra.

Identification of the lesion on plain radiographs is difficult. If seen, a small lucent lesion is usually surrounded by sclerosis. Bone scan will show increased uptake in the lesion. CT scans can be useful in precisely locating the nidus within the vertebra (Fig. 6).

Treatment of osteoid osteomas is usually surgical excision. First, however, a trial of nonsteroidal anti-inflammatory medications should be undertaken, as pain improves with medical management in a small percentage of patients. Complete surgical excision produces near immediate relief of the pain, but if associated scoliosis has been present for longer than 15 months, the spinal deformity may persist.

Osteoblastomas do have a predilection for the spine, with 40% of osteoblastomas involving the vertebrae. Like osteoid osteomas, they occur most often in the lamina or pedicle but may extend into the vertebral body. They also produce back pain, but the pain may not be as intense as in an osteoid osteoma. Because of their size, neurologic complaints such as radiculopathy are more common with osteoblastomas than with osteoid osteomas.

Scoliosis is present in 40% of children with osteoblastomas. Plain radiographs often identify the lesions, and CT is helpful in determining the extent of the tumor and guiding surgical excision. Treatment is surgical resection, with a recurrence rate of approximately 10%.

Aneurysmal Bone Cysts   Aneurysmal bone cysts usually originate in the posterior elements of the spine, but they can extend into the anterior column. Seen as expansile lucent lesions on radiographs, they may have a bubbly or blown-out appearance.

CT is used to determine the extent of the cyst. Treatment is surgical curettage with grafting. As the lesions are very vascular, preoperative angiography with embolization can be of great benefit. Recurrences are not uncommon.

Malignancies   Children with malignant tumors of the spine or spinal cord may present with back pain. It is usually constant and worsens in severity with time. Tumors that may involve the spine include Ewing's sarcoma (with a predilection for the sacrum), osteogenic sarcoma, chordoma, metastatic neuroblastoma, and leukemia. The most frequent spinal cord tumor is astrocytoma.

Back pain is the presenting complaint in 6% of children with acute lymphocytic leukemia. A high index of suspicion is necessary to make this unusual diagnosis. Systemic complaints such as lethargy, pallor, bruising, fever, and bleeding suggest a generalized condition. A laboratory investigation with a complete blood count (elevated white cell count), platelet count (often decreased), and sedimentation rate (increased) supports the diagnosis. Definitive diagnosis is made by bone marrow aspiration.

Visceral Etiologies
Several intra-abdominal processes may produce back pain. A careful history and physical examination may lead

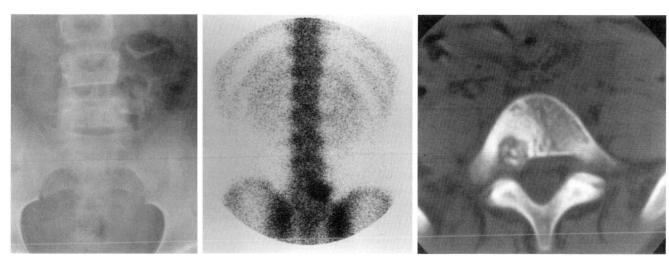

Fig. 6 **Left,** Plain radiograph of a 10-year-old male with complaints of back pain. The AP view demonstrates asymmetry of the L5 pedicles. **Center,** The bone scan shows increased uptake in the L5 pedicle. **Right,** CT scanning was used to localize the lesion (osteoid osteoma) to the posterior vertebral body and pedicle.

to a diagnosis of urinary tract infection, hydronephrosis, ovarian cysts, or inflammatory bowel disease. Thoracic back pain can be produced by pneumonia. A history of pain during the menstrual period is rarely of orthopaedic origin.

Psychologic Etiologies
Although most young children with back pain can be assigned a specific medical diagnosis after a thorough evaluation, there is a subset of patients with back pain who have

negative diagnostic work-ups. The diagnosis of psychosomatic pain can be made only after a complete evaluation has been performed, and all other etiologies of pain have been ruled out. Detailed questioning of these children often uncovers a social history of discord within the family. Often there are other family members who have similar complaints of back pain. Older adolescents are more likely to have psychosomatic back pain than are young children. Intensive counseling and a team approach with therapists, physicians, and psychologists can be helpful in relieving this form of back pain.

Annotated Bibliography

History
King H: Back pain in children, in Weinstein SL (ed): *The Pediatric Spine: Principles and Practice.* New York, NY, Raven Press, 1994, vol 1, pp 173–183.

This is an excellent review of the incidence and etiologies of back pain in children. Conversion reaction leading to back pain is a diagnosis of exclusion, but does occur in certain children. Diagnostic evaluation is indicated for all children with persistent back pain or neurologic findings.

Thompson GH: Back pain in children, in Schafer M (ed): *Instructional Course Lectures 43.* Rosemont, IL, American Academy of Orthopaedic Surgeons, 1994, pp 221–230.

The author reviews the examination, diagnostic workup, and common etiologies of back pain in the young patient.

Causes of Back Pain
Boriani S, Capanna R, Donati D, et al: Osteoblastoma of the spine. *Clin Orthop* 1992;278:37–45.

Thirty adults and children with osteoblastoma were reviewed. Continuous pain was the predominant symptom, and was not more severe at night. Scoliosis was present in 40% of the patients. The lesions could be visualized on plain radiographs.

Conrad EU III, Olszewski AD, Berger M, et al: Pediatric

spine tumors with spinal cord compromise. *J Pediatr Orthop* 1992;12:454–460.

Fifty-five percent of children with spinal tumors and canal compromise complained of back pain. Sarcomas were most often associated with pain.

Crawford AH, Kucharzyk DW, Ruda R, et al: Diskitis in children. *Clin Orthop* 1991;266:70–79.

Thirty-four children with diskitis were reviewed. All had an elevated erythrocyte sedimentation rate, but only 72% had a positive bone scan. CT and MRI were very sensitive in establishing the diagnosis. Bed rest was useful treatment. Antibiotic therapy was recommended for children whose symptoms do not resolve.

DeLuca PF, Mason DE, Weiand R, et al: Excision of herniated nucleus pulposus in children and adolescents. *J Pediatr Orthop* 1994;14:318–322.

Eighty-eight children with herniated disks were reviewed. Of patients treated surgically, 91% had excellent or good results, whereas 75% of patients who did not have surgery went on to poor results. At presentation, 94% of patients had low back pain, usually accompanied by sciatica. Neurologic findings were less common.

Harvey J, Tanner S: Low back pain in young athletes: A practical approach. *Sports Med* 1991;12:394–406.

Overuse syndromes, spondylolysis, fractures, and muscle strains can be seen in young athletes. Sports that have a high risk for producing back injuries are football, gymnastics, wrestling, dance, and diving. There is a good discussion of rehabilitation program to return athletes to their sports.

Ring D, Johnston CE II, Wenger DR: Pyogenic infectious spondylitis in children: The convergence of discitis and vertebral osteomyelitis. *J Pediatr Orthop* 1995;15:652–660.

Forty-seven patients with pyogenic infectious spondylitis (diskitis) were reviewed to determine the spectrum of disease.

MRIs were obtained in nine patients and were found to be identical to MRI findings in adult vertebral osteomyelitis. This provides strong evidence for an infectious process in diskitis. The investigation confirmed the usually benign course of spine infections in children but also emphasized the potential for serious sequelae. Symptoms were resolved more rapidly with intravenous antibiotics than they were with oral antibiotics or no antibiotics.

Ring D, Wenger DR: Magnetic resonance imaging scans in discitis: Sequential studies in a child who needed operative drainage. *J Bone Joint Surg* 1994;76A:596–601.

The authors present a case report of a child with diskitis who developed a psoas abscess diagnosed by MRI. Routine administration of intravenous antibiotics is advocated for the treatment of diskitis, regardless of the presence or absence of constitutional symptoms.

Yamane T, Yoshida T, Mimatsu K: Early diagnosis of lumbar spondylolysis by MRI. *J Bone Joint Surg* 1993; 75B:764–768.

Seventy-nine children with back pain underwent MRI and CT. Early detection of spondylolysis was discovered on MRI prior to visualization of a bony defect on CT. The pars interarticularis was hypointense in T1-weighted images, indicating a prefracture stage of spondylolysis.

Yancey RA, Micheli LJ: Thoracolumbar spine injuries in pediatric sports, in Stanitski CL, DeLee JC, Drez DD (eds): *Pediatric and Adolescent Sports Medicine.* Philadelphia, PA, WB Saunders, 1994, vol 3, pp 162–174.

This chapter discusses in detail the injuries sustained by the thoracolumbar spine of the adolescent athlete, in particular spondylolysis and spondylolisthesis, herniated disks, and slipped vertebral apophyses. The biomechanical etiologies, presenting symptoms, treatment regimens, and return to sport are all covered.

3
The Ambulatory Child With Cerebral Palsy

Introduction

Cerebral palsy, a nonprogressive disorder of the central nervous system secondary to a perinatal insult, results in varying degrees of motor milestone delay and dysfunction. Classification systems are based on the pattern of extremity involvement and type of motor dysfunction. For example, patients with hemiplegia have ipsilateral upper and lower limb involvement, and those with diplegia have involvement of all four limbs with the upper extremities only mildly affected. Because advances in perinatal care have decreased the incidence of athetosis, the predominant motor dysfunction in patients is spasticity, which is defined as velocity-dependent tone. Cognitive involvement varies, depending on the severity of central nervous system involvement. The incidence varies from 3% to 5% of live births, depending on the definition of cerebral palsy and diagnostic criteria.

The goals of treatment in patients with cerebral palsy are improvement of their functional abilities in self-care skills and promotion of functional independence. The four major types of treatment methods are physical therapy, orthoses, control of spasticity, and orthopaedic surgery. The indications and results for these methods are controversial. Often, all four methods are used together in various combinations. The orthopaedist plays a vital role in treatment by prescribing therapy and orthotics in addition to performing appropriate surgical procedures. Appropriate goal setting and realistic parental expectations are necessary to ensure parent and patient satisfaction with the treatment outcome.

Early Detection

Continued advances in the prevention and early detection of neuromuscular abnormalities have been made through the years. Advancing technology, with its improved imaging techniques, has increased the sensitivity of detection. In a study of high-risk infants followed prospectively for the development of neurologic disorder, ultrasound proved to be a practical diagnostic tool for the early detection of anatomic abnormalities, while magnetic resonance imaging (MRI) was the most sensitive radiographic technique.

Numerous systems to evaluate motor function have been developed to detect early clinical signs of cerebral palsy. The Movement Analysis of Infants (MAI) is used to identify early predictive signs for cerebral palsy in infants as young as 4 months of age. The MAI has proven to be a very sensitive tool, predicting the development of cerebral palsy in 73.5% of patients in a high-risk population at 4 months of age. Four specific signs are important: neck hyperextension tone, weightbearing through the arms in a prone position, head control in the sitting position, and hypertonia.

Physical Therapy

In a prospective study to examine the role of physical therapy in the development of motor skills, intensive neurodevelopmental therapy did not show superior results in the development of motor activities when compared with an approach based on a cognitive learning activity. Although previous claims of cure or prevention of neurologic involvement have been largely unsubstantiated, physical therapy continues to play an important role in the treatment of the patient with cerebral palsy.

The physical and occupational therapists provide services in many different areas of clinical importance. They provide a general physical fitness program that can incorporate muscle strengthening and stretching through specific exercises and general play activities, which can be done at school and at home, with parental supervision. The therapist evaluates the equipment needs of the patient and recommends the appropriate adaptive equipment and assistive devices, which are designed to improve function in the patient's activities of daily living (ADL) and to maximize function in the home and community. Because this equipment can be quite costly, it is important to purchase the appropriate equipment. The direct financial impact on families may be substantial as medical insurance policies cover less durable medical equipment. The indirect cost to society as a whole also may be great.

The therapist is an integral part of the management and treatment of the patient in the postoperative period. The initial mobilization after osteotomies or muscle procedures requires special care because of stiffness, pain, and weakness. The transition to improved function rests mainly on the therapist and efforts of the patient. Appropriate range of motion and muscle strengthening/stretching programs help the patient during this period. The initial use of mobility devices helps to progress and improve gait. By appropriate goal setting, the degree and timing of therapy can be regulated to provide an optimal outcome.

By coordinating the patient's care and needs, the therapist acts as a liaison among caretakers and the community. This includes interaction with the school therapy program, equipment needs, as well as being a general resource for the family.

Management of Spasticity

Ambulation is a complex neuromuscular function. Balance, muscle control, strength, functional joint motion, and sensory input are important factors influencing the patient's level of function. Although ambulatory function is not solely related to muscle tone, spasticity is the most easily identifiable clinical characteristic recognized by patients and family. Because most patients with cerebral palsy have spasticity, clinicians have focused their efforts toward its reduction. By diminishing spasticity, patients may theoretically perform integrated muscle movement, develop muscle strength, and function at a higher level. Three approaches have recently gained popularity. These include selective dorsal rhizotomy, intrathecal baclofen, and botulinum-A toxin.

Peacock has been responsible for the reintroduction and popularization of the neurosurgical approach, selective dorsal rhizotomy. This procedure addresses spasticity by the selective sectioning of abnormal dorsal rootlets. These are identified intraoperatively by observation of electromyographic (EMG) patterns and muscle activity through electric stimulation. A midline lumbar approach medial to the facet joints to avoid long-term structural abnormalities, (eg, scoliosis) allows exposure of the dorsal lumbar rootlets. Approximately 30% to 50% of the dorsal rootlets at levels L2-S1 are sectioned. The amount of rootlets transected varies, depending on the patient's clinical evaluation and intraoperative findings. Some centers section the rootlets at the L1 level. Following surgery, a combination of physical and occupational therapy four times per week is recommended for approximately 1 year. The results reported in the literature have been encouraging. All patients have significantly reduced spasticity as measured by a standardized scoring system (modified Ashworth scale). Evaluation of the patients 1 year after surgery shows improved lower extremity sagittal plane motion during gait.

The ideal candidate for selective dorsal rhizotomy is a patient with spastic diplegia who has not had previous orthopaedic procedures, is aged 4 to 8 years, has minimal to no contractures, has good muscle control, strength, and balance, has no extrapyramidal signs, and is a free ambulator. However, concerns have been raised regarding the potential for postoperative weakness, rapid hip subluxation, and hyperlordosis in the lumbar spine. Additionally, a significant number of patients may still require orthopaedic procedures after selective dorsal rhizotomy. The question remains as to the advantage rhizotomy offers the patient over traditional orthopaedic procedures, as similar improvements have been reported in this patient population after muscle lengthening procedures. With the long-time commitment to therapy thought to be necessary and the potential long-term complications after rhizotomy, its future role in the treatment of these patients still remains to be determined. As spasticity commonly remains after orthopaedic procedures, patients may best be treated with a combination of neurosurgical and orthopaedic procedures because one addresses spasticity, the other muscle contractures and fixed deformities.

The second approach to reduce spasticity is continuous infusion of intrathecal baclofen through an implantable pump. The pharmacologic action of this γ-aminobutyric acid (GABA) agonist is through inhibiting the release of excitatory neurotransmitters at the level of the spinal cord. Reports of its clinical effectiveness as an oral muscle relaxant have been mixed, but, when delivered directly into the intrathecal space, its action is localized to the specific neurologic levels and its systemic side effects (eg, drowsiness) can be minimized. Initial studies done with single or multiple intrathecal injections confirmed the clinical reduction of spasticity. These encouraging preliminary studies led Albright to perform clinical trials with 37 patients, who received continuous infusions of intrathecal baclofen. The dose of medication was titrated to achieve the desired reduction in spasticity. Patients had significant improvement in both upper and lower extremity muscle tone with improved upper extremity function and ADLs. Significant complications occurred, including catheter problems and infections. Eight patients have required pump removal at the time of their report. Despite the complications, the advantages of regulation of spasticity reduction through a titratable continuous delivery system were believed to hold clinical promise. The functional improvements achieved through spasticity reduction by each patient provide the necessary feedback to guide the clinician in dosage regulation.

The newest alternative takes advantage of the pharmacologic action of botulinum-A toxin. Reduction of spasticity occurs through the action of botulinum-A toxin at the myoneural junction. Acting at the presynaptic cholinergic terminal, the toxin inhibits the exocytosis of acetylcholine and produces its paralyzing effect. Selected muscles can be injected with the toxin in multiple sites to reduce spasticity. Two recent studies have documented the results of its use in clinical trials. The reduction in spasticity led to subjective improvement in observed gait patterns. Reported advantages include relatively painless injection (25- to 27-gauge needle), reversibility, and minimal side effects (injection site irritation). The spasticity reduction may last up to 6 months with patients requiring further injections to continue its beneficial effects, if desired. However, a recent report has shown that despite short-term improvements, most patients still require muscle lengthening for permanent correction. The role of botulinum-A toxin in the treatment of the patient with spastic cerebral palsy may be to delay surgical management or as a therapeutic trial to determine the effects of a specific proposed surgical treatment plan.

General Orthopaedic Procedures

Although specific deformities will be discussed in the following sections, it is imperative that the treating surgeon have a thorough knowledge of the complex effect each deformity has on other lower extremity joints. No deformity can be taken in isolation because each deformity has an impact on adjacent muscles and joints. Physicians must not fall into the well-known trap of "birthday" surgery, in which all of the deformities are addressed in multiple sequential surgeries rather than at a single surgical setting. However, this requires that the surgeon be able to distinguish between primary deformities, which need treatment, and compensatory ones, which will improve without intervention. With a thorough knowledge base, clinical experience, and advances in technology, such as gait analysis, treatment decisions can be made more confidently by the treating physician and more predictably for the patient. Although the surgical procedures may not be as technically demanding as some other orthopaedic procedures, the impact on the child's daily function can be significant.

The Hip

Dynamic gait deformities require surgical treatment more frequently than structural deformities, because concerns of hip subluxation are uncommon in the walking patient with diplegia. A common dynamic pattern is scissoring and excessive hip flexion with associated lumbar lordosis. This pattern restricts the advancement of the swing limb and contributes to instability of the stance phase limb. The excessive hip flexion may cause secondary compensations at the knee, ankle, and trunk. Scissoring gait can be approached by either adductor release or posterior transfer. Both procedures improve the adduction deformity. Studies have not shown a difference in hip radiographic measurements when comparing adductor transfer to adductor release. The rate of adductor pull-off after transfer is significant, reported as 33%. The concern of possibly producing asymmetric gait if only one side detaches has led some surgeons to perform tenotomies rather than transfers. The necessity of spica cast immobilization for transfers also makes this approach less appealing. The addition of an iliopsoas recession (or resection) to the adductor release improves hip extension and patient walking skills when compared to those undergoing just adductor release.

The Knee

Determining whether a particular knee posture is a primary or compensatory abnormality continues to be a focus of significant interest for clinicians treating these ambulatory patients. A better understanding of the function of the muscles around the knee, specifically the rectus femoris and the hamstrings, is being gained through kinetic analysis and computer modeling. The rectus femoris plays a significant role in the pathogenesis of stiff knee gait. EMG analysis has documented nonphasic activity of the rectus femoris during swing phase in patients with stiff knee gait. This is manifested by decreased knee flexion in swing phase, decreased total arc of knee motion, and delayed timing of peak knee flexion in swing phase (timing

abnormality). Surgical options include proximal release, distal release, and distal transfer. In a study that compared distal rectus transfer with simple proximal release, the former was reported to improve peak knee flexion (16.2° versus 9.1°, $p < 0.02$). It was concluded that distal rectus femoris transfer (medially to the sartorius) is the recommended surgical choice for the treatment of stiff knee gait in this patient population.

Crouched gait is an easily recognized gait abnormality in the walking diplegic population. Recent articles document improved knee extension with hamstring lengthening, although some recurrence of the deformity has been noted at 3-year follow-up. Some patients lose posterior pelvic stability after hamstring lengthening as manifested by increased anterior pelvic tilt and increased hip flexion. Gait analysis and computerized muscle length determinations have established that some patients with crouching at the knee may actually have elongated or normal hamstring muscle length due to simultaneous flexion of the hip. Hamstring lengthening in this particular group of patients may cause significant weakness in hip extension. The role of hamstring transfer to the femur to maintain hip extension power and concomitant hip flexor release is presently being investigated. Although hamstring lengthening is a proven procedure to achieve knee extension, caution should be taken to avoid postoperative stiff knee gait or hyperlordotic hip posture. Determining which antagonistic muscles need simultaneous intervention requires awareness and careful analysis.

The Foot and Ankle

Although not the most prevalent foot deformity, an equinovarus foot deformity may require treatment in the patient with spastic diplegia. Two distinctly different techniques for correction of this abnormality have been described. The approaches differ in the way they address the dominant deforming force, the posterior tibialis tendon. Fine wire EMG analysis has attempted to define the role of the posterior tibialis tendon in the pathogenesis of the deformity. Kaufer described the split posterior tibial tendon transfer with the lateral half placed posterior to the interosseous membrane and attached to the peroneus brevis. This transfer balances the forces across the subtalar joint by realigning its once dominant inverting force and allows better positioning of the foot by addressing the pathologic tendon through balancing its effect. Excellent results have recently been reported.

The other treatment approach proposes a split anterior tibial tendon transfer with posterior tibial tendon lengthening. This addresses the "over pull" of the posterior tibial tendon by lengthening it and the dorsiflexion/eversion of the foot is augmented by the lateral transfer of half of the anterior tibial tendon. Another recent study has also reported excellent results using this technique. Neither of these studies used gait analysis or fine wire EMG to help select the appropriate surgical procedure. Provided there is a passively corrected foot and a strong anterior tibial tendon, either procedure will be successful. Those with poor anterior tibial function are better treated with a split posterior tibial tendon transfer. For those patients with fixed deformity, osteotomy is indicated to correct the deformity because the majority of poor results in either group were in those patients with fixed deformity.

An equinovalgus foot is the most frequent foot deformity seen in the patient with spastic diplegia. It is commonly associated with a contracted Achilles tendon and secondary talonavicular subluxation. This becomes a clinical problem when pain or brace intolerance occurs secondary to pressure medially over the prominent talar head. Unlike the equinovarus foot, muscle balancing procedures are not available for this deformity. One proven approach to achieving permanent correction is subtalar arthrodesis. The problems of malunion and nonunion so prevalent with the classic Green-Grice procedure have been addressed with improved success. Although various methods are described, common to each technique is the use of internal fixation to maintain the corrected position and cancellous bone graft to assure fusion. Lengthening of the heel cord is often needed also.

Mosca has recently introduced his modification of the Evans procedure of calcaneal neck lengthening. This procedure theoretically preserves subtalar motion with its inherent advantages. He altered the skin incision, position and direction of the osteotomy, shape of the graft, management of the soft tissues, and use of internal fixation. The placement of a trapezoidal wedge in the distal oblique osteotomy of the calcaneus to elongate the lateral column and support the talar head appears to provide good correction. Placement of a wire for internal fixation and appropriate muscle and soft-tissue balancing procedures produced satisfactory results in 29 of 31 feet. Six patients with cerebral palsy were included in this report. All of these patients required lengthening of the peroneal tendons to balance the muscle forces and achieve correction of the deformity. Mosca's subjective evaluation showed maintenance of subtalar motion with adequate clinical correction of the deformity. This may prove to be an attractive alternative to subtalar arthrodesis in the treatment of the valgus foot in this patient population.

Despite reports of poor results in long-term follow-up of triple arthrodesis in patients without cerebral palsy (eg, Charcot-Marie-Tooth), it appears to be a valuable salvage procedure to obtain a plantigrade foot for the rigid deformity in the patient with cerebral palsy. Studies have reported good functional results up to 30 years after surgery. Because of the diminishing physical activity level of this patient group with age, a relatively symptom-free foot can be maintained in long-term follow-up, despite the development of radiographic changes of adjacent joint arthritis.

The Gastrocnemius-Soleus Complex

Many patients with spastic cerebral palsy walk on their toes. Treatment of dynamic deformities should be by bracing or by appropriate spasticity reduction using techniques described earlier. Fixed equinus deformity may be corrected through serial casting or treated with surgery. As heel cord lengthening has been performed using many techniques over the years, most physicians feel comfortable with its technical aspects. Lengthening of the Achilles tendon in dynamic deformities should be undertaken with caution because overlengthening with resultant calcaneal deformity can occur. This deformity is difficult to correct and has significant detrimental effects because this complex contributes a significant amount of power generation during gait.

The obvious need to maintain the gastrocnemius-soleus complex strength has led to careful evaluation of the contribution of each muscle to function. As muscles that span two joints appear to be particularly involved in cerebral palsy, there has been recent enthusiasm for performing only the isolated gastrocnemius intramuscular fascial slide. The gait analysis kinetic data gathered in a study of 20 patients support the maintenance of ankle push-off power with this procedure, thus avoiding the possible weakening effect of tendon lengthening (both muscle groups). This procedure may be indicated in patients with dynamic ankle equinus or an isolated gastrocnemius contracture as push-off power is maintained. Of importance in this study, the associated knee flexion was treated with hamstring lengthening on 22 of 24 sides in these patients. The frequency of heelcord lengthenings (both muscle groups) may diminish as the importance of its function and its interaction with other joint abnormalities is better understood.

Upper Extremity in Cerebral Palsy

Most procedures for the upper extremity in cerebral palsy have been directed at the flexed pronated wrist. One modification of Green's transfer of the flexor carpi ulnaris to the extensor carpi radialis brevis has had encouraging results. In this modified technique, the tension of the transfer is altered by holding the wrist in a neutral position rather than at 45° of dorsiflexion. By doing so, the potential complication of overcorrection is avoided. The single most important prognostic factor for the success of this surgery is the presence of at least some helper function of the hand. Although stereognosis was not a predicator of outcome, 80% of patients had improvement if it was present. Cosmetic improvement was seen in 88% of patients. Better results are obtained in patients younger than 12 years of age.

Postoperative Management

In the past, patients were immobilized for prolonged periods of time after soft-tissue surgery. A recent trend, however, focuses on rapid postoperative mobilization to quickly return patients to a functional level. Patients ambulate in casts or knee immobilizers in the early postoperative period (within 1 week). The length of time needed for immobilization depends on the functional improvements of the patient. In many patients, casts may be replaced by braces after only 1 week following soft-tissue procedures. Specific bracing during the day and at night is required to maintain the gains obtained through surgery.

Orthotics

Orthotic management in the patient with cerebral palsy includes predominantly the ankle-foot orthosis (AFO) and night bracing. The AFO has undergone many modifications as a better understanding of ankle biomechanics has fostered designs incorporating new lighter weight materials. Rigid AFOs have given way to braces with varying degrees of ankle motion. Many of these have 90° plantarflexion stop and free dorsiflexion settings. The added ankle motion appears to provide improved function as patients can ascend and descend stairs more easily. However, there are theoretic concerns as to whether each step provides either passive stretching of the gastrocnemius-soleus complex, or just triggers the stretch reflex, causing the patient to "fight" the brace. In addition, the role of the ankle plantarflexion-knee extension couple in these patients requires some limitation of ankle dorsiflexion. The ideal brace then must have a limited arc of motion, be positioned to prevent foot drop, and allow a reasonable amount of dorsiflexion for functional activities, yet be limited to maintain the ankle plantarflexion-knee extension couple.

An ideal brace would support joint position passively and store the kinetic energy generated by forward momentum. It would release this energy at the appropriate time during gait at push-off. Advancements in technology and materials have permitted the development of designs that claim characteristics of energy absorption and power generation. However, recent investigation has shown that the power generation of the posterior relief spring orthosis is minimal.

The use of a knee-ankle-foot orthosis (KAFO) has diminished greatly due to its weight and the difficulty in walking stiff-legged when the braces are locked.

Postoperative nighttime splinting is important in maintaining the benefits of muscle lengthenings. This includes the use of posterior KAFO night splints to maintain knee extension after hamstring lengthening along with an abduction pillow after adductor releases. Some authors recommend their use until the patient reaches skeletal maturity in order to prevent the recurrence of muscle shortening that can occur with skeletal growth. Knee immobilizers provide an attractive alternative to KAFOs. Their softness and ease of application increases compliance. If only one extremity is splinted, alternating sides each night allows the patient some freedom of movement in the bed, improving patient tolerance of the brace.

Hemiplegia

Winters and Gage identified four patterns of gait in patients with hemiplegic involvement. These patterns define a spectrum of involvement beginning with distal abnormalities, progressing to the more proximally involved patients. The type I pattern is characterized by a functional drop foot in swing phase. This results in initial toe contact with normal ankle dorsiflexion in stance phase. This swing phase dropfoot is best treated with an AFO with a 90° plantarflexion stop.

The type II pattern has ankle plantarflexion in both swing and stance phase. Associated hyperextension of the knee and hip occur secondary to the contracted Achilles tendon. Treatment with heel cord lengthening restores normal ankle kinematics. The exact type of surgical lengthening depends on the surgeon's experience and patient's physical examination. If residual drop foot persists after surgery, an AFO is utilized.

The type III pattern has a type II ankle pattern, but with a differing knee pattern consisting of crouch and stiff knee pattern. Treatment of this condition is approached with similar ankle surgery with an associated hamstring lengthening to improve knee extension and distal rectus femoris transfer to improve the stiff knee gait abnormality.

The type IV pattern has all the features of type III, but with associated hip flexor and adductor involvement. This is manifested by an adduction deformity at the hip with increased anterior pelvic tilt in late stance phase hip flexion. Treatment is as in type III patients with the additional adductor release and iliopsoas lengthening.

Outcome Measures

As part of the health care reform agenda, emphasis has been placed on standardized methods to critically evaluate outcomes of treatment. Two major areas of interest for documentation of outcome have included gait analysis and standardized functional assessments.

Gait Analysis

Recent technical developments have made three-dimensional gait analysis much more accessible and understandable to physicians. Systems are now available that are user friendly and are capable of producing accurate data with relative ease. Developments in the kinetic aspects of gait (moments and powers) have furthered the understanding of the pathomechanics of gait and of the effects of surgery. Gait analysis offers at a minimum an accurate measurement tool for documentation of treatment outcome, whether surgical or nonsurgical; however, debate still exists regarding its role in diagnostic and pretreatment therapeutic decisions and whether it is absolutely necessary in the treatment of ambulatory patients with cerebral palsy. As more systems develop a user-friendly interface requiring less technical understanding of the data acquisition and interpolation, the question of accreditation and personnel qualifications must also be addressed. Its use to document outcome has become quite prevalent in the recent literature and is the measurement tool of gait in many papers listed in the annotated bibliography. Its future clinical relevance is dependent on its usefulness in predicting outcome and its ability to clarify the causes of pathologic gait through advances in technologic-assisted research, such as moments and powers.

Functional Outcome Measures

Other important measures of functional needs and improvements must also be incorporated. The Gross Motor Performance Measure, Pediatric Evaluation of Disability Inventory, and WeeFIM are examples of standardized tests that have been used to measure these functional tasks. These are useful in the evaluation of any treatment, including orthopaedic procedures and physical therapy. By incorporating these measures in goal setting for each patient, realistic expectations and parental satisfaction can be achieved with any proven intervention. One comprehensive review of the published evaluation tools categorized strengths and weaknesses for each test and provides a basis for the interested investigator on the available standardized tests, with specific explanations of the appro-

priate applications. Correlation of gait analysis with these other outcome measurements will be of distinct use in the future.

Conclusion

Treatment of the ambulatory patient with cerebral palsy is a continuing challenge to the orthopaedist. With recent advancements in technology, especially in gait analysis, the evaluation and treatment of the patient has become more sophisticated and complex. Subtle deformities and concerns of maintenance of power in these particular patients requires careful evaluation before intervention is performed. As in any neuromuscular patient, function can be measured at multiple levels and it is imperative that the operating surgeon does not lose sight of the goal of treatment, which is to improve the "function" of the patient in daily living and integration into society. Through the use of therapy, orthotics, and selected orthopaedic procedures, these goals are achievable in the majority of patients.

Annotated Bibliography

Incidence

Nelson KB, Ellenberg JH: Epidemiology of cerebral palsy. *Adv Neurol* 1978;19:421–435.

The authors review the findings of the National Institute of Neurological and Communicative Disorders and Stroke Collaborative Perinatal Project on the incidence of cerebral palsy. The incidence depends on definition and criteria for perinatal insult.

Early Detection

Harris SR: Movement analysis: An aid to early diagnosis of cerebral palsy. *Phys Ther* 1991;71:215–221.

This article provides a review of recent literature regarding the use of movement signs as predictors of cerebral palsy. The authors evaluated 229 infants and compared their results with those of a larger collaborative study to determine the early predictive signs for cerebral palsy at 4 months. The author used movement assessment of infants (MAI) and identified the best predictors as neck hyperextension tone, weightbearing through the arms in prone position, head control in the sitting position, and hypertonia.

Keeney SE, Adcock EW, McArdle CB: Prospective observations of 100 high-risk neonates by high-field (1.5 Tesla) magnetic resonance imaging of the central nervous system: II. Lesions associated with hypoxic-ischemic encephalopathy. *Pediatrics* 1991;87:431–438.

One hundred infants were examined prospectively for risk of neurologic handicaps. The criteria for inclusion included Apgar less than 6, metabolic acidosis, sustained bradycardia and

hypoxemia (PaO_2 < 30 mm Hg). Thirty-three infants with 37 lesions were identified by MRI. Ultrasound showed 77% of these lesions, while CT showed only 41%. The authors recommend ultrasound at the bedside with MRI for further investigation as indicated.

Swanson MW, Bennett FC, Shy KK, et al: Identification of neurodevelopmental abnormality at four and eight months by the movement assessment of infants. *Dev Med Child Neurol* 1992;34:321–337.

The authors studied 160 infants with low birth weight to determine the predictive value (sensitivity and specificity) of the MAI scale. The sensitivity was 83% at 4 months of age and 96% at 8 months of age. The specifity was 78% at 4 months of age and 65% at 8 months. The authors concluded this assessment could be an excellent screening tool because its sensitivity was quite high. The Bayley motor scale was more specific at each age level when compared to the MAI, although its sensitivity is quite low.

Physical Therapy

Palmer FB, Shapiro BK, Wachtel RC, et al: The effects of physical therapy on cerebral palsy: A controlled trial in infants with spastic diplegia. *N Engl J Med* 1988;318:803–808.

Forty-eight infants were randomly assigned to two therapy protocols. Group A had 12 months of neurodevelopmental therapy (NDT), group B had 6 months of infant stimulation (cognitive and learning activities not focused on abilities to right oneself and maintain equilibrium), followed by 6 months of NDT. Patients were evaluated at 6 and 12 months. The significant finding was a significantly lower motor quotient in group A as compared to group B. The authors question the role of intensive NDT in affecting motor development. However, it did appear that pretreatment motor and cognitive abilities were more powerful determinants of outcome, strongly outweighing any effect of treatment.

Management of Spasticity

Albright AL, Barron WB, Fasick MP, et al: Continuous intrathecal baclofen infusion for spasticity of cerebral origin. *JAMA* 1993;270:2475–2477.

Based on the authors' previous favorable experience with a single injection of baclofen, a GABA agonist, to reduce spasticity, the study was extended to placement of a subcutaneous pump to deliver a continuous titratable dose intrathecally to patients with spastic cerebral palsy. The 37 patients presented had significant decrease in spasticity in the upper ($p = 0.04$) and lower ($p = 0.001$) extremities. Hamstring motion, upper extremity function, and activities of daily living improved in the 25 patients capable of self-care. Complications have been related to the catheter (five) and infection (four). Eight pumps had to be removed in total. The authors believe this treatment option has promise for treatment because of its ability to titrate the amount of spasticity reduction and its relation to clinical improvement and functional gains.

Boscarino LF, Ounpuu S, Davis RB III, et al: Effects of selective dorsal rhizotomy on gait in children with cerebral palsy. *J Pediatr Orthop* 1993;13:174–179.

Three-dimensional gait analysis showed significant improvement in sagittal joint motion in 19 ambulatory patients with spastic cerebral palsy 1 year after selective dorsal rhizotomy (rootlet levels L2-S1). A greater incidence of plantigrade foot position in stance was noted. Gait parameters revealed an increase in stride length. Some increase in anterior pelvic tilt was noted. The authors concluded that the reduction in spasticity noted by measurement of muscle tone and ankle clonus translated to gait kinematic improvements in the sagittal plane toward normal in this patient population.

Cosgrove AP, Corry IS, Graham HK: Botulinum toxin in the management of the lower limb in cerebral palsy. *Dev Med Child Neurol* 1994;36:386–396.

The initial clinical trials of BOTOX® injection by this group notes reduced spasticity and improved joint motion after injection. Twenty-six patients with 1- to 2-year follow-up had various muscles injected. The gastrocnemius-soleus, hamstrings, and posterior tibialis were the selected muscle groups. In ambulatory patients, an increase in ankle dorsiflexion of $11°$ ($p < 0.05$) with a $22°$ gain ($p < 0.01$) in knee extension was documented with electrogoniometric gait analysis. At 6 months, ankle motion gains diminished, but knee gains were maintained. The authors conclude that BOTOX® has promise for spasticity reduction in the treatment of dynamic deformities in patients with spastic cerebral palsy.

Koman LA, Mooney JF III, Smith B, et al: Management of cerebral palsy with Botulinum-A toxin: Preliminary investigation. *J Pediatr Orthop* 1993;13:489–495.

Twenty-seven patients underwent multiple injections of selected muscles with BOTOX® at the myoneural junction to reduce spasticity. Of the ambulatory patients, 16 were injected in the gastrocnemius-soleus; six of these patients were also injected in the posterior tibialis muscle. The desired effect was noted 12 to

72 hours after injection. A gait rating scale (maximum number of points, 14) revealed a significant change from a preinjection value of 5.3 to postinjection value of 10.3. The frequency of side effects included soreness in 45% (transient 1 to 2 days), fatigue in 13%, and transient weakness in 6%. The authors conclude that BOTOX® can provide spasticity reduction with improved walking.

McLaughlin JF, Bjornson KF, Astley SJ, et al: The role of selective dorsal rhizotomy in cerebral palsy: Critical evaluation of a prospective clinical series. *Dev Med Child Neurol* 1994;36:755–769.

Thirty-four consecutive patients with cerebral palsy underwent selective dorsal rhizotomy (SDR). Ten spastic quadriplegia and 24 spastic diplegia patients were evaluated at 3-month intervals with neurologic evaluation, deep tendon reflexes, presence of orthopaedic deformities, range of motion, spasticity (as measured on the Ashworth scale), and the Gross Motor Performance Measure (GMPM), a criterion-referenced evaluative assessment tool. No significant complications were noted. Muscle spasticity, deep tendon reflexes, and clonus were reduced in all patients. Two of ten patients with hip subluxation required surgical intervention, while eight patients stabilized. GMPM score improved by 9% ($p < 0.0001$) in spastic quadriplegia and 9.8% ($p < 0.0001$) in spastic diplegia. The authors conclude that functional changes were seen after SDR, but were hesitant to attribute these improvements solely to spasticity reduction. Other assessments of outcome (gait analysis, O_2 consumption) and a randomized/controlled study were recommended to better assess the specific effect that SDR therapy, motivation, and spontaneous developmental change have on outcome.

Price R, Bjornson KF, Lehmann JF, et al: Quantitative measurement of spasticity in children with cerebral palsy. *Dev Med Child Neurol* 1991;33:585–595.

The authors describe a measurement device that moves the ankle in a $5°$ arc at certain frequencies while recording torque. Nine children were tested and the variation of elastic and viscous stiffness over a spectrum of frequency was independent of the passive elastic elements secondary to contracture. By appropriate corrections, aging can be eliminated as an important variable. This device provides a quantitative measurement tool to evaluate the effects of treatment directed at spasticity reduction.

General Orthopaedic Procedures

The Hip

Aronson DD, Zak PJ, Lee CL, et al: Posterior transfer of the adductors in children who have cerebral palsy: A long-term study. *J Bone Joint Surg* 1991;73A:59–65.

Forty-two patients with 78 adductor transfers were evaluated an average of 5.7 years after surgery. Surgical indications included an adduction contracture and/or reducible hip subluxation in a patient with spastic cerebral palsy between the ages of 4 and 12. Eighty-eight percent achieved hip stability, hip abduction, extension, and functional walking. Those patients with simultaneous iliopsoas release improved hip extension by $25°$ as opposed to $11°$ in those without tenotomy ($p < 0.01$). Abduction improved by $12°$ or more if the iliopsoas was also tenotomized ($p < 0.005$). Walking improved, based on the Hoffer grading system, from a preoperative score of 1.3 to a postoperative score of 2.0. Significant radiographic improvement of the center edge angle and acetabular index were noted. The recommended treatment was adductor longus, gracilis transfer with iliopsoas tenotomy and placement in above knee casts with an abduction bar for 4 weeks as spica cast immobilization offered no measurable improved outcome.

Buckley SL, Sponseller PD, Magid D: The acetabulum in congenital and neuromuscular hip instability. *J Pediatr Orthop* 1991;11:498–501.

Nine nonambulatory patients with global neuromuscular deficiencies at an average of 9.1 years of age were evaluated by CT. The patients had less than 50% head coverage on the anteroposterior radiograph and had no previous surgery. Using four radiographic measurements, these patients displayed significant posterior insufficiency, although anterior deficiency was also present though to a lesser degree. The authors conclude that surgical stabilization must include careful preoperative and intraoperative evaluation to provide adequate coverage where needed.

Loder RT, Harbuz A, Aronson DD, et al: Postoperative migration of the adductor tendon after posterior adductor transfer in children with cerebral palsy. *Dev Med Child Neurol* 1992;34:49–54.

A review of 33 hips revealed that 11 (33%) transfers had pulled loose from their original position. Eight of 11 occurred after cast removal, with more occurring in the ambulatory patient with diplegia (nine of 20) than patients with spastic quadriplegia (two of 13). No specific gait alterations or deleterious effects were noted though three-dimensional gait analysis was not performed. The authors believed that the forces placed on the hip for walking were more significant than the spastic pull in the nonambulator because ambulatory patients had a higher rate of pull-off. The authors believed that gait analysis may provide information to determine the significance of pull-off, which was not clinically relevant in this study. As transfer requires more surgical time and more extensive immobilization, its efficiency as a transfer and relationship to outcome is questioned.

Zimmermann SE, Sturm PF: Computed tomographic assessment of shelf acetabuloplasty. *J Pediatr Orthop* 1992;12:581–585.

Eleven cerebral palsy patients underwent shelf acetabuloplasty for subluxation with preoperative and postoperative CT. Significant anterior acetabular deficiencies were noted, although no significant posterior deficiency was noted using the same measurements as Buckley. This study and that by Buckley and associates point out the need to identify specific deficiencies in these patients so that appropriate reconstructive/salvage procedures can be performed.

The Knee

Hoffinger SA, Rab GT, Abou-Ghaida H: Hamstrings in cerebral palsy crouch gait. *J Pediatr Orthop* 1993;13:722–726.

The authors review 16 patients with spastic diplegia and crouch gait with anterior pelvic tilt. With the use of three-dimensional gait analysis and a computer modeling program for muscle origin and insertion, the authors revisit the role of the hamstrings in crouch gait. By correlating EMG activity and hamstring length, some patients are concentrically contracting their hamstrings, thus generating hip extension power. These patients, though in crouch gait, may not benefit from hamstring lengthening because it may weaken their hip extension power. They conclude that careful evaluation of crouch gait is necessary to prevent a poor result secondary to loss of hip extension power.

Sutherland DH, Santi M, Abel MF: Treatment of stiff-knee gait in cerebral palsy: A comparison by gait analysis of distal rectus femoris transfer versus proximal rectus release. *J Pediatr Orthop* 1990;10:433–441.

All patients had evidence of stiff knee gait (decreased maximum knee flexion in swing, decreased dynamic knee range of motion, and delay in peak knee flexion) and abnormal rectus EMG activity during swing phase. No other soft-tissue release was performed. Gait analysis revealed improved peak knee flexion with proximal release of 9.1° versus 16.2° with distal transfer ($p < 0.02$). Improved knee arc of motion was seen in both groups and the transfer group appears to have a greater effect on the timing of peak knee flexion, although it was not statistically significant ($p < 0.07$). No ill effects on hip motion were noted. The authors conclude that distal rectus transfer improves knee motion to a greater degree than the proximal release and is the recommended treatment for stiff knee gait in this select group of patients.

The Foot and Ankle

Barnes MJ, Herring JA: Combined split anterior tibial-tendon transfer and intramuscular lengthening of the posterior tibial tendon: Results in patients who have a varus deformity of the foot due to spastic cerebral palsy. *J Bone Joint Surg* 1991;73A:734–738.

Twenty-two limbs in 20 patients with spastic cerebral palsy were reviewed with the split anterior tibial tendon transfer and intramuscular posterior tibial lengthening. Eighteen of 22 feet had good or excellent results. Three failures were secondary to preoperative fixed varus deformity and one failure was secondary to a weak anterior tibial tendon. The authors modified the original technique by stabilizing the lateral half of the transfer with a bone block and passing it under the extensor retinaculum. If a patient has dynamic varus and a passively correctable foot with good anterior tibial strength, a good result can be expected. The authors believe that preoperative electromyography is not necessary because their results were obtained through careful clinical evaluation and assessment. They believe that a better balance to the foot can be achieved with this surgery because it addresses both muscles by lengthening/weakening the posterior tibial tendon and augmenting dorsiflexion/eversion by split anterior tibial tendon transfer.

Mosca VS: Calcaneal lengthening for valgus deformity of the hindfoot: Results in children who had severe, symptomatic flatfoot and skewfoot. *J Bone Joint Surg* 1995;77A:500–512.

Thirty-one severe, symptomatic valgus deformities of the hindfoot in 20 children were treated with calcaneal lengthening. The author's modifications of the Evans procedure are described, including a detailed description of the surgical procedure. Additional midfoot and muscle balancing procedures are performed concomitantly. Twenty-nine of 31 feet had clinically and/or radiographically satisfactory results. Six patients (eight feet) had cerebral palsy. The author concluded that the procedure is an alternative to arthrodesis in the valgus foot because it corrects the deformity while preserving subtalar motion.

Rose SA, DeLuca PA, Davis RB III, et al: Kinematic and kinetic evaluation of the ankle after lengthening of the gastrocnemius fascia in children with cerebral palsy. *J Pediatr Orthop* 1993;13:727–732.

Twenty patients with spastic cerebral palsy underwent gastrocnemius fascial release on a total of 24 sides. The patients were evaluated before surgery and 1 year after surgery with three-dimensional gait analysis, including kinetic data. Passive ankle dorsiflexion with knee extension improved by 7° ($p <$

0.0001) and dynamic single stance ankle dorsiflexion improved by 8° ($p < 0.0003$), with no significant increase in total energy absorbed. No adverse knee effects were noted (ie, crouch), although the large majority (22 of 24 sides) had concomitant hamstring lengthening. The authors concluded that gastrocnemius fascia lengthening improves ankle motion, does not produce weakening, and improves ankle push-off power generation.

Synder M, Kumar SJ, Stecyk MD: Split tibialis posterior tendon transfer and tendo-Achilles lengthening for spastic equinovarus feet. *J Pediatr Orthop* 1993;13:20–23.

Twenty-one patients with a minimum follow-up of 2 years constitute the population reviewed. Of the 18 ambulatory patients, 15 had excellent or good results. Twelve patients did not require bracing postoperatively. The three failures were due to technical factors and patient selection because some had a fixed bony varus deformity. The transfer balances the forces across the subtalar joint. The authors recommend this procedure for the varus/supinated foot in stance that is passively correctable. They believed gait analysis was not necessary for the preoperative evaluation because clinical examination sufficed in this series.

Tenuta J, Shelton YA, Miller F: Long-term follow-up of triple arthrodesis in patients with cerebral palsy. *J Pediatr Orthop* 1993;13:713–716.

With an average follow-up of 17.8 years, 24 patients (35 feet) showed continued good functional results from triple arthrodesis. Nineteen of 24 patients were pleased with the results, with only two patients having occasional pain and one patient with frequent pain. Although degenerative arthritis of the tibiotalar joint was seen in 43% of patients and pseudarthrosis was noted in 14%, these findings did not correlate with greater symptoms. The authors concluded that triple arthrodesis is still an excellent salvage for the severely deformed foot in patients with cerebral palsy as long-term follow-up shows continued good to excellent functional results in the majority of patients.

Upper Extremity

Beach WR, Strecker WB, Coe J, et al: Use of the Green transfer in treatment of patients with spastic cerebral palsy: 17-year experience. *J Pediatr Orthop* 1991;11: 731–736.

A review of 40 patients with an average follow-up of 5 years and 3 months (range, 12 months to 12 years) from a Green transfer revealed 88% with a cosmetic improvement and 79% with a functional improvement. The authors modified the technique by tension of the graft to hold the wrist at neutral against gravity and immobilized at 5° of dorsiflexion and 45° of supination. No increased arc of motion was noted, rather it was shifted toward dorsiflexion. Supination improved 22° with a further improvement of 60° with additional pronator surgery. Quadriplegia or a component of athetosis was not a contraindication. Good stereognosis was not a necessary prerequisite to a good result. The authors conclude that with proper tensioning of the transfer and appropriate splinting, cosmetic improvement resulted in 88% of patients. If the extremity functions at minimum as a helper hand, functional improvement can be expected because those patients with no improvement had hands that functioned poorly preoperatively.

Hemiplegia

Winters TF Jr, Gage JR, Hicks R: Gait patterns in spastic hemiplegia in children and young adults. *J Bone Joint Surg* 1987;69A:437–441.

The authors described four major patterns of gait in the patient with spastic hemiplegia. The degree of involvement progressed from distal to proximal. Each described pattern has a recommended treatment plan. Of interest in type III and type IV is the pelvic femoral relationship, which may be very difficult to distinguish without the use of gait analysis.

Outcome Measures

Russell DJ, Rosenbaum PL, Cadman DT, et al: The gross motor function measure: A means to evaluate the effects of physical therapy. *Dev Med Child Neurol* 1989;31:341–352.

This article describes a standardized motor assessment tool that has been validated in patients with motor disability. The measure is scored based on the ability of patients to perform certain motor tasks. This criterion-based scoring system may provide a basis for assessment of treatments meant to change function in patients with cerebral palsy and will be widely used in the future. One criticism is that the scoring does not account for the *quality* of the performance of the motor task. This is addressed in the Gross Motor Performance Measure (GMPM).

Young NL, Wright JG: Measuring pediatric physical function. *J Pediatr Orthop* 1995;15:244–253.

An excellent review of the available standardized assessments of pediatric physical function are presented. The specific information to be gained from each specific test is reviewed, along with the strengths and deficiences of the listed inventories. This provides a nice resource for any investigator interested in the functional assessments of patients after intervention.

Gait Analysis

Gage JR: The clinical use of kinetics for evaluation of pathological gait in cerebral palsy. *J Bone Joint Surg* 1994;76A:622–631.

This excellent review builds on the article by Ounpuu and associates discussed below and specifically discusses the implications of power generation/absorption in providing insight into the mechanics of pathologic gait. The ankle rocker concept is explained in detail and is related to the kinetic data generated. A specific case example is presented for illustrative purposes.

Ounpuu S, Gage JR, Davis RB: Three-dimensional lower extremity joint kinetics in normal pediatric gait. *J Pediatr Orthop* 1991;11:341–349.

This article reviews the theoretical basis for the calculations and determinants of joint moments and power in normal children. Thirty-one patients form the database. It was found that 54% of the power generation for gait occurs at the hip; 10%, at the knee; and 36%, at the ankle. Power absorption is greatest at the knee (56%); at the hip and the ankle, power absorption equals 22% at each site.

4

Rotational and Angular Deformities of the Lower Extremities

Metatarsus Adductus

In the child with metatarsus adductus, the forefoot is adducted and the lateral border of the foot is convex. Normally, a line bisecting the weightbearing surface of the heel should traverse the web space between the second and third toes. The medial aspect of the foot with metatarsus adductus is concave, and a deep medial crease may be present. This deformity is differentiated from clubfoot in that the heel is not in the equinovarus position. In most cases of metatarsus adductus, the natural history tends to be one of spontaneous improvement; in approximately 85% of infants with metatarsus adductus, the deformity resolves without treatment.

However, an appreciable number of patients have a persistent clinical abnormality that may be responsive to treatment in infancy. In evaluation of the foot, the flexibility must be assessed. If the deformity is completely correctable passively, treatment is rarely needed. Parents may perform stretching exercises, and use of a reverse last shoe can be considered. If the feet are not passively correctable to neutral alignment, the child should be treated with serial manipulations and casting weekly until the deformity is fully corrected. Once correction is achieved, reverse last shoes will help maintain it. Best results are achieved when this treatment regimen is initiated before 8 months of age. However, there still may be improvement with the use of casting up until the age of 2 years. With the stretching and casting techniques, the hindfoot must be stabilized in the neutral position with one hand, while the opposite hand applies lateral pressure to the first metatarsal head and neck. Improper casting or use of an abduction bar with shoes may apply valgus force to the hindfoot as well as the forefoot, resulting in a planovalgus foot. When forefoot adduction recurs, it usually does so within the first few months following cessation of casting. This recurrence usually responds to an additional series of correcting casts.

Clinically, metatarsus adductus should be distinguished from the so-called "skewfoot," in which there is a combination of forefoot adduction, lateral translation of the midfoot, and hindfoot valgus. The parents should be counseled that skewfoot is significantly more difficult to treat. It will require a more prolonged period of casting and may require surgery.

Radiographs of the foot are not routinely indicated for assessment of metatarsus adductus. In patients for whom conservative management has failed or who are being assessed for the possibility of skewfoot, radiographs of the feet should be taken in the weightbearing position.

Previous articles have raised concerns about an association between metatarsus adductus and acetabular dysplasia. Studies have reported a 10% prevalence of dysplasia in infants with adductus. Recently, this relationship has been questioned. Pelvic radiographs are necessary only if there is a positive physical finding on the hip examination.

A number of surgical procedures have been advocated for treatment of persistent metatarsus adductus, including release of the abductor hallucis, medial release, and extensive tarsometatarsal capsulotomies (the Heyman-Herndon procedure). However, long-term poor results have been recorded in up to 50% of patients treated with the Heyman-Herndon technique. In the rare older child with severe deformity, multiple metatarsal osteotomies can be considered (with care being taken not to injure the physis of the first metatarsal). Alternatively, a lateral closing wedge osteotomy of the cuboid with an opening wedge osteotomy of the first cuneiform could be performed.

It must be emphasized that patients who have a mild to moderate deformity are generally asymptomatic over the long term and do not have an increased incidence of hallux valgus. Surgical intervention is rarely indicated, even in the older child.

Torsional Deformities

Rotational conditions of the lower extremities are extremely common in infants and children. They are a frequent cause of anxiety in parents and a common cause of referral to the orthopaedic surgeon. Nearly always, the orthopaedist can reassure the family by explaining the etiology and natural history of these torsional malalignments. Intrauterine molding is commonly responsible for the rotational appearance. In utero, the hips may be held flexed and laterally rotated. This may result in a mild flexion and external rotation contracture of the hip, which resolves with time. The in utero molding effect may rotate the feet medially, resulting in medial rotation of the tibia (and also metatarsus adductus). With the passage of time, medial and lateral rotation of the hip become more symmetric and medial rotation of the tibia resolves.

In evaluating a patient with a rotational abnormality, begin by assessing the rotational profile. This allows one to measure the severity of the rotational problem. This consists of assessment of the foot-progression angle during gait, evaluation of hip rotation (with the patient in the prone position and the knee flexed 90°), assessment of the thigh-foot angle, and evaluation of the foot. The foot-progression angle is quantified in degrees and is the average amount of in toeing or out toeing. Hip rotation in the prone position should be symmetric. Medial rotation greater than 70° indicates a diagnosis of medial femoral torsion. The thigh-foot angle is the difference between the axis of the foot and the axis of the thigh. The shape of the foot also should be noted. Medial rotation of the hips tends to be greatest in early childhood (after 12 to 18 months) and then declines until adulthood. From middle childhood on, medial rotation of the hip is roughly 50°, and lateral rotation is about 45°. The thigh-foot angle in newborns is directed a few degrees medially; with time, this changes to a lateral thigh-foot angle of 10°. In the older child, in-toeing gait is commonly caused by femoral antetorsion (exhibited by increased medial rotation of the hip) or medial tibial torsion (with a medial thigh-foot angle).

The natural history for both tibial and femoral torsion is one of spontaneous improvement. Parents and pediatricians should be educated about this natural untreated improvement. No form of conservative management has been shown to have any effect on tibial or femoral torsion. There is a less than 1% chance that a significant functional problem will remain in late childhood, at which point a rotational osteotomy could be performed.

Rotational osteotomies should not be performed before the age of 10, because spontaneous improvement of excessive femoral anteversion can occur up to this age. In the patient with cosmetically disabling femoral antetorsion, computed tomography (CT) can be used preoperatively to assess the deformity. This will quantitate the severity of the femoral anteversion and aid in planning the amount of derotation. To consider a rotational osteotomy of the femur, the child should have 80° of medial rotation of the hips clinically, and CT should indicate femoral anteversion of over 50°. For children who have persistent tibial torsion in late childhood and who may have a severe functional abnormality because of this, surgical correction at the supramalleolar level can be considered. The tibial deformities should exceed a medial thigh-foot angle of greater than 10° or a lateral thigh-foot angle of greater than 35°. Very rarely, a patient may present with a combination of severe medial femoral torsion and lateral tibial torsion. This combination can complicate the management of patients, who may have knee discomfort or patellar instability and may require correction of both the femoral and tibial torsion.

Bowlegs and Knock Knees

Bowlegged and knock-knee deformities in young children are a common concern with parents. As with torsional deformities, an explanation of the natural history of these usually benign deformities is essential. However, the orthopaedist must rule out pathological conditions, such as infantile tibia vara, metaphyseal chondrodysplasia, rickets (particularly hypophosphatemic rickets), and focal fibrocartilaginous dysplasia.

Normal knee alignment is approximately 10° to 15° of varus at birth, which progresses to neutral alignment at about 18 months of age. The child then develops genu valgum, which is most noticeable in the 30- to 36-month old child (Fig. 1). Radiographs are not routinely necessary. If a young child has severe angular deformity, is significantly short in stature, has asymmetric involvement, or has a positive family history, standing anteroposterior (AP) radiographs at the lower extremities should be taken. In the patient with persistent genu varum after the age of 18 to 24 months, radiographs of the knee are helpful in assessing infantile tibia vara (infantile Blount's). A metaphyseal-diaphyseal angle of greater than 11° has been reported as predictive for the development of infantile tibia vara. A more recent study reports that this angle should be 16° or greater to be considered predictive of impending infantile Blount's.

Infantile tibia vara results from abnormal growth of the medial and posterior aspect of the proximal tibial physis. Overweight children who are early walkers seem to be those most likely to develop tibia vara, possibly because of excessive compressive forces on the medial aspect of the physis. Over time, the abnormality in the medial aspect of the physis progresses, resulting in potentially severe varus deformity of the proximal tibia. The Langenskiöld radiographic staging classification reflects the progression of tibia vara in untreated cases (Fig. 2). For stages I and II, bracing may be effective in correcting the deformity. By stages III and IV, a proximal tibial valgus osteotomy is required in an effort to correct this condition. In stages V or VI, a medial physeal bar has developed. Therefore, an osteotomy plus other procedures such as bar resection, elevation of the medial tibial plateau and lateral physeal arrest may be necessary.

Brace management for tibia vara in patients younger than 3 years old may be successful in correcting the mild deformity. Bracing must be used during walking or weight-bearing to be effective. Therefore, nighttime bracing is not thought to be helpful. The orthosis must be a long leg brace with a cuff at the knee providing a valgus force. If improvement has not occurred, then by age 4 early tibial valgus osteotomy should be performed. With this, overcorrection into 5° to 10° valgus angulation (beyond normal) should be the goal.

Tibia vara may also develop in juveniles or adolescents. In the adolescent whose tibial physes are open and who is calculated to have significant remaining growth, a lateral hemiepiphysiodesis may provide correction. If significant remaining growth is not present, a proximal tibial valgus osteotomy is indicated. It is difficult to achieve a tibial femoral angle within 5° of normal in these patients due to their obesity.

The pathology of late onset tibia vara is similar to that of infantile tibial vara, which shows fissuring and clefts in the physis along with cartilaginous repair at the physeal-metaphyseal junction and evidence of necrotic cartilage. However, because growth at the tibia is closer to maturity

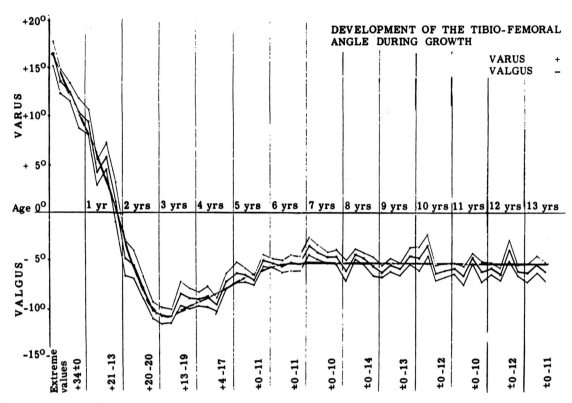

Fig. 1 Development of the tibiofemoral angle during growth. (Reproduced with permission from Salenius P, Vankka E: The development of the tibiofemoral angle in children. *J Bone Joint Surg* 1975;57A:260.)

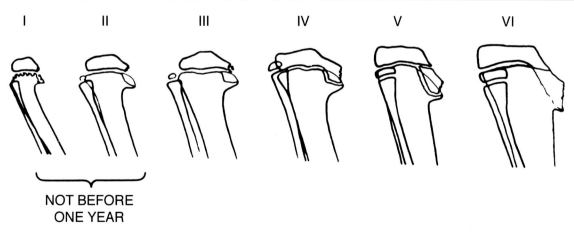

Fig. 2 Langenskiöld classification of tibia vara. (Reproduced with permission from Langenskiöld A, Riska EB: Tibia vara [osteochondrosis deformans tibiae]: A survey of seventy-one cases. *J Bone Joint Surg* 1964;46A:1405–1420.)

in the adolescent, the recurrent deformities that are seen in the infantile variety following surgical intervention are unlikely to occur following surgical correction in the adolescent. Recent prevalence studies indicate that late onset tibia vara appears to be more common than previously thought. This may be related to an increase in the prevalence of morbid obesity.

Focal fibrocartilaginous dysplasia is an unusual, recently described condition, which may be confused with tibia vara. These patients demonstrate indentation of the medial aspect of the tibia at the junction of the metaphysis and diaphysis. A period of observation is recommended, because spontaneous resolution is common.

In the older child with excessive genu valgum, conservative management is not helpful. If there is an underlying metabolic abnormality, it must be corrected before surgery is considered. If marked genu valgum persists, correction may be performed either by hemiepiphysiodesis or stapling of the medial physis. The goal of surgery is to create a horizontal knee joint for weightbearing. Neither procedure should be performed before the age of 10 years.

A minimally displaced proximal tibial metaphyseal fracture may develop marked valgus deformity over time. Parents certainly must be informed of this possibility at the time of initial injury. This deformity should be observed for 3 to 4 years, as there is often a strong tendency towards spontaneous correction. A corrective osteotomy may be associated with recurrent deformity.

Annotated Bibliography

Metatarsus Adductus

Farsetti P, Weinstein SL, Ponseti IV: The long-term functional and radiographic outcomes of untreated and non-operatively treated metatarsus adductus. *J Bone Joint Surg* 1994;76A:257–265.

This long-term study evaluated 31 patients (45 feet) with metatarsus adductus, with an average follow-up of 32 years. Patients with a passively correctable deformity had no treatment, those with a more rigid deformity had application of corrective plaster casts. The results were good in all untreated feet, and in 90% of the patients treated with casting. There were no poor results. In most patients with mild to moderate residual deformities, surgical intervention is not warranted.

Torsional Deformities

Eckhoff DG, Kramer RC, Alongi CA, et al: Femoral anteversion and arthritis of the knee. *J Pediatr Orthop* 1994;14:608–610.

Numerous studies have shown that no correlation exists between femoral anteversion and osteoarthritis of the hip. The degree of osteoarthritis present within the knee was correlated with the degree of femoral anteversion in this study, and the authors found that the degree of arthritis of the distal femur increased as the degree of femoral anteversion decreased. Cadaveric femur specimens from Africa were used as study material.

Katz K, Naor N, Merlob P: Rotational deformities of the tibia and foot in preterm infants. *J Pediatr Orthop* 1990; 10:483–485.

This study showed that preterm infants have external tibial torsion and everted or normal feet at birth. This supports the theory that postural deformities (such as medial tibial torsion and metatarsus adductus) occur during the later weeks of pregnancy, as the volume of amniotic fluid decreases and intrauterine molding occurs.

Payne LZ, DeLuca PA: Intertrochanteric versus supracondylar osteotomy for severe femoral anteversion. *J Pediatr Orthop* 1994;14:39–44.

The authors compared 34 derotational osteotomies using a supracondylar technique with cross pin fixation with 51 osteotomies using an intertrochanteric osteotomy with a blade-plate fixation. The complication rate was 15% with the supracondylar osteotomy technique, but there were no complications with the intertrochanteric osteotomy technique.

Staheli LT: Rotational problems in children: Office pediatric orthopaedics, in Schafer M (ed): *Instructional Course Lectures 43*. Rosemont, IL, American Academy of Orthopaedic Surgeons, 1994, pp 199–200.

The author emphasizes the importance of using the rotational profile in assessing and following children with torsional abnormalities of the lower extremities, and he emphasizes the responsibility of the orthopaedic surgeon to educate the parents regarding the benign natural history of most of these problems and to resist parental pressures towards overtreatment. Persistent or rigid metatarsus adductus, however, should be treated with casting. The likelihood of persistence of torsional deformity of the lower extremity is less than 1%.

Bowlegs and Knock Knees

Dietz FR, Merchant TC: Indications for osteotomy of the tibia in children. *J Pediatr Orthop* 1990;10:486–490.

The authors evaluated the amount of angulation in the tibia that was consistent with good long-term function without degenerative arthritis. In patients with a mean 29 years of follow-up, angular deformities up to 10° to 15° are well tolerated.

Feldman MD, Schoenecker PL: Use of the metaphyseal-diaphyseal angle in the evaluation of bowed legs. *J Bone Joint Surg* 1993;75A:1602–1609.

The accuracy of the metaphyseal–diaphyseal angle in predicting tibia vara was assessed. The authors thought that bracing for potential early tibia vara was indicated only if the metaphyseal–diaphyseal angle was more than 16°. Bracing would be considered with a metaphyseal–diaphyseal angle from 9° to 16° if instability on walking was present.

Heath CH, Staheli LT: Normal limits of knee angle in white children: Genu varum and genu valgum. *J Pediatr Orthop* 1993;13:259–262.

The clinical parameters of the knee angle, the intermalleolar distance, and the intercondylar distance were measured in 196 white children aged 6 months to 11 years. The knee angle was determined by evaluation of a photograph where a line was drawn between the anterior superior iliac spine and the center of the patella and then between the center of the patella at a point midway between the medial and lateral malleoli. Clinical bowleg after the age of 2 years was found to be abnormal. Children between 2 and 11 years had genu valgum up to 12°, and an intermalleolar distance up to 8 cm.

Henderson RC, Greene WB: Etiology of late-onset tibia vara: Is varus alignment a prerequisite? *J Pediatr Orthop* 1994;14:143–146.

Two case studies illustrate that adolescent tibia vara can develop in patients with a neutral mechanical axis. In a grossly obese patient, the large thigh circumference may require increased abduction of the extremity resulting in varus forces at the knee; there may be other factors in the pathogenesis of adolescent late-onset tibia vara that would also tend to explain its predilection for the black race and for males.

Henderson RC, Kemp GJ, Hayes PR: Prevalence of late-onset tibia vara. *J Pediatr Orthop* 1993;13:255–258.

One hundred forty teenage males who weighed at least 210 pounds were evaluated for varus alignment. The result of the screening study revealed two males with late onset tibia vara. The number of reported cases of late onset tibia vara has increased significantly, probably related to the increase in prevalence of obesity.

Henderson RC, Kemp GJ Jr, Greene WB: Adolescent tibia vara: Alternatives for operative treatment. *J Bone Joint Surg* 1992;74A:342–350.

Patients with adolescent tibia vara are often very obese, and it is very difficult to accurately assess the mechanical axis intraoperatively. This series showed a high incidence of unsatisfactory results with proximal tibial osteotomies. The authors recommend a lateral hemiepiphysiodesis of the proximal tibia as an alternative for patients with adolescent tibia vara who have open proximal tibial physes. This achieved acceptable correction in five of ten extremities (eight patients) followed to skeletal maturity.

Johnston CE II: Infantile tibia vara. *Clin Orthop* 1990;255:13–23.

The author noted that even in patients with grade IV Langenskiöld disease, there is a very high tendency toward recurrent deformity. As the recurrence rate is significant, the author suggests that physeal resection and placement of an interposition material be done to help prevent recurrent deformity.

Kariya Y, Taniguchi K, Yagisawa H, et al: Focal fibrocartilaginous dysplasia: Consideration of healing process. *J Pediatr Orthop* 1991;11:545–547.

Two patients are presented with focal fibrocartilaginous dysplasia who had improvement in their mechanical axis without treatment. The authors recommend a trial of conservative management before considering surgical intervention.

Kline SC, Bostrum M, Griffin PP: Femoral varus: An important component in late-onset Blount's disease. *J Pediatr Orthop* 1992;12:197–206.

The authors identified six patients with adolescent tibia vara with femoral varus deformity of greater than 10°. There is a need to check for the presence of significant femoral varus in order to make appropriate preoperative planning.

Langenskiöld A: Editorial: Tibia vara. *J Pediatr Orthop* 1994;14:141–142.

Slight overcorrection of the varus deformity when performing a corrective osteotomy is critical in order to achieve a successful result in children younger than 7 years of age. Operation at a later age than this often results in recurrent deformity.

Langenskiöld A: Tibia vara: A critical review. *Clin Orthop* 1989;246:195–207.

For correction of tibia vara, the author recommends a dome-shaped osteotomy that is performed subperiosteally (with the convexity in the diaphyseal fragment). The lateral aspect of the osteotomy should be slightly more proximal than the medial. The distal fragment is slid medially, the varus is then corrected to valgus alignment, and a long-leg cast is applied.

Loder RT, Schaffer JJ, Bardenstein MB: Late-onset tibia vara. *J Pediatr Orthop* 1991;11:162–167.

The authors review 15 children with late onset tibia vara (9 years of age or older). Results following surgical correction with tibial osteotomies were good in 15, fair in two, and poor in six. Difficulties in achieving the appropriate mechanical axis in these large, obese patients are discussed.

Scheffer MM, Peterson HA: Opening-wedge osteotomy for angular deformities of long bones in children. *J Bone Joint Surg* 1994;76A:325–334.

The treatment results of angular deformities with the use of an opening wedge osteotomy technique and insertion of an autogenous tricortical iliac bone graft was presented for 31 osteotomies. The technique was found to have low morbidity with rapid time to union and was successful in correcting angular deformities of 25° or less. The predicted limb length discrepancy for this technique should be less than 25 mm at skeletal maturity for this to be used as an isolated technique.

Schoenecker PL, Johnston R, Rich MM, et al: Elevation of the medial plateau of the tibia in the treatment of Blount disease. *J Bone Joint Surg* 1992;74A:351–358.

Patients with severe tibia vara (Langenskiöld grade V or VI) have a significant depression of medial tibial plateau. The authors recommend that the depressed articular surface of the medial portion of the tibia be elevated to correct the distorted anatomy of the knee in addition to correction of the proximal tibial varus. The authors also note that there may be a secondary valgus deformity in the distal end of the femur, which may be sufficiently severe to justify a femoral osteotomy.

Stricker SJ, Edwards PM, Tidwell MA: Langenskiöld classification of tibia vara: An assessment of interobserver variability. *J Pediatr Orthop* 1994;14:152–155.

Interobserver agreement for the Langenskiöld classification was good for early and late stages but poor for the intermediate stages. This classification system may be difficult to apply in the clinical situation in these intermediate stages.

5

Pediatric Orthopaedic Infections

Introduction

Musculoskeletal infections remain a common challenge for the orthopaedic surgeon, even though morbidity and mortality have dropped significantly since the advent of antibiotics. Nearly all pediatric orthopaedic infections may be cured and deformity and disability prevented with early diagnosis, appropriate antibiotic therapy, and surgical intervention when required. Infection should be suspected in any child who presents with pain, swelling, or tenderness in the limbs, spine, or pelvis.

Osteomyelitis

Overview

Osteomyelitis is a potentially devastating disease that can be examined from several different perspectives, including patient age (neonatal, childhood, or adult), causative organism (pyogenic or granulomatous), nature of onset (acute, subacute, or chronic), and route of infection (hematogenous, direct inoculation, or contiguous spread).

Acute Hematogenous Osteomyelitis

The incidence of acute hematogenous osteomyelitis (AHO) has decreased over recent decades; however, the need for prompt diagnosis and treatment remains unchanged. The differential diagnosis is extensive and may include rheumatic fever, septic arthritis, cellulitis, malignancy (Ewing's sarcoma and leukemia), thrombophlebitis, sickle-cell crisis, Gaucher's disease, and toxic synovitis.

Pathogenesis The causes of AHO remain unknown. Infection begins in the metaphyseal venous sinusoids (Fig. 1). As the infection spreads, the medullary vessels thrombose and prohibit the inflow of white blood cells (WBCs) and therefore the WBCs must slowly migrate from the medullary cavity. Thus, this early phase in osteomyelitis is called the "cellulitic" phase, because pus has not been produced. In this stage, antibiotic treatment alone may be adequate to fight the infection. Without such treatment, however, pus forms. To lessen the intraosseous buildup of pressure, the pus exits the bone through the porous metaphyseal cortex, elevating the periosteum and forming a subperiosteal abscess. The most common microorganisms found in neonates, infants, and children are listed in Table 1.

Diagnosis The physician should have a high index of suspicion for osteomyelitis when examining the child with fever and unexplained bone pain. Nearly half of these patients have a history of recent or concurrent infection. They may refuse to move the limb, have tenderness over the involved bone, and demonstrate a decreased range of motion in adjacent joints. Swelling, erythema, and warmth over the involved metaphysis occur later. Recent series have demonstrated, however, that a significant number of children do not fit this classic stereotype.

The WBC count may not be a reliable indicator of infection because it is not always elevated. The erythrocyte sedimentation rate (ESR), which is elevated in over 90% of cases, is believed to be a reliable indicator of infection. Exceptions may include the neonate with osteomyelitis, the child with sickle-cell anemia, and the child who is taking steroids. Blood cultures are positive in 40% to 50% of cases. Plain radiographs may show soft-tissue swelling within 3 days of infection, but bone changes do not appear for 7 to 14 days.

Aspiration of the affected site is essential if osteomyelitis is suspected. The aspirate should be Gram stained and should undergo a routine culture, as well as cultures for anaerobic bacteria, acid-fast bacilli (AFB), and fungi. Several authors have suggested that fine-needle bone biopsy using an 11-gauge bone marrow biopsy needle be performed at the same sitting to obtain material for histologic examination. This procedure requires sedation.

If the diagnosis remains uncertain, additional studies may be required. Bone scans may be used to locate the area of involvement in difficult sites, such as the pelvis or spine. Bone scans are also useful in patients with multiple sites of involvement, particularly in the neonate. However, because bone scans may be falsely negative in the first month of life, they are rarely used to establish the diagnosis. Bone aspiration will not affect the results of bone scans if the study is performed within 48 hours of aspiration; therefore, aspiration should not be delayed. Gallium scans are rarely indicated. They take 24 to 48 hours to complete and require a much higher dose of irradiation. Furthermore, they rarely add information beyond that provided by a two- or three-phase bone scan. Computed tomography (CT) has not been useful for establishing the diagnosis of acute osteomyelitis, but it has been used to evaluate primary epiphyseal bone abscesses. It also may help in differentiating osteomyelitis from other lucent lesions, especially chondroblastoma and osteoid osteoma. Finally, CT is useful for identifying extraosseous collections of pus. Magnetic resonance imaging (MRI) is very sensitive, but not specific, for osteomyelitis. It can be used to differentiate between the acute and chronic forms of the disease. Ultrasound is useful in localizing a subperio-

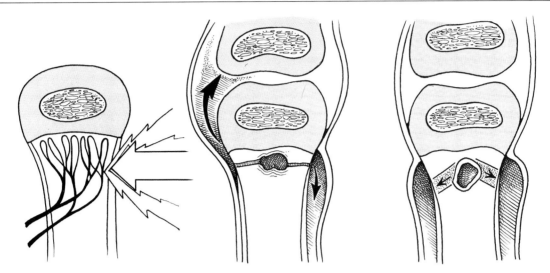

Fig. 1   Left, The combination of bacteremia and trauma favors the development of infection in the metaphyseal venous sinusoids. **Center,** The infection will eventually track through the porous metaphyseal cortical surface and elevate the surrounding periosteum. If the metaphysis is intra-articular, the infection will break into the joint and cause concurrent septic arthritis. **Right,** The elevated periosteum lays down new bone initially (involucrum), and the dead medullary (or cortical) bone becomes a sequestrum. (Reproduced with permission from Dormans JP, Drummond DS: Pediatric hematogenous osteomyelitis: New trends in presentation, diagnosis, and treatment. *J Am Acad Orthop Surg* 1994;2:333–341.)

Table 1. Bacterial analysis: Osteomyelitis

Neonates	*Staphylococcus aureus*, Group B *Streptococcus*, gram-negative coliforms
Infants and Children	*S aureus*

steal abscess in the child with diffuse tenderness and swelling of an extremity. Ultrasound cannot penetrate dense bone, but it can show early changes in soft tissue. In a recent study of 29 children with acute hematogenous osteomyelitis, 26 showed characteristic ultrasound findings. These findings include (1) thickening of the periosteum with hypoechogenic zones, both superficial and deep, which give the appearance of a "sandwich;" (2) elevation of the periosteum by more than 2 mm; or (3) swelling of overlying muscle or subcutaneous tissue with altered echogenicity of the tissue, depending on the angle of scan. These changes were detectable on ultrasound within 24 hours of the onset of symptoms. When the periosteum had lifted off the bone by 2 mm or more, pus usually was present.

Treatment   The principles of treatment include identification of the microorganism, selection of the correct antibiotic, delivery of the antibiotic in sufficient concentrations and for sufficient duration, and arrest of tissue destruction.

Antibiotics are started as soon as all cultures have been obtained. When pus is absent, the infection may still be in the early stages, and antibiotic therapy alone may be adequate. In the neonate, pending culture results, oxacillin, in combination with cefotaxime or gentamicin, is used as initial empiric therapy. Oxacillin is also the primary drug used in infants and children. Cefazolin is used if the patient is allergic to penicillin; clindamycin or vancomycin is recommended if the patient is allergic to both penicillin and cephalosporin.

The appropriate duration of intravenous antibiotics and the time allowed before switching to oral medication remain debatable. The patient's clinical response determines the duration of therapy and is judged by monitoring the patient's temperature and ESR, and by clinical examination. The fall in ESR following treatment may lag behind clinical improvement. C-reactive protein has been shown to be elevated in 98% of patients with osteomyelitis and to decrease rapidly following treatment. Although it is believed by some authors to be a more sensitive indicator of the effectiveness of therapy than ESR, it has not generally replaced the ESR. In the neonate, the C-reactive protein level is believed to be helpful in making the initial diagnosis, because some infants cannot mount an ESR but do have an elevated C-reactive protein. However, many authors believe that the C-reactive protein level returns to normal too quickly and that it may be misleading to use it to determine the duration of therapy.

If the patient is unable to swallow or retain medications, the microorganism has not been identified, bactericidal levels of oral antibiotics have not been obtained, or the infection is caused by a microorganism for which no effective oral antibiotic exists, intravenous antibiotic administration must be continued. Once oral antibiotics can be started, the usual choices are dicloxacillin or cephalexin.

An abscess is drained, generally by opening the periosteum and drilling the cortex, although some authors question the need to drill the cortex. Dead or avascular bone must also be removed.

Osteomyelitis in the Neonate

In the neonate, several unique anatomic features affect the course of bone and joint infections. The metaphyseal vessels communicate with the epiphyseal vessels in the cartilaginous precursor of the ossific nucleus, thus permitting a route for infection to spread. As the child matures, the epiphysis develops a separate blood supply, and communication with the metaphyseal vessels ceases. Because of the epiphyseal–metaphyseal communication in the neonate, septic arthritis and AHO often occur together. The metaphyses of the hip, proximal humerus, proximal radius, and distal lateral tibia are intra-articular; thus, pus from osteomyelitis can track under the capsule into the joint. Thrombosis of the vessels may cause ischemia of the epiphyseal growth plate, and infection may cause subsequent lysis of the growth plate. Complete ischemia and lysis of the physis before ossification of the femoral head may result in necrosis and reabsorption of the femoral head and neck. Finally, because the immune system of the neonate is immature, the inflammatory response is compromised and infection may be caused by microorganisms not typically seen in the older child.

Soft-tissue swelling and pseudoparalysis are hallmarks of AHO in neonates; however, detection of the infection is often delayed. The child may have only minimal symptoms, such as malaise or failure to gain weight. There may be no fever, and the WBC count and ESR may be normal. Multiple sites of infection occur in nearly 40% of cases. It is important to aspirate and culture all bones and joints that appear abnormal. Historically, *Staphylococcus aureus* has been the most prevalent microorganism, but recently group B *Streptococcus* has emerged as the most common cause of this infection.

Long-term complications of osteomyelitis in the neonate include osteonecrosis of the epiphyses, joint dislocation, and premature physeal arrest. The clinical effect of infection on the physis is often not appreciated for many years. Long-term follow-up is strongly recommended.

Subacute Hematogenous Osteomyelitis

Subacute hematogenous osteomyelitis (SHO) is the cause of nearly one third of primary bone infections. Its presentation differs strikingly from that of acute osteomyelitis and is characterized by an insidious onset, mild symptoms, longer duration, and inconclusive laboratory data (Table 2).

A modified classification of the radiographic abnormalities in subacute osteomyelitis is seen in Figure 2. Although SHO can cross the growth plate, it rarely causes permanent damage.

The findings for SHO are similar to those of chronic recurrent multifocal osteomyelitis, although the natural history of the two conditions differs. SHO is less likely to recur and is more responsive to antibiotic treatment than is chronic recurrent osteomyelitis. SHO may also be confused with neoplasms such as Ewing's sarcoma, metastatic neuroblastoma, malignant round cell tumors, and osteoid osteoma.

A biopsy is usually required to rule out tumor and provide a definitive diagnosis. Cultures are frequently negative. *Staphylococcus* species is the most common microorganism. Most patients respond to a single course of antibiotics and curettage, although a longer course of intravenous therapy is generally required for SHO than for AHO. A positive culture or failure to respond to antibiotics indicates the need for curettage, drainage of abscesses, and sequestrectomy.

Chronic Multifocal Osteomyelitis

Chronic multifocal osteomyelitis is a rare condition of unknown etiology. The onset is insidious; patients present with vague constitutional symptoms and localized bone pain. Presenting features may range from bone lesions (alone or in combination with arthritis), palmoplantar

Table 2. Comparison of acute and subacute hematogenous osteomyelitis

	Subacute	Acute
Pain	Mild	Severe
Fever	Few patients	Majority of patients
Loss of function	Minimal	Marked
Prior antibiotic therapy	Often (30% to 40% of patients)*	Occasionally
Elevated WBC count	Few	Majority of patients
Elevated ESR	Majority of patients	Majority of patients
Blood cultures	Few positive	50% positive†
Bone cultures	60% positive	85% positive
Initial radiographs	Frequently abnormal	Often normal
Site	Any location (may cross physis)	Usually metaphysis

*Unger E, Moldofsky P, Gatenby R, et al: Diagnosis of osteomyelitis by MR imaging. *Am J Roentgenol* 1988;150:605–610.
†Jackson MA, Nelson JD: Etiology and medical management of acute suppurative bone and joint infections in pediatric patients. *J Pediatr Orthop* 1982;2: 313–323.
(Reproduced with permission from Dormans JP, Drummond DS: Pediatric hematogenous osteomyelitis: New trends in presentation, diagnosis, and treatment. *J Am Acad Orthop Surg* 1994;2:333–341.)

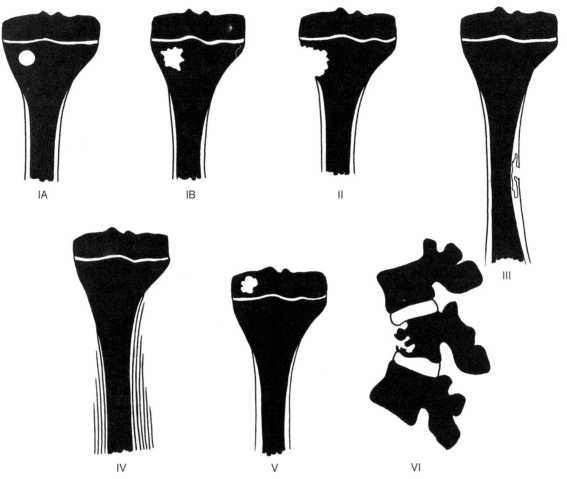

Fig. 2 Modified classification of subacute osteomyelitis. Type IA is characterized by a punched-out radiolucency suggestive of eosinophilic granuloma. Type IB is similar but has a sclerotic margin and represents a classic Brodie's abscess. Type II is a metaphyseal lesion associated with loss of cortical bone. Type III is a diaphyseal lesion with excessive cortical reaction. Type IV is a lesion associated with onionskin layering of subperiosteal bone. Type V is a concentric epiphyseal radiolucency. Type VI is an osteomyelitic lesion of a vertebral body. (Reproduced with permission from Dormans JP, Drummond DS: Pediatric hematogenous osteomyelitis: New trends in presentation, diagnosis, and treatment. *J Am Acad Orthop Surg* 1994;2:333–341.)

pustulosis, or psoriasis. The lesions, which may occur sequentially, are symmetrically located, predominantly in the metaphyses of long bones. Plain radiographs usually reveal features suggestive of osteomyelitis. The diagnosis can be made only when more than one lesion is present. Bone scan establishes the diagnosis and may be useful in identifying lesions that have no clinical manifestations. The WBC count is usually normal; however, the ESR is elevated in most patients. Culture results usually are negative. Biopsy is generally done to exclude other diagnoses such as tumor or histiocytosis. An initial course of antibiotics is commonly prescribed, but the effectiveness of such an approach is controversial. Nonsteroidal anti-inflammatory agents are used to provide symptomatic relief of pain. Steroids have been used but are generally avoided because of the detrimental side effects. The symp-

toms of chronic multifocal osteomyelitis may last up to 5 years, and relapse is common. The prognosis is generally good.

Chronic Osteomyelitis

Despite adequate drainage of pus and intensive antibiotic therapy, some children with acute osteomyelitis, particularly those who present late, develop chronic osteomyelitis with cavities, sequestra, and sinuses. *S aureus* is most commonly associated with this outcome. CT should be used to identify the number and extent of infected cavities and the location of sequestra. As with adults, surgical intervention is required to remove sequestra and to open cavities widely. The Papineau procedure of bone grafting has been used in the past; however, methods that allow wound closure are preferred in children. One such method includes muscle transfer into the cavity.

Septic Arthritis

Overview

Septic arthritis (SA) requires urgent treatment. The duration of symptoms prior to treatment is the most important prognostic factor for outcome and prevention of growth anomalies; therefore, it is essential to recognize this condition and initiate appropriate treatment quickly.

The differential diagnosis includes transient synovitis, rheumatic fever, hemarthrosis, juvenile arthritis, cellulitis, osteomyelitis, hemophilia, chondrolysis, Henoch-Schönlein purpura, Lyme disease, and sickle-cell crisis. If the complaint is at the hip, Legg-Calvé-Perthes disease, slipped capital femoral epiphysis, and pelvic, sacroiliac, and vertebral osteomyelitis must also be considered.

Diagnosis

Septic arthritis is more common in boys than in girls and occurs most commonly in children younger than 2 years of age. Patients generally have a temperature of 38° to 40° C and physical signs that include restricted joint motion, tenderness, and joint warmth and effusion. In the infant, however, physical signs may be restricted to limited spontaneous motion or asymmetric posturing of the extremity. The knees, hips, ankles, and elbows, in descending order, account for 90% of affected joints.

The WBC count is elevated in 30% to 60% of patients, with a left shift in 60% of those with an elevated count. The ESR is a more sensitive test and is usually higher in patients with septic arthritis than in those with osteomyelitis; however, it is unreliable in the neonate, the child with sickle-cell anemia, and the patient taking steroids. Return of the ESR to normal values is much slower than the clinical improvement of the patient and, therefore, is of limited use in monitoring resolution of infection. C-reactive protein may be more useful, particularly in identifying children with AHO who have concurrent SA. Blood cultures are positive in 40% to 50% of patients with septic arthritis.

Plain radiographs are frequently normal. Changes are subtle and may include widening of the joint space (usually found in younger children), obliteration of fat planes, soft-tissue swelling, and, after 7 to 14 days, bone destruction. Widening of the joint space is an indication of increased joint fluid and pressure that may lead to subluxation, dislocation, or ischemic necrosis of the capital epiphysis.

The definitive test for septic arthritis is needle aspiration, which should not be delayed if SA is suspected. If no fluid is found during aspiration of a hip lesion, an arthrogram should be performed to confirm that the needle has entered the joint. If infection is present, the joint fluid is usually cloudy, the WBC count is usually 50,000 or greater (except in neonates and infants, in whom it may be lower), and polymorphonucleocytes predominate. Aspirates from infected joints yield positive cultures 54% to 68% of the time. Aspiration has been shown to have no effect on the results of subsequent bone scans. Gram stain demonstrates a microorganism in 30% to 40% of cases.

Additional studies may be of benefit; however, technetium bone scan is less effective in the diagnosis of SA than of AHO. This is particularly true in the neonate, in whom the inflammatory response is limited. In patients with SA and osteomyelitis, the bone scan may miss the site of joint sepsis. Some reports state that bone scan findings do not correlate specifically with the presence or absence of joint sepsis, and that they are not useful in differentiating infectious from noninfectious arthropathy.

A bone scan can be helpful, however, in the pelvis, hip, spine, scapula, shoulder, and swollen foot and ankle, where the exact location of infection can be difficult to identify. It may also identify multiple sites of infection in the neonate.

The role of ultrasound remains controversial. Although it is more sensitive than plain radiography in diagnosing an effusion, it is not specific. A more important factor is that it is not immediately available in most institutions. Because outcome has been clearly tied to delay in treatment, prompt aspiration must take priority.

Haemophilus influenzae B has been reported as the most common pathogen associated with SA in young children (Table 3). A number of epidemiologic studies have documented a decline in *H influenzae B* systemic disease in children since the development of a vaccine for *H influenzae B*. Use of the vaccine may eventually lead to a decrease in the incidence of *H influenzae B* as a contributing factor in SA; however, no decrease has yet been reported.

Treatment

Treatment of SA should not begin until all of the necessary culture materials have been obtained because the positive yields from blood cultures and aspirations are diminished in the presence of antibiotics. Surgical incision and drainage of the joint are required to remove the microorganisms, host and bacterial enzymes, and particulate debris in nearly all patients with SA. Open debridement is required for hip involvement in patients with gonococcal arthritis; however, in patients with gonococcal arthritis who have involvement in other locations, joint aspirations, rather than surgery, is sufficient. The role of arthroscopy remains unclear.

Antibiotic treatment should begin as soon as blood, synovial fluid, and other appropriate culture materials have been obtained. Results of synovial fluid Gram stain offer the best guide to the selection of an appropriate initial antibiotic. If the Gram stain identifies no microorganisms, the antibiotic should be chosen on the basis of the child's age, immune competency, the joint involved, and local epidemiology. Young children may also have meningitis (particularly with *H influenzae B*); therefore, spinal fluid examination should be considered before starting the antibiotic, because an antibiotic that crosses the blood–brain barrier

Table 3. Bacterial analysis-Septic arthritis

Neonate	Group B *Streptococcus* species, *Staphylococcus aureus*, gram-negative coliforms
Infants and children up to age 4	*Staphylococcus aureus*, pneumococcus Group A *Streptococcus*, *Haemophilus influenzae B*
Children over age 4	*Staphylococcus aureus*
Adolescents	Consider gonococcus

may be required. In this situation, consultation with a specialist in pediatric infectious disease may be helpful. Antibiotic therapy in the neonate consists of oxacillin in combination with gentamicin or cefotaxime as initial empiric therapy, pending culture results. In the child younger than 4 years of age, oxacillin and cefotaxime or cefuroxime are used. In the child older than 4 years of age, oxacillin alone is usually adequate. Oxacillin and ceftriaxone may be needed in the immunocompromised patient or in cases in which microorganisms other than traditional gram-positive organisms (*S aureus,* pneumococcus, group A *Streptococcus*) are suspected.

Sequelae

Most patients with SA generally will have a normal outcome following appropriate treatment. Several factors contribute to a poor prognosis, including delay in treatment, patient age younger than 6 months, prematurity (particularly if the child has required an umbilical catheter or developed respiratory distress syndrome), *Staphylococcus* species infection, or concomitant osteomyelitis.

There are several reasons why a delay in treatment is the most common cause of a poor outcome. First, delay allows the toxins produced by the bacteria to destroy the hyaline cartilage. Second, a sustained increase in intracapsular pressure may cause occlusion and thrombosis of the retinacular vessels that supply the femoral head, leading to ischemia of the capital epiphysis. Further, the increased intracapsular pressure may distend the joint and lead to subluxation or dislocation, which may cause furthur vascular embarrassment.

Patients with concomitant osteomyelitis also have a poorer prognosis. In infants and children, the metaphyses of the hip, proximal humerus, proximal radius, and distal lateral tibia are intra-articular; thus, pus from osteomyelitis may decompress into the joint. Nearly 15% of children with septic arthritis have coexisting osteomyelitis; of these, significant problems have been reported in more than half. In general, the children who have both septic arthritis and osteomyelitis are younger and have been symptomatic for a longer period of time prior to hospital admission than those who only have SA.

A radiographic classification system has been developed to describe deformities at the hip found on long-term follow-up studies. This classification system can help predict functional outcome and the need for surgical intervention. Type I deformities include those caused by transient ischemia that resolved; mild coxa magna developed in some of these hips. Type II deformities include deformity of the epiphysis, physis, and metaphysis. These hips are at risk for subluxation. Type III deformity involves malalignment of the femoral neck and type IV deformity includes destruction of the femoral neck and head.

Specific Infections and Conditions

Diskitis

Diskitis is an inflammation of the intervertebral disk with an uncertain etiology. It is usually a disorder of younger children and the onset is generally gradual. Typically, a parent reports that a child has progressed from being irritable to limping to refusing to sit or stand. This progression is noted over a 2- to 4-week period. Fewer than half of these patients have a fever.

The child's age frequently correlates with the presenting symptoms and signs. One review reported that in children younger than 3 years of age, the most common findings were hip irritability in extension (positive log roll test) and reluctance to ambulate. Only half of these children had tenderness over the the lumbar spine. Thirty percent complained of abdominal pain. In children between the ages of 3 years and 9 years, the most frequent complaint was abdominal pain; only 30% complained of back pain. Seventy-five percent were reluctant to ambulate and 50% had tenderness in the spinal region. All children older than 9 years of age complained of back pain, yet only 10% complained of associated symptoms, eg, abdominal pain or reluctance to ambulate. Physical findings varied and included decreased lumbar lordosis, positive straight leg raise sign, positive log roll, and paravertebral muscle spasm.

Laboratory findings are nonspecific. The WBC count is usually normal or mildly elevated. The ESR is almost always elevated. Blood cultures are generally negative, except in patients with an acute form of the disease.

Plain radiographs may be unremarkable early in the course of the disease. At 2 to 6 weeks, however, a narrowing of the intervertebral disk space may be accompanied by decreased vertebral height and demineralization. Four to 8 weeks after the onset of diskitis, there may be irregular erosion of the adjacent vertebral plates. The disk sometimes "balloons" into the plates. After 3 months, gradual repair occurs; residual sclerosis of the vertebral end plates is sometimes evident. The height of the disk space may be partially restored, but rarely returns to normal. Previous studies have indicated that bone scan is very sensitive for diskitis; however, one recent review found it to be only 72% sensitive.

Biopsy and aspiration are positive in as many as 60% of patients. However, because positive cultures nearly always reveal *S aureus,* biopsy or aspiration should be reserved for patients with recurrent disease. A skin test for tuberculosis is essential.

The management of diskitis is not settled. Because most children improve with rest and traction, or traction alone, many authors believe that antibiotics may not be required. A recent review that included a case of diskitis which progressed to form an abscess requiring drainage, however, strongly supports the need for antibiotic therapy. The authors point out that the 60% rate of positive cultures in children with diskitis is comparable with the 70% rate of positive cultures in adults with vertebral osteomyelitis. The authors suggest that sampling error, culture technique, and previous antibiotic treatment may explain the small difference between the two groups. Because one cannot predict which infections will progress, there is potential danger in withholding antibiotic treatment from patients with diskitis.

Hemophilia

Although septic arthritis is rare in patients with hemophilia, it has recently been reported in individuals who are positive for human immunodeficiency virus (HIV). A report of four HIV-positive individuals with hemophilia and SA revealed that the knee was involved in three cases and the elbow, in one case. Causative organisms were *S pneumoniae* and *S aureus* (one patient each) and *Salmonella* species (two patients). Two patients developed acquired immunodeficiency syndrome (AIDS) after diagnosis of SA. A painful swollen joint mimicking hemarthrosis can actually be SA. This condition should be suspected if factor replacement fails to relieve symptoms and fever persists.

In this situation, joint aspiration and culture are mandatory. The procedures commonly used to manage a septic joint are appropriate for these patients. Septic arthritis may serve as a clinical marker for immunosuppression in patients with hemophilia.

Human Immunodeficiency Virus (HIV)

As of December 1995, more than 500,000 persons in the U.S. have been diagnosed with AIDS and over 60% have died. Compared with that of adults, the number of AIDS cases among children and adolescents is small, and the source of infection differs. The male-to-female ratio of new AIDS cases among adolescents is 2:1, compared with a 3:1 ratio in adults. The diagnosis of HIV infection is now close to 1:1 among adolescent males and females, compared with the adult ratio of 7:1. Forty-three percent of new AIDS cases in adolescent males that were reported to the Centers for Disease Control from June 1993 to July 1995 occurred in young men with coagulation disorders; 33% occurred in homosexual men. Only 6% occurred in intravenous drug users and 5% occurred in men who were intravenous drug users and homosexual. In adolescent females, 16% of cases occurred in intravenous drug users and 53% in heterosexuals. In women aged 20 to 24 years, 33% of cases occurred in intravenous drug users and 50% occurred in heterosexuals. Nearly all cases of AIDS in children result from in utero transmission of HIV. Thus,

efforts to reduce AIDS in children have been aimed at discouraging intravenous drug use and high-risk sexual activities in women of childbearing age. Ironically, AIDS cases in children fell in 1995 even though the disease developed in more women during this time. This scenario may be the result of increased use of azidothymidine by pregnant women to prevent transmission of the disease.

Septic arthritis in HIV-infected intravenous drug users is not uncommon. *S aureus* is the most commonly isolated microorganism. Clinical profiles and laboratory findings at the time of onset, such as the presence of fever, peripheral blood leukocyte count and ESR, and type of infecting microorganism, are the same in HIV-positive and -negative patients.

Lyme Disease

Lyme disease is a complex, multisystem disease caused by the tick-borne spirochete *Borrelia burgdorferi*. The illness, which closely mimics several other rheumatic diseases, usually occurs in stages, each of which is characterized by different clinical manifestations and by remissions and exacerbations. Correct diagnosis is important because the condition is usually curable with appropriate antibiotic therapy. Lyme disease has been recognized in 47 states in the United States and in 18 other countries on four continents. The distribution correlates primarily with the geographic ranges of certain Ixodes ticks. It is prevalent in New England states, New York, New Jersey, areas of the mid-Atlantic and Midwestern states.

Lyme disease consists of three stages. The first stage is early localized infection. A red mark may form at the site of the bite. The rash, erythema migrans, may then spread to the patient's entire back or leg. The rash has been reported in 18% to 72% of those infected and often disappears within a few days. It probably is not noticed or is forgotten in many cases. Flu-like symptoms, such as fatigue and nausea, are often present. The second stage is early disseminated infection. A rash may appear and the heart muscle may become inflamed, leading to possible arrhythmias. Bell's palsy may occur. The third stage is persistent infection. Arthritis may develop up to 16 weeks after infection. Joints most commonly infected include the knee, shoulder, elbow, ankle, and wrist, in that order. The temporomandibular joint also may be infected. This disease is particularly difficult to diagnose because individuals may proceed from the early stage to the persistent phase without symptoms.

A review of 44 children with Lyme arthritis found marked clinical and serologic variability. Only 43% of patients presented with "classic" Lyme arthritis, namely, episodic synovitis of one to four joints for periods of several days, separated by asymptomatic intervals of at least 2 weeks. Acute pauciarticular arthritis, ie, continuous involvement of one to four joints for less than 4 weeks, occurred in 36% of patients. Thirteen percent had chronic pauciarticular persistent arthritis, with "pauci-juvenile rheumatoid arthritis (JRA)-like" symptoms, in one to four joints for more than 4 weeks. Migratory involvement of three or more joints in a sequential pattern (in which one "hot" joint predominated at any given time), occurred in 4% of patients, and 4% had involvement of five or more joints.

With the exception of classic intermittent arthritis, the remaining patterns of Lyme arthritis mimic those of other pediatric rheumatic diseases. Patients with the acute form of Lyme arthritis may be suspected of having septic arthritis or toxic synovitis. Children with the chronic form of the disease have symptoms similar to those of patients with pauciarticular juvenile rheumatoid arthritis. A positive antinuclear antibody test (ANA), usually thought to be a confirmatory test for JRA, occurs in 30% of patients with Lyme disease.

In endemic areas, Lyme disease is a common cause of acute arthritis in children. It produces a positive enzyme-linked immunosorbent assay (ELISA) test result, but other forms of chronic arthritis and/or spondyloarthropathies may produce a false-positive ELISA test result. A clinical diagnosis may be supported by the presence of extra-articular manifestations; however, these are uncommon. Erythema migrans has been detected in as few as 18% of patients. Bell's palsy and aseptic meningitis are very rare.

Although 10% of adults with Lyme arthritis eventually develop chronic or recurrent synovitis despite antibiotic therapy, the prognosis for children is much better. The rate of chronic arthritis in children appears to range from 0 to 2%.

Thus, Lyme disease should be considered in any child from an endemic area who presents with arthritis, regardless of the articular pattern.

Puncture Wounds of the Foot

A puncture wound of the foot, often caused by stepping on a nail, is a common problem in children. Its peak incidence occurs between May and October. The majority of children who sustain these injuries do well with minimum treatment and do not develop infectious complications. Initial treatment of a nail puncture wound should include tetanus prophylaxis, excision of devascularized skin flaps, and irrigation of the puncture tract. Antibiotic coverage for gram-positive organisms generally is given only if there is evidence of cellulitis or soft-tissue infection.

Infectious complications include cellulitis, soft-tissue abscess, osteomyelitis–osteochondritis, and pyarthrosis. Although cellulitis is the most frequent complication, *Pseudomonas aeruginosa* osteomyelitis–osteochondritis is the complication of greatest concern to the orthopaedic surgeon, with an estimated incidence of 0.6% to 1.8% of children who present with plantar puncture wounds. *P aeruginosa* accounts for as many as 93% of all cases of puncture wound osteomyelitis. The true incidence of complications of puncture wounds is not known because many children who sustain these injuries do not seek medical care.

A nail is the most common penetrating object associated with osteomyelitis caused by *Pseudomonas* species,

and the majority of children affected are wearing sneakers at the time of their injury. *Pseudomonas* species reside in the foam rubber contained within the soles of the sneakers. A nail that pierces the sole of a contaminated sneaker may introduce pieces of material containing *Pseudomonas* species deep into the wound. If this material is not removed during initial wound care, it may serve as a nidus of infection that may eventually lead to osteomyelitis.

A child with osteomyelitis from a puncture wound typically presents with pain around the puncture site, swelling, and a decreased ability to bear weight on the affected foot. The dorsal aspect of the foot may be swollen. The patient may be afebrile and nontoxic. Purulent drainage is rare. The WBC count may be normal but the ESR is typically mildly to moderately elevated. Changes on plain radiographs generally do not appear for 10 to 14 days; however, bone scans are very sensitive and may show changes sooner. MRI shows abnormalities on both the T1 and T2 images.

Pseudomonas species appear to have a propensity to invade the cartilaginous structures of the foot; thus, the physes and the cartilaginous joint surfaces are at particular risk. Septic arthritis adjacent to an intraosseous abscess occurs frequently, and recurrence of the signs and symptoms of infection has been attributed to missed SA; consequently, all suspicious joints should be aspirated. Surgery should include careful exploration for foreign bodies, debridement of dead tissue, and extensive lavage. The forefoot may need to be approached from the dorsal aspect. After vigorous surgical debridement, a 7-day course of parenteral antibiotics is usually sufficient, but longer treatment is suggested if osteochondritis caused by the *Pseudomonas* organism is present.

Pyomyositis

Pyomyositis, a bacterial infection of muscle caused by *S aureus,* is found most commonly in persons living in tropical regions. Patients typically present with general malaise, muscle ache, fever, decreased range of motion, and tenderness in the involved area. The ESR is generally elevated. MRI is the preferred diagnostic tool. Most patients require surgical debridement, followed by antibiotics. If the patient does not respond quickly, careful evaluation for a secondary abscess should be made. The possibility of multiple abscess sites should always be considered prior to debridement.

Sickle-Cell Disease

Although osteomyelitis is uncommon in the patient with sickle-cell disease, it is still more prevalent in these individuals than in the general population. Differentiation between acute bone infarction and acute osteomyelitis is difficult; fever, localized or generalized bone pain, localized erythema, tenderness, and swelling are characteristic of both conditions, as are an elevated ESR and a high WBC count. In general, radionucleotide studies are not helpful; however, some authors feel that a "cold" bone scan indicates infarction, while normal or increased uptake indicates infection. A positive blood culture is consistent with osteomyelitis, and aspiration of purulent material from bone confirms the diagnosis. Most studies report that *Salmonella* species is the most common causative microorganism, but a recent report found that *S aureus* dominated. Salmonellae probably enter through the gastrointestinal tract.

Aggressive management is recommended for all patients with sickle-cell disease in whom osteomyelitis is suspected. Management should include (1) careful preoperative preparation, which includes exchange transfusions to raise the level of hemoglobin A to 60% and vigorous intravenous hydration to avoid vascular stasis secondary to increased viscosity of the blood; (2) prompt decompression of all abscesses; (3) avoidance of tourniquets to prevent vascular stasis and decreased oxygenation; (4) careful collection of culture materials prior to initiation of antibiotics; and (5) parenteral antibiotics for 6 to 8 weeks. A prolonged course of antibiotics is required because of the weakened immune system and compromised vascularity to the affected bone. The antibiotics of choice include oxacillin in conjunction with ampicillin, and chloramphenicol or cefotaxime.

Syphilis

The incidence of syphilis, caused by the spirochete *Treponema pallidum,* has undergone a resurgence. In 1990, the incidence of primary and secondary cases reported in the United States peaked at 20.3 cases per 100,000, its highest level since 1949. In 1992, however, the incidence dropped to 13.7 per 100,000. The increase in reported cases occurred primarily in heterosexual teenagers and adults. In addition, the rise in cases of congenital syphilis is linked to AIDS, drug abuse, exchange of sex for drugs, teenage pregnancy, limited health care access, and poor prenatal care.

Signs and symptoms of active congenital syphilis include temperature instability, mucocutaneous lesions, rhinorrhea, hepatomegaly, splenomegaly, adenopathy, anemia, hydrops fetalis, pathologic jaundice, and pseudoparalysis. In early infancy, the usual radiographic finding is syphilitic metaphysitis (metaphyseal lucent bands, erosions, or a wide zone of provisional calcification), which has been reported in more than 90% of infants with symptomatic congenital syphilis. The incidence of these findings in asymptomatic newborns in the present epidemic is unknown.

A positive serology is frequently found in asymptomatic newborns. At present, there are no means to differentiate whether this represents occult disease or passive transfer of maternal antibodies. Therefore, a presumptive diagnosis of active congenital syphilis in seropositive asymptomatic newborns depends on demonstrating abnormalities in the long-bone films, spinal fluid, or other laboratory tests, such as a change from a negative result to a positive result of the rapid plasma reagin (RPR) test. A recent study demonstrated abnormal long-bone radiographs consisting of radiolucent and radio-opaque lines in the metaphysis, metaphyseal destruction, osteitis, and/or periostitis, in approximately 20% of asymptomatic seropositive newborns. This indicates occult disease that must be treated. A single anteroposterior film of the lower extremities should be obtained to rule out occult disease in all newborns with a positive perinatal serology. In addition, all of these children should be monitored as they grow, because even those treated remain at risk for developing late sequelae of congenital syphilis.

Tuberculosis

Physicians must maintain a high index of suspicion for diagnosis of tuberculosis and skeletal tuberculosis because of increased occurrence of these infections over the past decade. Radiographic findings of tuberculosis include joint effusion, periarticular osteopenia, joint space narrowing, cortical irregularity, radiolucencies, periosteal new bone formation, and advanced epiphyseal maturity. When the hip is involved, subluxation is common because of joint distention.

Spinal deformity resulting from tuberculosis is a management challenge. It has long been assumed that an anterior arthrodesis (following resection of the infection) at an early age would cause progressive kyphotic deformity during subsequent growth. For this reason, posterior spinal fusion has been advocated. A recent study, however, concluded that prophylactic posterior spinal fusion in childhood may not be needed, because progressive kyphosis was not observed.

Annotated Bibliography

Osteomyelitis

Carr AJ, Cole WG, Roberton DM, et al: Chronic multifocal osteomyelitis. *J Bone Joint Surg* 1993;75B:582–591.

This report describes 22 patients with chronic multifocal osteomyelitis between the ages of 4 and 14 years. It reviews the presenting symptoms, natural history, radiographic and laboratory findings, and treatment.

Cole WG: The management of chronic osteomyelitis. *Clin Orthop* 1991;264:84–89.

This article classifies chronic osteomyelitis into two groups: nonspecific and specific. The specific group includes children with chronic osteomyelitis because of mycobacteria or mycoses. The nonspecific group includes children with chronic osteomyelitis as a sequel to acute osteomyelitis plus individuals with chronic unifocal and chronic multifocal osteomyelitis. Natural history and treatments for each group are discussed.

Correa AG, Edwards MS, Baker CJ: Vertebral osteomyelitis in children. *Pediatr Infect Dis J* 1993;12: 228–233.

Craigen MA, Watters J, Hackett JS: The changing epidemiology of osteomyelitis in children. *J Bone Joint Surg* 1992;74B:541–545.

In this article, the authors note that osteomyelitis is becoming a rarer disease, with a 50% decrease in prevalence. The proportion of cases involving long bones has decreased from 84% to 57%, and those involving *Staphylococcus aureus* infection have dropped from 55% to 31%.

Daoud A, Saighi-Bouaouina A, Descamps L, et al: Hematogenous osteomyelitis of the femoral neck in children. *J Pediatr Orthop Part B* 1993;2:83–295.

Dormans JP, Drummond DS: Pediatric hematogenous osteomyelitis: New trends in presentation, diagnosis, and treatment. *J Am Acad Orthop Surg* 1994;2:333–341.

Ezra E, Khermosh O, Assia A, et al: Primary subacute osteomyelitis of the axial and appendicular skeleton. *J Pediatr Orthop Part B* 1993;1:148–152.

This article is a retrospective review of 28 cases, emphasizing the difficulties in diagnosing this condition due to scarcity of symptoms and signs and the lack of noninvasive laboratory tests.

Hoffman EB, de Beer JD, Keys G, et al: Diaphyseal primary subacute osteomyelitis in children. *J Pediatr Orthop* 1990;10:250–254.

Six cases in which the radiographic picture was indistinguishable from that of a round cell tumor were discussed. Diagnoses required surgical exploration and biopsy.

Jacobs NM: Pneumococcal osteomyelitis and arthritis in children: A hospital series and literature review. *Am J Dis Child* 1991;145:70–74.

Mustafa MM, Saez-Llorens X, McCracken GH Jr, et al: Acute hematogenous pelvic osteomyelitis in infants and children. *Pediatr Infect Dis J* 1990;9:416–421.

Nelson JD: Acute osteomyelitis in children. *Infect Dis Clin North Am* 1990;4:513–522.

This is a review of 398 cases that have been treated over 30 years. Fourteen children (3.5%) developed chronic infection; relapses or chronicity occurred in less than 5%. Pathologic fractures occurred in four patients.

Nelson JD: Skeletal infections in children. *Adv Pediatr Infect Dis* 1991;6:59–78.

Peters W, Irving J, Letts M: Long-term effects of neonatal bone and joint infection on adjacent growth plates. *J Pediatr Orthop* 1992;12:806–810.

Children with neonatal osteomyelitis must be followed to skeletal maturity to observe the adjacent physis for late tethering. Growth abnormalities and physeal bars may not be clinically evident for several years after the initial infection has been treated.

Petty RE: Septic arthritis and osteomyelitis in children. *Curr Opin Rheumatol* 1990;2:616–621.

Roy DR, Greene WB, Gamble JG: Osteomyelitis of the patella in children. *J Pediatr Orthop* 1991;11:364–366.

Scott RJ, Christofersen MR, Robertson WW Jr, et al: Acute osteomyelitis in children: A review of 116 cases. *J Pediatr Orthop* 1990;10:649–652.

Many patients have a normal WBC count and no temperature elevation, making bone tenderness and an elevated ESR of paramount importance in making a diagnosis.

Tudisco C, Farsetti P, Gatti S, et al: Influence of chronic osteomyelitis on skeletal growth: Analysis at maturity of 26 cases affected during childhood. *J Pediatr Orthop* 1991;11:358–363.

The authors review long-term outcome of 26 cases, four of which showed shortening and angular deformity of the affected limb. Irreversible damage of the growth plate, due to the virulence of the pathogen or inappropriate surgical treatment, was responsible for the deformities.

Wang EH, Simpson S, Bennet GC: Osteomyelitis of the calcaneum. *J Bone Joint Surg* 1992;74B:906–909.

Septic Arthritis

Abernethy LJ, Lee YC, Cole WG: Ultrasound localization of subperiosteal abscesses in children with late-acute osteomyelitis. *J Pediatr Orthop* 1993;13:766–768.

Asmar BI: Osteomyelitis in the neonate. *Infect Dis Clin North Am* 1992;6:117–132.

Bennett OM, Namnyak SS: Acute septic arthritis of the hip joint in infancy and childhood. *Clin Orthop* 1992;281:123–132.

The authors of this report emphasize the need for rapid diagnosis and surgical management. It also notes that almost all children treated within 4 days of symptoms had a satisfactory outcome. The authors reiterate that concomitant osteomyelitis of the proximal femur produced a far worse prognosis than if the infection was confined to the hip joint.

Betz RR, Cooperman DR, Wopperer JM, et al: Late sequelae of septic arthritis of the hip in infancy and childhood. *J Pediatr Orthop* 1990;10:365–372.

Bohay DR, Gray JM: Sacroiliac joint pyarthrosis. *Orthop Rev* 1993;22:817–823.

In a review of six cases with this rare infection, the most common symptom was fever and the most common physical findings were elevated temperature and limited ipsilateral hip motion. The most specific imaging study was technetium bone scan.

Choi IH, Pizzutillo PD, Bowen JR, et al: Sequelae and reconstruction after septic arthritis of the hip in infants. *J Bone Joint Surg* 1990;72A:1150–1165.

In this article, the residual deformity and late treatment of 34 hips in 31 children who had septic arthritis when they were less than 1 year old were reviewed. Hips were classified into four groups on the basis of radiographic changes.

Connor E, McSherry G: Treatment of HIV infection in infancy (review). *Clin Perinatol* 1994;21:163–177.

Dagan R: Management of acute hematogenous osteomyelitis and septic arthritis in the pediatric patient. *Pediatr Infect Dis J* 1993;12:88–92.

Frederiksen B, Christiansen P, Knudsen FU: Acute osteomyelitis and septic arthritis in the neonate: Risk factors and outcome. *Eur J Pediatr* 1993;152:577–580.

In a review of 22 neonates with acute osteomyelitis or septic arthritis, fever was rare and WBC count was generally normal. Plain radiographs were more efficient than bone scan. Risk factors included prematurity, respiratory distress, and umbilical artery catheterization.

Howard CB, Einhorn M, Dagan R, et al: Fine-needle bone biopsy to diagnose osteomyelitis. *J Bone Joint Surg* 1994;76B:311–314.

Howard CB, Einhorn M, Dagan R, et al: Ultrasound in diagnosis and management of acute haematogenous osteomyelitis in children. *J Bone Joint Surg* 1993;75B: 79–82.

The authors demonstrated the usefulness of ultrasound in distinguishing between early cases of osteomyelitis, which deserve a trial of conservative management, and more advanced cases, which require immediate surgical drainage.

Jackson MA, Burry VF, Olson LC: Pyogenic arthritis associated with adjacent osteomyelitis: Identification of the sequela-prone child. *Pediatr Infect Dis J* 1992;11:9–13.

Sixteen percent of children in this series who presented with pyogenic joint infection had coexisting bone disease. Significant sequelae occurred in 57% of those cases. Children with adjacent osteomyelitis tended to be younger, were symptomatic more than 7 days, and had received prior antibiotics.

Jacobs RF, Darville T, Parks JA, et al: Safety profile and efficacy of cefotaxime for the treatment of hospitalized children. *Clin Infect Dis* 1992;14:56–65

Knudsen CJ, Hoffman EB: Neonatal osteomyelitis. *J Bone Joint Surg* 1990;72B:846–851.

The authors reviewed 34 neonates with osteomyelitis. The hip was the most common site involved; swelling and pseudoparalysis were the most significant local signs.

Nelson JD, Norden C, Mader JT, et al: Evaluation of new anti-infective drugs for the treatment of acute hematogenous osteomyelitis in children: Infectious Diseases Society of American and the Food and Drug Administration. *Clin Infect Dis* 1992;15(suppl 1):S162–S166.

Prober CG: Current antibiotic therapy of community-acquired bacterial infections in hospitalized children: Bone and joint infections. *Pediatr Infect Dis J* 1992;11:156–159.

Tuson CE, Hoffman EB, Mann MD: Isotope bone scanning for acute osteomyelitis and septic arthritis in children. *J Bone Joint Surg* 1994;76B:306–310.

The authors discuss the accuracy of bone scan.

Wopperer JM, White JJ, Gillespie R, et al: Long-term follow-up of infantile hip sepsis. *J Pediatr Orthop* 1988; 8:322–325.

Nine hips in eight patients were reviewed in this article with the suggestion that reconstructive efforts following sepsis of the hip-joint may not yield results comparable to nonsurgical treatment.

Specific Infections and Conditions

Brion LP, Manuli M, Rai B, et al: Long-bone radiographic abnormalities as a sign of active congenital syphilis in asymptomatic newborns. *Pediatrics* 1991;88:1037–1040.

This study found that approximately 20% of asymptomatic newborns with positive perinatal treponemal serology had abnormal long-bone radiographs. As it is difficult to determine whether positive treponemal serology represents occult disease or passive transfer of maternal antibodies, a presumptive diagnosis of active congenital syphilis can be made on the basis of long-bone films. With the increasing incidence of congenital syphilis, radiologic studies should be performed on all newborns with a positive serology.

Crawford AH, Kucharzyk DW, Ruda R, et al: Diskitis in children. *Clin Orthop* 1991;266:70–79.

The authors present a thorough review of 36 patients, which suggests that antibiotics are appropriate if the child fails to respond to immobilization.

Epps CH Jr, Bryant DO III, Coles MJ, et al: Osteomyelitis in patients who have sickle-cell disease: Diagnosis and management. *J Bone Joint Surg* 1991;73A:1281–1292.

Early diagnosis of osteomyelitis in patients who have sickle-cell disease requires a high index of suspicion, careful physical examination, and accurate interpretation of laboratory and radiographic studies. *Staphylococcus aureus* was the causative agent more frequently than was *Salmonella*.

Frey C: Marine injuries: Prevention and treatment. *Orthop Rev* 1994;23:645–649.

This is a review of penetrating wounds, stings, and inoculation of venom, which are common marine injuries to unwary walkers during the summer. A must-read article for anyone who enjoys the beach.

Gardiner JS, Zauk AM, Minnefor AB, et al: Pyomyositis in an HIV-positive premature infant: Case report and review of the literature. *J Pediatr Orthop* 1990;10:791–793.

Gregg-Smith SJ, Pattison RM, Dodd CA, et al: Septic arthritis in haemophilia. *J Bone Joint Surg* 1993;75B:368–370.

Although septic arthritis is a rare complication in patients with hemophilia, the diagnosis should be considered when an episode of hemoarthrosis does not respond to coagulation therapy and joint immobilization. The authors of this paper describe six cases, of which four were seropositive for HIV.

Jacobs JC, Li SC, Ruzal-Shapiro C, et al: Tuberculous arthritis in children: Diagnosis by needle biopsy of the synovium. *Clin Pediatr* 1994;33:344–348.

The increasing frequency of tuberculosis in the United States and the need for greater awareness of the risk of tuberculous arthritis in childhood is underscored in this article. It also demonstrates a case of tuberculosis synovitis during the early weeks of infection when the tuberculin skin test may be negative and suggests a needle biopsy of the synovium in all children with monoarticular arthritis and a positive tuberculin skin test.

Jacobs RF, McCarthy RE, Elser JM: Pseudomonas osteochondritis complicating puncture wounds of the foot in children: A 10-year evaluation. *J Infect Dis* 1989;160: 657–661.

Seventy-seven cases of microbiologically proven *Pseudomonas* osteochondritis and septic arthritis following nail puncture wound to the foot were reviewed. Most children had been wearing tennis shoes. All cases were treated with surgical debridement and antibiotics. Treatment failure was attributed to previously undetected septic arthritis.

Jarvis JG, Skipper J: Pseudomonas osteochondritis complicating puncture wounds in children. *J Pediatr Orthop* 1994;14:755–759.

The authors review 15 cases of *Pseudomonas* osteochondritis in children with puncture wounds to assess the current approach to diagnosis and treatment. This uncommon complication can lead to significant permanent sequelae in the growing child. A high index of suspicion, coupled with aggressive medical and surgical treatment, is required for a satisfactory outcome.

Merchan EC, Magallon M, Manso F, et al: Septic arthritis in HIV-positive haemophiliacs: Four cases and a literature review. *Int Orthop* 1992;16:302–306.

Septic arthritis has rarely been reported in hemophiliacs. The authors of this article present four patients who had painful, swollen joints that failed to respond rapidly to factor replacement, suggesting that septic arthritis may serve as a clinical marker for immunosuppression in hemophiliacs.

Piehl FC, Davis RJ, Prugh SI: Osteomyelitis in sickle cell disease. *J Pediatr Orthop* 1993;13:225–227.

In this review of 16 cases of osteomyelitis in 15 patients, 13 were due to *Salmonella* species and support earlier findings that *Salmonella* species is the most common microorganism in sickle-cell disease.

Renwick SE, Ritterbusch JF: Pyomyositis in children. *J Pediatr Orthop* 1993;13:769–772.

The authors emphasize that pyomyositis should be considered in the differential diagnosis of children who appear septic and those complaining of joint pain or muscle aches. MRI is more reliable in making the diagnosis. The possibility of multiple abscess sites must be ruled out.

Ring D, Johnston CE II, Wenger DR: Pyogenic infectious spondylitis in children: The convergence of discitis and vertebral osteomyelitis. *J Pediatr Orthop* 1995;15:652–660.

Forty-seven patients with pyogenic infectious spondylitis (diskitis) were reviewed to determine the spectrum of disease. MRIs were obtained in nine patients and were found to be identical to MRI findings in adult vertebral osteomyelitis. This provides strong evidence for an infectious process in diskitis. The investigation confirmed the usually benign course of spine infections in children but also emphasized the potential for serious sequelae. Symptoms were resolved more rapidly with intravenous antibiotics than they were with oral antibiotics or no antibiotics.

Ring D, Wenger DR: Magnetic resonance-imaging scans in discitis: Sequential studies in a child who needed operative drainage. A case report. *J Bone Joint Surg* 1994;76A:596–601.

In this article the authors discuss possible risks associated with withholding antibiotic treatment of diskitis.

Rose CD, Fawcett PT, Eppes SC, et al: Pediatric Lyme arthritis: Clinical spectrum and outcome. *J Pediatr Orthop* 1994;14:238–241.

The authors describe the rheumatologic features, serologic findings, and articular outcomes of children treated for Lyme arthritis. They demonstrated that Lyme disease should be considered in any child from an endemic area who presents with arthritis, regardless of the articular pattern.

Upadhyay SS, Saji MJ, Sell P, et al: Spinal deformity after childhood surgery for tuberculosis of the spine: A comparison of radical surgery and debridement. *J Bone Joint Surg* 1994;76B:91–98.

Radical surgery and grafting produced a reduction in kyphosis and deformity; however, in debridement surgery there was an increase in deformity. There was no evidence to suggest that disproportionate posterior spinal growth contributes to progression of deformity after anterior spinal fusion in children.

US Department of Health and Human Services: *HIV/AIDS Surveillance Report* 1995;7:3–30.

6

Acute Pain Management

Pain management in children is a complex and inadequately studied problem. Limited cognitive and language skills in young children frequently lead to underestimation of pain intensity and, consequently, undertreatment. Pain is known to induce neuroendocrine responses that may affect postoperative outcome. In the surgical patient, inadequate postoperative pain control has been associated with disruptions of eating and sleep cycles, slower recovery, and poor outcomes after surgery. Thus, the quality of analgesia may influence length of hospital stay and the incidence of complications, thereby affecting hospital costs and appropriate utilization of health care resources.

The inherent difficulty of assessing pain in children, concerns regarding opioid-induced respiratory depression, and the potential for addiction are responsible in part for the undertreatment of pain. This chapter discusses assessment of pain using physiologic, self-report, and behavioral measures; and the management of pain using systemic analgesia, regional analgesia, and nonpharmacologic interventions.

Pain Assessment

Appropriate management of pain depends upon its accurate assessment and measurement. This can be done using physiologic measures, observation of behaviors, and self-report.

Physiologic Measures

Changes in heart rate, respiratory rate, and blood pressure are often used to identify the presence of pain. Most studies of physiologic measures have involved infants and have established the validity of changes in heart rate, transcutaneous Po_2, sweating, and EEG in identifying pain. These indicators are also altered by other stress-arousal events and disease complications and, therefore, they should be used in conjunction with other measures of pain.

Behavioral Observations

Behavioral observation is the primary approach for the assessment of pain in children with limited verbal and cognitive skills. Specific behaviors such as vocalization (crying or groaning), facial expression, body tension, rigidity, and inability to be consoled are used by clinicians and parents to estimate a child's pain intensity. Several scales based on behaviors have been designed for clinical use. These tools offer a valuable guide for the observation and evaluation of postoperative pain. The Children's Hospital of Eastern Ontario Pain Scale (CHEOPS) consists of six categories of behavior. The Objective Pain Scale (OPS) incorporates four behavioral categories with blood pressure. These scales are difficult to memorize and use in a busy clinical setting. The FLACC scale (Table 1) includes five categories of behavior (face, legs, activity, cry, and consolability). The acronym FLACC facilitates recall of the categories. Preliminary studies have established its validity, interrater reliability, and ease of use in the clinical setting. Reliability and validity of behavioral assessment tools are highest with moderate to severe pain and with the short sharp pain associated with procedures. Children cry and withdraw not just in response to pain but also in response to other types of distress, such as hunger or anxiety. Use of behavioral observations to guide analgesic administration requires consideration of the context of the child's behaviors.

Self-Report

As with adults, self-report provides the most reliable indication of the location and intensity of pain in children. Simple self-report methods can be used in children 4 years and older who can verbalize. The pain vocabulary avail-

Table 1. Assessment of pain intensity: FLACC scale

Behavior Category	0	1	2
Face	No particular expression, or smiling	Occasional grimace or frown, withdrawn, disinterested	Frequent to constant clenched jaw, quivering chin
Legs	Normal position or relaxed	Uneasy, restless, tense	Kicking, or legs drawn up
Activity	Lying quietly, normal position, moves easily	Squirming, shifting back and forth, tense	Arched, rigid, or jerking
Cry	No crying-awake or asleep	Moans or whimpers, occasional complaint	Crying steadily, screams or sobs, frequent complaints
Consolability	Content, relaxed	Reassured by occasional touching, hugging, or "talking to," distractable	Difficult to console or comfort

WONG/BAKER FACES RATING SCALE

Fig. 1 The Faces Pain Scale. The child chooses which face depicts the degree of pain intensity experienced at a given time. (Reproduced with permission from Wong DL: *Whaley & Wong's Nursing Care of Infants and Children,* ed 5. St. Louis, MO, Mosby-Year Book, 1995.)

Word-Graphic Rating Scale

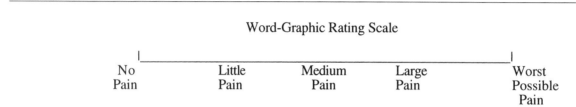

Fig. 2 The Word-Graphic Rating Scale uses a straight horizontal line with the end points identified as "no pain" or "worst possible pain." The child is instructed to draw a straight vertical line anywhere along the horizontal line to demonstrate the intensity of pain. (Reproduced with permission from Savedra MC, Tesler MD, Holzemer WL, et al: *Adolescent Pediatric Pain Tool (APPT) Preliminary User's Manual.* San Francisco, CA, University of California, 1989.)

able to a 5 year old is limited to a few simple words such as bad, hurting, and ouch. This vocabulary increases to about 26 words by 12 years of age. A young child can point to an area of pain but the precision of indicating the location of pain increases with the age of the child. Assessment scales such as the Oucher, Poker Chip Scale, and the Faces scale can be used by young children to express the intensity of their pain. Advance preparation greatly facilitates the use of these scales by children. Studies indicate that young children prefer to use the Faces scale (Fig. 1). A Number scale and a Word Graphic scale (Fig. 2) can be used by children who understand the concepts of numbers and order. Most children over 7 years of age are able to use number scales.

Routine assessment and documentation is critical for effective pain management. Sleeping and withdrawn behavior can be misinterpreted as the absence of pain, while in fact the child may be attempting to control pain by limiting activity and interactions. A child sleeping quietly who awakens with jerky body movements and is unable to settle may be having muscle spasms. Extremity pain following injury or surgery that is unrelieved by a 50% increase in the dose of opioid and increases significantly with movement of the extremity or digits may indicate the beginning of a compartment syndrome. Escalating opioid doses would not be effective or indicated in either of these situations. Agitation and dysphoria may occur as side effects of opioids; for example, meperidine may cause irritability and result in sleep disturbances and muscle twitching.

Although the objective assessment of pain in children can be a challenge, the utilization of more than one measure helps the clinician to understand the source of pain and provide effective treatment.

Pain Management

Pain after orthopaedic surgery can be intense, regardless of the age of the patient. Fortunately, recent advances in pain management techniques have provided a scientific foundation for rational treatment in children. Traditional regimens of intramuscular opioid injections have been conclusively shown to be ineffective in 50% of postoperative patients and are rapidly becoming obsolete. These regimens resulted in delays in administration of pain medication and fluctuating plasma drug levels due to unpredictable intramuscular absorption, leading to either excessive sedation or uncontrolled pain. This technique is particularly unsuitable in children because of their fear of frequent injections. This section will discuss the clinical pharmacology and treatment options relevant to pain management after orthopaedic surgery.

Systemic Analgesia

Acetaminophen Acetaminophen is the most commonly used nonopioid analgesic in children. Its analgesic effect results from inhibition of prostaglandin synthetase centrally. Prostaglandins sensitize pain receptors to mechanical stimulation and to chemical mediators such as bradykinin and histamine. Acetaminophen can be administered orally in a dose of 15 to 18 mg/kg or rectally in a dose of 25 to 30 mg/kg every 4 hours either alone for minor pain or as an adjunct to opioids for more severe pain. In one study, a smaller dose of rectal acetaminophen (20 mg/kg) was found to be ineffective in children undergoing tonsillectomy.

Nonsteroidal Anti-Inflammatory Drugs   The advent of an injectable nonsteroidal anti-inflammatory drug (NSAID), ketorolac, has resulted in a renewed interest in the use of NSAIDs in children after surgery. The therapeutic effects of NSAIDs are derived from their ability to inhibit prostaglandin synthesis. NSAIDs decrease levels of inflammatory chemical mediators such as bradykinin, substance P, thromboxane, and prostaglandins at the site of tissue injury. NSAIDs may be used alone to treat mild or moderate pain. For severe pain, NSAIDs used in conjunction with opioids have an opioid dose-sparing effect. In addition, the concurrent use of opioids and NSAIDs frequently provides more effective analgesia than either of the drug classes alone. The side effects of NSAIDs include gastrointestinal upset, mucosal ulceration, altered renal function, and interference with platelet function, which prolongs bleeding time. The risk of bleeding may make these drugs unsuitable in the early postoperative period after some operations, although these concerns have not been adequately addressed in clinical studies.

Ketorolac tromethamine (Toradol) has been shown to be as effective as morphine or meperidine for short-term management of moderate to severe postoperative pain. In a large study of adult patients, intramuscular ketorolac (30 mg and 90 mg) was reported to be at least as effective in relieving postoperative pain as 12 mg of morphine administered intramuscularly, and the ketorolac had a significantly longer duration of action than morphine. This study involved gynecologic, abdominal, and orthopaedic procedures. Ketorolac may also be administered orally in a dose of 10 mg every 6 hours. It is only available as a 10-mg pill, the adult dose. If a child is able to tolerate oral medications, ibuprofen may offer greater flexibility in the dose as well as a significant cost saving. Ketorolac may be administered intramuscularly or intravenously in a dose of 0.5 mg/kg every 6 hours. It lacks the respiratory depressant effects of opioids but shares the potential side effects of NSAIDs. It is known to cause adverse nervous system effects, including somnolence, dizziness, and headache. Long-term administration of ketorolac has been reported to cause renal impairment in approximately 3% of patients and, therefore, it should be used with caution, if at all, in patients with renal disease. It is known to inhibit platelet adhesion and aggregation and to prolong bleeding time by approximately 3 minutes from baseline values. Unlike aspirin, this effect is transient with ketorolac, and platelet aggregation returns to normal within 24 to 48 hours after

therapy is discontinued. Adult studies have demonstrated that ketorolac does not produce excessive perioperative bleeding and that prolongation of bleeding time appears to be of little clinical importance in most patients. Its lack of respiratory depressant effects makes ketorolac a valuable drug used alone or as an adjunct to opioids in the management of postoperative pain. According to suggestions by the Food and Drug Administration, parenteral ketorolac should not be used for more than than 5 days.

Benzodiazepines   These drugs are frequently prescribed as adjuncts in pain management. They are most useful for sedation, anxiolysis, and amnesia for painful procedures. They provide no analgesia but their short-term use may be indicated when skeletal muscle spasms are the primary cause of pain. Benzodiazepines should be used with extreme caution in conjunction with opioids, because they potentiate the respiratory depressant effects of opioids.

Opioids   Opioids exert their effects by interacting with opioid receptors in the brain, spinal cord, and in the peripheral nervous system. In addition to four major receptors (mu, delta, kappa, and sigma), a number of minor subgroups have also been identified. Both endogenous substances (endorphins) and exogenous substances (opioid drugs) interact with these receptors. Some of the opioid drugs are pure agonist (morphine), some are antagonist (naloxone), and some are both (nalbuphine). The mu and delta receptors are related to analgesia, respiratory depression, euphoria, sedation, and physical dependence. The kappa receptor is located in the spinal cord and is primarily related to spinal analgesia and sedation. The sigma receptor is responsible for the psychotomimetic effects of opioids, such as hallucinations and dysphoria. Interaction of opioids with receptors in the brain results in activation of descending pathways that inhibit pain sensation.

Opioids are administered by several routes and pharmacokinetic differences account for the major differences in effect. Intravenous administration reliably achieves a desired opiate blood level; however, the same opiate blood level may exert different effects in different patients. With other routes of administration, additional factors such as absorption and first pass metabolism will affect blood levels. Based on adult data, the bioavailability of oral morphine and meperidine is 30% and that of codeine is 40% to 70% of the administered dose. Intramuscular administration of opioids leads to highly variable absorption and is no longer the preferred route for pain management. Epidural opioids are gaining increasing popularity in adults and children. When morphine is administered into the epidural space, it crosses the dura and binds with opiate receptors in the substantia gelatinosa of the spinal cord. Small doses of epidural morphine produce adequate analgesia because its effects are related to cerebrospinal fluid level rather than blood level. Yet another route of administration of opioids is transdermal fentanyl, which has been used primarily in adults with chronic pain. A single patch releases fentanyl at the rate of 25 μg/hr. Absorption is slow, but once therapeutic levels are reached, approximately 12 hours after application, fairly constant blood levels are maintained. After the patch is removed, a reservoir of opioid remains in the skin and effects persist for several hours. In children, its use has been primarily reserved for chronic pain in those with poor intravenous access, such as patients with malignancies. Oral transmucosal fentanyl citrate (fentanyl lollipop) has recently been approved by the Food and Drug Administration, but its use is restricted to monitored settings by personnel specifically trained in the use of anesthetics, airway management, and cardiorespiratory resuscitation.

The common side effects of opioids are nausea, vomiting, and itching. In addition, opioids can cause life-threatening respiratory depression in a dose-dependent manner. Initially, there is a depressed response to increased CO_2 followed by an increase in resting CO_2 due to decreased minute ventilation. Opioids also depress the hypoxic ventilatory drive, slow the respiratory rate, and lead to a decrease in tidal volume. Some opioids cause hypotension with or without bradycardia. Other side effects include urinary retention, constipation, and central nervous system (CNS) effects such as somnolence, sedation, euphoria, and dysphoria. Meperidine in high doses or with prolonged use may cause CNS excitation due to the accumulation of normeperidine. This results in tremors, twitching, and seizures. Opioids are known to produce tolerance and when used for longer than 7 days it is recommended that the dose of the opioids be tapered to prevent withdrawal symptoms. This group of drugs should be used with caution in infants younger than 3 months of age because clearance and protein binding are decreased, resulting in a greater free fraction of the drug. Immaturity of the blood-brain barrier in infants may contribute to enhanced passage of opioids into the CNS.

Patient-Controlled Analgesia   Patient-controlled analgesia (PCA) provides safe and effective analgesia in children as young as 5 years of age. It allows the patient to self-administer small preprogrammed doses of opioids via a microprocessor-controlled pump that is connected to the patient's intravenous tubing. This enables the patient to titrate an opioid blood level in response to the changing intensity of pain. The inherent safety of PCA lies in the fact that in the event of oversedation, the patient falls asleep and is unable to self-administer additional doses. It is well documented that most patients choose a dosage regimen that strikes a balance between adequate comfort and side effects such as sedation, nausea, vomiting, and pruritus. Other advantages of PCA include avoiding delays in administration of analgesics, safety, acceptability, patient satisfaction, and reduced nursing staff workload. Use of PCA does not obviate the need for frequent assessment of pain control and side effects by health care professionals. In children too young for PCA, nurse-controlled anal-

Table 2. Guidelines for initiation of PCA using morphine sulfate in children

PCA Method	Incremental Dose (mg/kg)	Lockout Interval (min)	Infusion Rate (mg/kg/hr)	Four Hour Limit (mg/kg)
Bolus doses only	0.02 to 0.03	8 to 15	0	0.25 to 0.3
Infusion and bolus doses	0.02 to 0.03	8 to 15	0.01 to 0.02	0.25 to 0.3

gesia has been used with success. This technique allows nursing staff the flexibility to titrate small incremental doses of analgesic medications on the basis of their assessment of pain or in anticipation of painful procedures, such as physical therapy and dressing changes.

Most PCA devices can deliver a continuous infusion of analgesics in addition to incremental boluses. Continuous infusions maintain therapeutic plasma opioid levels during sleep and prevent disruption of sleep, provide improved pain scores and patient satisfaction, and avoid side effects or excessive opioid use. When a continuous technique is used in conjunction with PCA, it commits the patient to receive a fixed amount of opiate regardless of the level of sedation. This may in some cases reduce the inherent safety of PCA, and close monitoring for oversedation may be required in patients on continuous opioid infusions. Morphine sulfate in vials containing 1 mg/ml is most suitable for PCA in children although meperidine and hydromorphone have also been used extensively. Guidelines for initiation of PCA using morphine are presented in Table 2 based on published literature and the authors' experience.

Regional Analgesia

Regional anesthetic techniques provide profound analgesia with decreased opioid requirements, a rapid and pain-free recovery, and early ambulation. Regional analgesia also provides greater patient acceptance of continuous passive motion and physical therapy. With careful patient selection, regional analgesia provides safe and effective pain relief in children.

Epidural Analgesia   A caudal block is an effective means of providing analgesia for operations below the diaphragm. This block is technically simple to perform in children younger than 8 years of age because the landmarks are easily identified. It is commonly indicated for lower extremity procedures such as clubfoot repair or for urologic or abdominal surgery. Bupivacaine in concentrations of 0.125% to 0.25% with 1 in 200,000 epinephrine provides effective analgesia. The duration of sensory blockade and quality of analgesia are similar with both concentrations, but the lower concentration produces significantly less motor blockade. Morphine sulfate in a dose of 50 to 75 μg/kg provides analgesia for 12 to 24 hours, but close monitoring for respiratory depression is required for 24 hours after injection.

Table 3. Guidelines for epidural analgesia in children and adolescents

Drug	Onset/Duration	Dose
Duramorph (single shot)	Onset 45 min Duration 6 to 24 (22) hrs	0.03 to 0.05 mg/kg
Duramorph infusion	Onset 45 min	3 to 4 mcg/kg/hr
Fentanyl infusion*	Onset 5 to 15 min	0.5 to 2.0 mcg/kg/hr
Bupivacaine infusion*	Onset 10 min	0.0625% or 0.100% 0.1 to 0.4 cc/kg/hr

*Frequently used in combination

In older children who weigh more than 20 kg, lumbar epidural analgesia is indicated because a smaller volume per kilogram of local anesthetic is required to reach the dermatome desired. Effective postoperative analgesia can be provided with local anesthetics, opioids, or a combination of the two classes of drugs. Epidural local anesthetics provide dose-related intense analgesia, prevent muscle spasm, and allow pain-free mobilization and physical therapy while they avoid the respiratory depressant effects of opioids. The disadvantages of epidural local anesthetics are related to motor and autonomic blockade, and the potential to mask perioperative complications, such as compartment syndrome and pressure sores. Use of dilute solutions of local anesthetics (0.125% bupivacaine) and vigilance by the nursing staff can minimize these risks. Epidural opioids have the advantage of providing analgesia without sympathetic, sensory, or motor blockade, but they carry the risk of adverse effects of respiratory depression, nausea, vomiting, and pruritus. Systemic opioids and sedative drugs, such as benzodiazepines, probably should not be used in conjunction with epidural opioids because of the risk of respiratory depression. A combination of epidural opioids and local anesthetics (eg, fentanyl and bupivacaine) blocks nociceptive pathways at different sites, allowing the use of lower doses of each agent with fewer side effects. The dosages of drugs administered by the epidural route are presented in Table 3.

The use of epidural opioids for spine surgery is gaining increasing popularity. A single dose of morphine injected intrathecally by the surgeon prior to wound closure has been shown to provide effective analgesia for 12 to 24 hours. Alternatively an epidural catheter is placed by the surgeon at the upper end of the incision and tunneled lateral to the incision prior to wound closure. The catheters are left in place for 72 hours and low-dose opioids are infused to provide effective analgesia. This technique requires close monitoring, including continuous pulse oximetry and hourly documentation of respiratory rate, until 24 hours after the infusion has been discontinued.

Peripheral Nerve Blocks   Peripheral nerve blockade with local anesthetic allows interruption of sensory transmission along specific nerves or nerve groups. The peripheral blocks pertinent to orthopaedic surgery include brachial plexus blocks for upper extremity surgery, intercostal blocks and intrapleural catheters for thoracic surgery; and femoral, sciatic nerve, and lumbar plexus blocks (3-in-1 block) for lower extremity surgery. As with any regional anesthetic technique, careful assessment of needle placement and prudent estimation of safe quantities of local anesthetic are required.

Regional analgesia is absolutely contraindicated if an infection is present at the site of needle puncture, in the presence of sepsis or bleeding disorders, and in patients on anticoagulants. Complications of regional anesthetics include inadvertent intravascular or subarachnoid injection, local anesthetic toxicity, medication errors, and pneumothorax or hemothorax from brachial plexus and intercostal blocks.

Preemptive Analgesia   Current literature suggests that sensory signals generated by tissue injury during surgery can trigger a prolonged state of increased excitability in the CNS that may contribute to hyperalgesia postoperatively. The theoretical basis of preemptive analgesia is that it prevents the development of this hyperexcitability by diminishing the barrage of nociceptive inputs during surgery. The underlying principle is that therapeutic intervention is made in advance of the pain rather than in reaction to it. Studies in adult patients have demonstrated a dramatic decrease in the incidence of phantom limb pain when epidural blockade is performed before amputation. Preemptive treatment could be directed at the periphery at inputs along sensory axons and/or at central neurons by using NSAIDs, local anesthetics, or opioids, singly or in combination.

Nonpharmacologic Interventions

Nonpharmacologic interventions are classified as cognitive-behavioral approaches and physical measures. Cognitive-behavioral approaches include education, relaxation, music distraction, hypnosis, and biofeedback. These measures help children understand their pain and take an active part in its assessment and management. Physical interventions that inhibit the transmission of impulses generated by noxious stimuli include application of heat and cold, massage, exercise, and immobilization. Counterstimulation techniques, such as transcutaneous electrical nerve stimulation (TENS) therapy, have been effective in reducing self-reported pain and analgesic use following abdominal, thoracic, and orthopaedic surgery. TENS is a method of applying controlled, low-voltage electrical stimulations to large, myelinated peripheral nerve fibers via cutaneous electrodes for the purpose of modulating stimulus transmission and relieving pain.

Summary

Pain in children contributes to emotional and physical suffering, longer recovery periods, and greater use of scarce health care resources, and it can compromise patient outcomes. A multidisciplinary approach, including all members of the healthcare team, with input from the patient and the patient's family, is essential for effective pain management.

Annotated Bibliography

Pain Assessment

Merkel S, Voepel-Lewis T, Shayevitz J, et al: FLACC pain assessment tool: Reliability and validation with existing tools. *Anesthesiology* 1994;81:A1359.

The inter-rater reliability and reproducibility of the FLACC pain assessment tool was demonstrated in this prospective study of 30 children in the postoperative period. In addition, its validity against existing tools (ie, the nurses' global ratings of pain and the objective pain scale) was established.

US Agency for Health Care Policy and Research: *Acute Pain Management: Operative or Medical Procedures and Trauma.* Rockville, MD, US Department of Health and Human Services, 1992 (AHCPR Publication No. 92-0032).

This clinical practice guideline was developed by an interdisciplinary panel of experts in pain management. It outlines the physiologic basis for acute pain, discusses pain assessment techniques, and reviews the literature that links effective pain management with improved patient outcomes. It also describes therapeutic practices and principles and emerging technologies that can minimize or eliminate acute pain.

Pain Management: Systemic Analgesia

Berde CB, Lehn BM, Yee JD, et al: Patient-controlled analgesia in children and adolescents: A randomized, prospective comparison with intramuscular administration of morphine for postoperative analgesia. *J Pediatr* 1991; 18:460–466.

This prospective study evaluates the efficacy, risks, and benefits of intramuscular morphine versus PCA with and without a continuous background infusion in 82 children undergoing orthopaedic surgery. Both PCA techniques provided lower pain scores and were better accepted than intramuscular injections, without increasing morbidity. The PCA group with continuous infusion had lower pain scores than the PCA group alone; however, there were no statistical difference between these groups. Overall, there was greater patient satisfaction with PCA than with intramuscular morphine.

Goodarzi M, Shier NH, Ogden JA: Epidural versus patient-controlled analgesia with morphine for postoperative pain after orthopedic procedures in children. *J Pediatr Orthop* 1993;13:663–667.

In this prospective, randomized study the adequacy of analgesia and the incidence and severity of side effects related to the use of epidural morphine versus PCA were compared in 40 children undergoing orthopaedic surgery. The pain scores were not statistically different in the two groups, but the morphine requirement was significantly greater in the PCA group. There was a higher incidence of drowsiness in the PCA group while the epidural group experienced nonrespiratory side effects, such as nausea, vomiting, pruritus, and urinary retention, more

frequently. Both analgesic techniques produced satisfactory analgesia with no respiratory complications.

Litvak KM, McEvoy GK: Ketorolac, an injectable nonnarcotic analgesic. *Clin Pharm* 1990;9:921–935.

The authors present an extensive review of the clinical studies of the injectable NSAID ketorolac. In addition the chemistry, pharmacology, drug interactions, and adverse effects of ketorolac are described. This article provides useful information regarding the efficacy, potency, and side effects of ketorolac in comparison with those of other NSAIDs, as well as the opioids.

O'Hara DA, Fragen RJ, Kinzer M, et al: Ketorolac tromethamine as compared with morphine sulfate for treatment of postoperative pain. *Clin Pharmacol Ther* 1987;41:556–561.

In this prospective, double blind study, 155 patients were randomly assigned to receive 10, 30, or 90 mg of ketorolac or 6 or 12 mg of morphine intramuscularly for pain relief after abdominal or orthopaedic surgery. Ketorolac 30 and 90 mg provided lower pain scores than morphine 6 mg and pain scores similar to those with morphine 12 mg. Ketorolac had a significantly longer duration of action than either dose of morphine. There were no serious side effects in any of the groups.

Polaner DM, Berde CB: Postoperative pain management, in Cote CJ, Ryan JF, Todres ID, et al (eds): *A Practice of Anesthesia for Infants and Children,* ed 2. Philadelphia, PA, WB Saunders, 1993, pp 451–470.

This detailed chapter on principles and techniques of postoperative pain management in children addresses pain assessment techniques, preoperative preparation, intraoperative anesthetic interventions that enable a patient to awaken free of pain, and pain management strategies, such as patient-controlled analgesia and regional blockade. An appendix of appropriate pain management in different clinical situations is included.

Tyler DC: Pharmacology of pain management. *Pediatr Clin North Am* 1994;41:59–71.

A detailed review of the mechanism of action, pharmacokinetics, and side effects of opioids and nonopioid analgesics is presented. The clinical use of opioids, NSAIDs, and tricyclic depressants is discussed, and expected risks and benefits are substantiated by extensive references.

Woolf CJ, Chong MS: Preemptive analgesia: Treating postoperative pain by preventing the establishment of central sensitization. *Anesth Analg* 1993;77:362–379.

In this extensive review, the concept of preemptive analgesia is introduced and mechanisms of central sensitization are discussed. Clinical trials of preemptive analgesia using difference analgesic interventions are extensively reviewed.

Pain Management: Regional Analgesia

Rice LJ: Regional anesthesia in the pediatric patient. *Intenational Anesthesic Research Society Review Course Lectures.* Cleveland, OH, International Anesthesic Research Society, 1994, pp 32–36.

This is a concise current review of the use of central and peripheral nerve blocks in children. The pharmacology and pharmacokinetics of local anesthetics in children are discussed, and appropriate dosing guidelines are suggested.

Wedel DJ: The pediatric patient: Regional anesthesia, in Wedel DJ (ed): *Orthopedic Anesthesia.* New York, NY, Churchill Livingstone, 1993, pp 129–149.

This chapter reviews the indications, advantages, and disadvantages of regional anesthetic techniques applicable to orthopaedic surgery. The pharmacology and dosing guidelines of local anesthetics are discussed. Practical suggestions for selection of blocks and local anesthetics and safety measures with individual blocks are included.

7

Musculoskeletal Neoplasms

Initial Evaluation

Evaluation of the child with a suspected neoplasm begins with a careful history and physical examination prior to extensive radiographic imaging. Often, clinical details regarding the presentation may rule out or suggest non-neoplastic etiologies, and the practitioner must consider a broad range of possibilities when evaluating the child with a suspected neoplasm.

History

Pain about the extremity is a common feature of both neoplasms and other maladies. Benign neoplasms may be asymptomatic and found incidentally, although this is rarely the case with malignancies. Pain may result from the neoplastic invasion itself, or it may be a consequence of structural weakening. A history of pain that is exacerbated by weightbearing may suggest a pathologic or impending pathologic fracture. Night pain, especially pain that awakens the patient or prevents sleep onset, may suggest a neoplastic etiology. Pain relieved by aspirin is most commonly associated with osteoid osteomas, but may be observed in other types of tumors. Younger children may be unable to report pain per se, and parents may note selective weightbearing on the well extremity or lack of use of the affected limb. Duration of pain and increasing or decreasing intensity may give additional clues as to the source as well; pain related to malignant tumors rarely diminishes without treatment.

Duration of swelling or mass, if any, and any reported growth should be identified. Rapidly enlarging lesions suggest malignancy, although some benign tumors can reach rapid growth rates. Lesions that fluctuate in size, becoming larger or smaller with the passage of time, are more likely to be cystic lesions or hemangiomas. Erythema and warmth are usually nonspecific indicators of increased blood flow to the area, but may also suggest infection or malignancy.

The practitioner must also search carefully for a history of systemic symptoms. Osteomyelitis is frequently in the differential diagnosis of pediatric tumors, and usually is associated with a history of fever, chills, and anorexia. A recent history of antibiotic usage with symptom improvement may indicate the possibility of a partially treated infection. Ewing's sarcoma may be associated with systemic flu-like illness even when apparently localized. Patients with metastatic malignancies may have considerable systemic illness or be relatively asymptomatic. Disseminated histiocytosis may present with constitutional symptoms.

Physical Examination

The physician must perform a careful physical examination of the child, noting both local and general findings. Inspection will identify obvious masses or swelling, as well as more subtle findings, such as skin color alterations seen in hemangiomas in light-skinned individuals. The affected limb should be palpated carefully to ascertain areas of tenderness and to localize maximally tender areas. Size and depth of any masses present should be noted, as well as any apparent involvement of adjacent or underlying structures. Although the majority of pediatric orthopaedic malignancies are spread hematogenously, regional lymph node examination can identify tender nodes in a patient with an infection. Painful range of motion of the affected joint suggests adjacent joint involvement or a possible pathologic fracture.

Radiographic Analysis

Radiographs of the affected area should be obtained in two planes and carefully evaluated. The location in the bone (diaphyseal, metaphyseal, epiphyseal, or a combination of these) should be noted. Eccentric or central placement in the bone should be observed as well. The margins of the lesion should be assessed; benign lesions in children are typically well marginated and usually unmineralized. Lesions that suggest malignancy should promptly be referred to centers specializing in their care, prior to obtaining additional studies or biopsy.

Staging

Correlating the history, physical examination, and the plain film findings, the practitioner usually can formulate a differential diagnosis that contains relatively few items. Occasionally, additional studies may be necessary. Bone scans can detect additional bone lesions with a high degree of sensitivity, and can identify the activity and extent of a lesion. Computed tomography (CT) scans give information about the degree of bone involvement and the presence of intralesional mineralization, which would suggest an osteoblastic or chondroid etiology of the tumor. Magnetic resonance imaging (MRI) is the study of choice for assessing soft-tissue involvement and bone-marrow involvement. Because the imaging of musculoskeletal neoplasms may employ techniques different from those usually used, every effort should be made to obtain additional studies at the center where the child is to be treated.

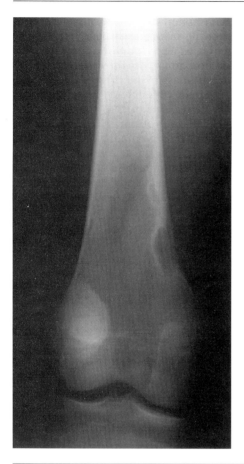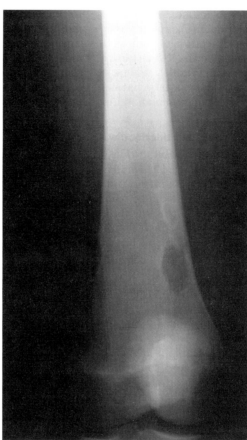

Fig. 1 Left, A classic nonossifying fibroma is seen in this anteroposterior plain radiograph of the distal femur of a 15-year-old previously asymptomatic boy who had suffered a knee sprain. The lesion is well-marginated, eccentric, and scalloped in the femoral metaphysis. **Right,** Slightly oblique view of the same patient demonstrates that nonossifying fibromas seen en face can appear as lytic lesions in the bone.

Patients presenting with bone lesions with the classical appearance of a benign, inactive tumor such as nonossifying fibroma or a fibrous cortical defect can be followed with serial radiographs. Lesions with a high likelihood of malignancy should be evaluated with CT, MRI, or both, a bone scan to detect remote lesions and assess local extent of activity, and a chest radiograph and chest CT to evaluate the possibility of pulmonary metastatic disease.

Patients presenting with large (greater than 5 cm), deep soft-tissue masses are at risk for a diagnosis of malignancy, and should be promptly referred to a musculoskeletal oncologist. Small, clearly subcutaneous masses may not require further imaging; however, larger deep lesions are best seen with an MRI. Preoperative staging of large deep masses may also include a chest radiograph and chest CT to determine whether there is evidence of pulmonary metastatic disease, and a bone scan can detect underlying bone involvement or the presence of remote metastatic disease.

Biopsy

Biopsy of suspected or possibly malignant lesions should be carried out only in centers equipped to perform defini-

tive treatment. Biopsy prior to referral has been demonstrated to result not infrequently in unnecessary amputations or other adverse outcomes in patients with malignancies. Controversy exists over whether open or closed biopsies are optimal. In the limbs, incisions usually should be longitudinally directed and should avoid neurovascular structures. Recommendations around limb girdles may be different.

Benign Bone Tumors

Nonossifying Fibroma/Fibrous Cortical Defect

These lesions are usually asymptomatic and can be found at any age in childhood. They are most frequently found when a child is radiographed following a trauma to rule out a fracture. Most commonly metaphyseal, they may be slightly expansile. They uniformly have a sharp, sclerotic rim, and are often located eccentrically in the bone. Multiple adjacent lesions may be present, or the lesion may appear multilocular. No further investigations are necessary for lesions with the classic appearance; however, they should be observed on serial radiographs in the growing child (Fig. 1). Because of the risk of pathologic fracture,

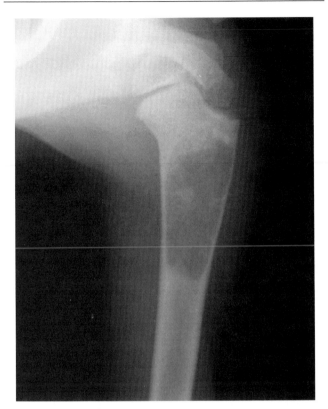

Fig. 2 Unicameral cyst in a 5-year-old boy shows the typical proximal humeral location, with modest expansion of the bone; the width of the lesion does not exceed the width of the adjacent physis.

curettage and bone grafting may be recommended in any lesions that occupy more than 50% of the cortex of a long bone.

Unicameral (Solitary) Bone Cyst

These lesions can occur at any age in the pediatric population. The majority of these tumors are asymptomatic; they most frequently come to medical attention when a pathologic fracture is sustained. Usually an antecedent history of trauma, which may be relatively minor, is followed by acute onset of pain and refusal to move the limb. The most common sites are in the proximal humeral and proximal femoral metaphyses (Fig. 2). Lesions generally appear modestly lytic and expansile, but do not exceed the width of the adjacent physis. The cortex is not broached unless there is fracture present. Lesions appear unilocular or, occasionally, multilocular. Actively growing lesions are found near the physis; latent ones will appear to grow away from the physis and be separated from it by a zone of normal-appearing bone. The etiology of the cyst formation is controversial, but recently bone resorptive factors have been found in the cyst fluid, which is typically clear. Treatment is usually by aspiration followed by injection of methylprednisolone. Fractures occur most commonly

in larger lesions, and healing is occasionally noted after fracture. Large lesions that are refractory to repeated injections may be treated with curettage and bone grafting or bone substitute packing.

Aneurysmal Bone Cyst

Aneurysmal bone cysts (ABCs) may occur at any age in childhood. Lesions most commonly involve the posterior elements of the spine and the long bones of the extremities, but they may occur in any bone. The involved bone typically has an expanded appearance. The lesion may be contained by a thin rim of bone only, or it may extend out beyond the confines of the attenuated cortex, and the appearance may be quite aggressive. Unresolved controversy continues regarding the etiology of the ABC. It may be found in association with other lesions, and some consider it to be a reactive lesion and not a true neoplasm. Treatment consists of curettage and bone grafting, or excision of involved expendable bones such as the fibula or rib. Local recurrence rate is dependent on the site and treatment modality, but in a recent large series was 21%. Aneurysmal bone cysts have been reported to recur more frequently in younger children.

Osteochondroma (Exostosis)

Pediatric patients with osteochondromas usually present with a long history of a mass that may have enlarged gradually. Although osteochondromas are not intrinsically painful, pain may result from pressure or irritation of nearby structures, or, less commonly, from a fracture through the lesion. They appear as exophytic masses usually extending away from the metaphysis of a long bone (Fig. 3). A constant radiographic finding is continuity of the marrow space of the involved bone with the center of the lesion. Osteochondromas have a cartilage cap, which may be quite large in children. Malignant transformation is rarely if ever seen in children, although in adulthood they may rarely transform to low-grade chondrosarcomas. Treatment consists of removal of the symptomatic osteochondroma only; the vast majority can be managed with observation. A small number of patients may have the hereditary multiple form of the disease (hereditary multiple exostoses), in which they have involvement of most of the long bones. Involvement may be mild or severe. Although there was initially reported to be a fairly high life-time risk of conversion to chondrosarcoma in these patients, a recent report suggests the risk is relatively low (1%). Associated deformities include short stature and limb length inequality. The forearm and the knee are most commonly affected with greatest severity.

Eosinophilic Granuloma (Histiocytosis X)

Eosinophilic granuloma appears as a lytic lesion in the bone of a child of nearly any age. The skull is most commonly affected, but any bone may be involved. Lesions are generally painful and there may be swelling of the overlying tissues. Although the lesion may present as an isolated

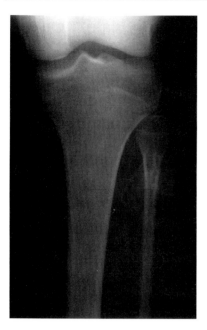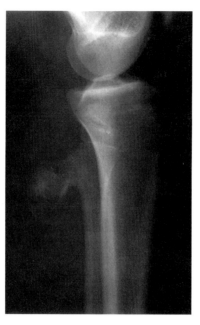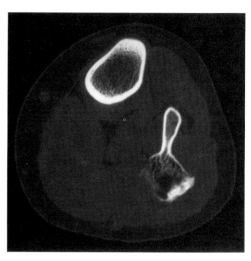

Fig. 3 Plain radiographs of the proximal fibula of a 15-year-old girl presenting with a painless, firm, lateral leg mass. **Left,** Anteroposterior view shows a well-marginated osseous lesion superimposed on the proximal fibula, but the lateral view **(center)** shows continuity of the medullary cavity of the long bone with the center of the lesion. **Right,** Computed tomography shows the medullary space in continuity with the lesion, and a small cartilage cap, both of which are characteristic of an exostosis.

bone lesion, systemic involvement is not infrequent and severity is usually greater in younger children. Bone lesions generally appear lytic, but the appearance is quite variable and hence eosinophilic granuloma frequently must be considered in the differential diagnosis of bone lesions in children. Systemic and visceral involvement may include a wide variety of manifestations, and children with a documented bone lesion should be referred to rule out other organ involvement.

Treatment has involved a wide variety of modalities in the past, including curettage and bone grafting and steroid injection. A recent report indicated that, because most osseous lesions heal spontaneously, intervention should be limited to symptomatic or easily accessible lesions.

Fibrous Dysplasia

Lesions from fibrous dysplasia are frequently asymptomatic, and may be found at any age in the pediatric population. Common sites include the skull, ribs, and long bones. The lesions have a characteristic "ground glass" appearance on radiographs owing to the intralesional woven bone formation that is seen histologically. Lesions are often surrounded by a thick sclerotic margin, and are commonly metaphyseal or diaphyseal. Although the majority of cases can be observed, bone deformity or pain (particularly involving the proximal portion of the femur) can occur, which may necessitate curettage and bone grafting,

surgical stabilization, or resection. Degeneration to malignancy is extremely rare, and, when it occurs, is often associated with radiation treatment of the lesion.

Chondroblastoma

Chondroblastoma is a rare tumor that most commonly presents as a painful lesion in the epiphysis or apophysis of a skeletally immature patient. Calcification within the matrix of the lesion is occasionally visible on plain films. When possible, curettage and bone grafting can be performed, although proximity to a joint or pathologic fracture may sometimes necessitate a more involved procedure.

Enchondroma

Enchondromas, generally asymptomatic intramedullary lesions, may occur in the metaphysis or diaphysis of a long bone, and are frequently seen in the bones of the hand. In adults they usually have punctate calcifications, but in children calcification may not be evident and the enchondroma may have the appearance of a unicameral bone cyst. The majority of enchondromas can be treated with observation. Multifocal lesions (Ollier's disease) often lead to lower limb length inequalities. Rare large or symptomatic lesions predisposed to fracture may be treated with curettage and bone grafting following healing of fracture if present.

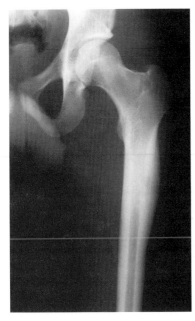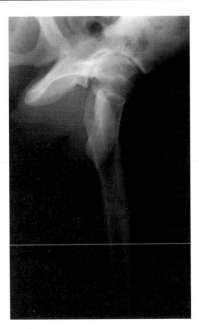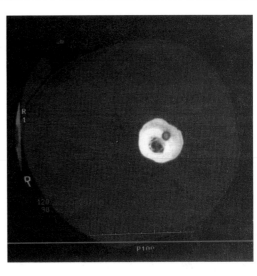

Fig. 4 **Left** and **center,** Radiographs of the proximal femur show an osteoid osteoma. Within a dense, sclerotic cortex of the lateral femur lies a small lucency. **Right,** Computed tomography shows that the small intracortical lucency actually contains a small nidus of mineralization.

Chondromyxoid Fibroma

Children with chondromyxoid fibroma usually present with pain and possibly swelling about the affected area. Radiographs show a well-marginated, usually eccentrically placed, lesion, which is most frequently located in the diaphysis of a long bone, often the proximal tibia. The lesion most commonly confused with a chondromyxoid fibroma is a nonossifying fibroma. The tumor responds to curettage and bone grafting, but en bloc resection may also be considered, if possible, because of the potential for local recurrence.

Osteoid Osteoma

Osteoid osteomas present as painful bone lesions, often with overlying soft-tissue swelling, in children of any age. Lesions may occur in nearly any bone, but commonly occur in the metaphysis or diaphysis of a long bone (Fig. 4). Classically, pain is worse at night and is relieved by aspirin, but this history may not be elicited. Radiographs characteristically show a dense, sclerotic cortex, within which lies a small lucency or nidus. CT may be necessary to show the central nidus.

Until recently, effective treatment consisted of en bloc resection of the tumor. Recently, some investigators have reported success with medical management of the tumor with anti-inflammatory medications; a high level of prostaglandins has been found in the central portion of the osteoid osteoma, and this may account for the success of medical treatment. Localization and removal of the central nidus at surgery is mandatory to obtain symptom relief, and techniques have been described using CT or bone scan localization to facilitate this. As an alternative to en bloc excision, a burr-down technique may be used to reduce operative morbidity. Very young patients with osteoid osteoma may be misdiagnosed because of inconclusive initial radiographs.

Osteoblastoma

Patients with osteoblastoma generally present with pain, usually in the dorsal elements of the spine. Radiographic appearance varies and may be similar to that of an osteoid osteoma or may be lytic. Treatment usually consists of curettage and bone grafting or en bloc resection. Spinal locations may require bone grafting or other measures for stabilization.

Malignant Bone Tumors

Ewing's Sarcoma

Ewing's sarcoma generally presents in children with pain about the diaphyses and metaphyses of long bones, as well as arising from flat bones such as the pelvis or scapula. Patients with Ewing's sarcoma typically have increasing pain about the affected bone, and may have soft-tissue swelling. Systemic symptoms of weight loss, fever, or malaise may be present even in the absence of detectable metastatic disease. Radiographs typically show an aggressive, permeative pattern, which may be confused with infection. A large soft-tissue mass is often seen adjacent to the bone as well (Fig. 5).

While Ewing's sarcoma previously carried a dismal prognosis, contemporary chemotherapy has markedly improved the survival rate, particularly in patients without metastatic disease at presentation. Chemotherapy regimens for Ewing's now include multiple agents. Hematopoietic and leukocyte growth factors, as well as antiemetics, have allowed for significant dose escalations and less toxicity when compared with drug regimens in the past.

With improved survival of patients with Ewing's, issues of local control have become more important. Additional concerns have been raised with the use of radiation, as increasing numbers of secondary malignancies are identified in Ewing's survivors. Although a randomized, prospective study of radiation versus surgery is lacking, several recent reports have identified slightly improved local control with surgery, and surgery is now advocated for accessible lesions, particularly in expendable bones.

Osteosarcoma

Osteosarcoma classically occurs in the metaphyses of long bones, particularly about the knee and in the proximal humerus. Patients usually present with gradually increasing pain and occasionally with pathologic fracture. Radiologically, these poorly marginated lesions demonstrate blastic areas, although they may on occasion be purely lytic.

The five-year survival rate for patients with conventional osteosarcoma undergoing standard therapy regimens is about 70%. Treatment usually involves a combination of chemotherapy and surgery. Improved adjuvant therapy has allowed for more limb-sparing surgery, and the majority of patients receive neoadjuvant or preoperative chemotherapy followed by limb-sparing surgery. In a recent retrospective multi-institutional study, there was no difference in survival rates in patients undergoing limb salvage versus amputation for osteosarcomas of the distal femur, although patients who had limb salvage had a higher reoperation rate.

A high rate of tumor necrosis following preoperative chemotherapy has been associated with a better prognosis and new imaging modalities such as MRI and thallium scanning are being explored for their accuracy in predicting histologic tumor response.

Parosteal osteosarcomas are a rare, low-grade variant of osteosarcoma, which occurs most frequently in the posterior distal femur. Because the radiologic appearance is usually diagnostic, biopsy of the lesion is rarely indicated, and may compromise further limb-sparing treatment. Chemotherapy is not indicated, and the prognosis is more favorable than for conventional osteosarcoma.

Leukemia

Leukemia may present as a painful bone lesions in children, and the radiographic appearance is quite variable.

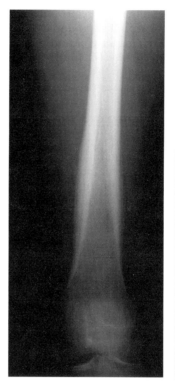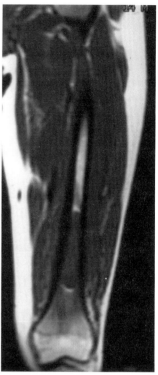
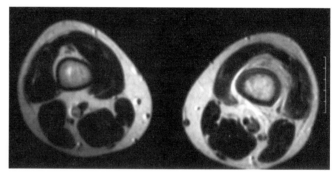

Fig. 5 A 15-year-old boy presented with pain in the femur of 6 months duration. **Top left,** Plain anteroposterior radiograph shows classic onion-skin periosteal reaction of the distal femoral diaphysis. **Top right,** T1-weighted coronal magnetic resonance image of the thighs clearly outlines the extent of marrow abnormality. **Bottom,** T2-weighted axial magnetic resonance image shows soft-tissue mass and edema adjacent to the bone. Biopsy confirmed Ewing's sarcoma.

Diagnosis usually can be made on peripheral blood smears, and surgery is rarely indicated. Bone lesions generally respond to systemic therapy. Because of the wide variety of presentations, a high index of suspicion for this diagnosis should be maintained when evaluating children with bone lesions.

Limb Salvage in the Skeletally Immature

Major advances in the medical management of malignant bone tumors in children have allowed limb salvage to be performed with increased frequency. Reconstruction in the skeletally immature patient presents additional difficulties, including the need to accommodate future growth and the small size of the patient.

A standardized functional evaluation system has been widely used to allow comparisons between different types of salvages. In general, options for limb salvage include endoprostheses, large segment allografts, autografts, and rotationplasty. Expandable prostheses can accommodate growth, are available in essentially limitless quantities, and can be customized. However, they have been reported to have a high rate of expansion failure and a high revision rate. Allografts may provide better options for soft-tissue reattachment, but allograft-related complications include infection, nonunion, and fracture. The Van Ness rotationplasty offers the option of converting an above-knee amputation into a more functional amputation stump, but complications include fracture, wound problems, and vascular occlusion. Psychosocial adjustment has been reported to be good, but patient and families may choose other alternatives because of the appearance of the stump.

Benign Soft-Tissue Tumors

Intramuscular hemangiomas may present as soft-tissue masses with minimal overlying skin abnormality. Controversy exists as to whether these lesions are actual benign neoplasms or are a response to trauma. Plain radiographs are usually normal but may show phleboliths and soft-

tissue mass. Arteriography, particularly in conjunction with CT, may be helpful in determining the diagnosis, and MRI can show the extent of the lesion. Simple removal may be carried out for accessible lesions. Eradication of diffuse lesions may be quite difficult. Treatment options include sclerosing therapy and surgical excision; radiation has been suggested by some investigators.

Malignant Soft-Tissue Tumors

Rhabdomyosarcoma

Rhabdomyosarcoma is the most common type of malignant soft-tissue tumor in children. Presentation is generally that of a mass, although symptoms vary according to location of the lesion. While rhabdomyosarcomas of the head and neck and genitourinary sites tends to occur in young children, extremity rhabdomyosarcoma is most often diagnosed in adolescents. Treatment of these tumors involves a multimodality approach, involving surgery, chemotherapy, and radiation.

Synovial Sarcoma

Synovial sarcomas usually present as slow-growing soft-tissue masses. Masses about the lower extremities may initially be confused with benign processes. About a third of synovial sarcomas will show the classic speckled soft-tissue calcification within the mass. Diagnosis can be made by either needle or open biopsy. Treatment of these lesions may involve a combination of chemotherapy, surgery, and radiation. Even lesions that are relatively small at diagnosis present a significant risk for metastatic disease.

Annotated Bibliography

Staging

Simon MA, Finn HA: Diagnostic strategy for bone and soft-tissue tumors. *J Bone Joint Surg* 1993;75A:622–631.

The importance of a systematic evaluation of both bone and soft-tissue tumors is described, and a outline given. Emphasis is on initial evaluation of plain films and patient presentation as a guide to further workup strategy.

Biopsy

Simon MA, Biermann JS: Biopsy of bone and soft-tissue lesions. *J Bone Joint Surg* 1993;75A:616–621.

General considerations regarding the biopsy of musculoskeletal tumors are reviewed. The importance of prebiopsy evaluation and staging as well as appropriate prebiopsy referral are stressed. Biopsy incision placement, considerations regarding open versus closed biopsy, and biopsy techniques are addressed.

Benign Bone Tumors

Ahn JI, Park JS: Pathologic fractures secondary to unicameral bone cysts. *Int Orthop* 1994;18:20–22.

Seventy-five children who had unicameral bone cysts and who had sustained 52 pathologic fractures were reviewed retrospectively. In all cases of fracture, the percentage of bone occupied by the cysts was more than 85% on both anteroposterior (AP) and lateral radiographs. In most cases the cysts recurred after fracture.

Burgess RC, Cates H: Deformities of the forearm in patients who have multiple cartilaginous exostosis. *J Bone Joint Surg* 1993;75A:13–18.

AP and lateral radiographs of 35 children with multiple cartilaginous exostoses were evaluated. The authors found proportional shortening of the radius and ulna, contradicting the previously widely held theory regarding ulna tethering as the etiology of wrist deformity. However, large negative ulnar variance was predictive of subsequent radial head dislocation.

Campanacci M, Capanna R, Picci P: Unicameral and aneurysmal bone cysts. *Clin Orthop* 1986;204:25–36.

One hundred and seventy-eight cases of unicameral bone cysts treated with curettage and bone grafting were compared to 141 cases treated with cortisone injections and found to have comparable end results. Follow-up was available for 166 cases of ABC; 91 were treated with curettage and bone grafting, the treatment of choice, with a local recurrence rate of 21%. Radiotherapy was used in 23 patients with a 22% recurrence rate.

Freiberg AA, Loder RT, Heidelberger KP, et al: Aneurysmal bone cysts in young children. *J Pediatr Orthop* 1994;14:86–91.

Seven patients, all under the age of 11, with aneurysmal bone cysts were reviewed. Local recurrences occurred following curettage and bone grafting in five of seven children (71%) at an average of 8 months from the first procedure.

Inoue O, Ibaraki K, Shimabukuro H, et al: Packing with high-porosity hydroxyapatite cubes alone for the treatment of simple bone cyst. *Clin Orthop* 1993;293:287–292.

Twenty-three patients with simple bone cysts were treated with curettage, followed by packing with cubes of high-porosity hydroxyapatite. Complete healing without cyst recurrence occurred in 18 cases (78%); two cases showed incomplete healing without recurrence.

Kaweblum M, Lehman WB, Bash J, et al: Osteoid osteoma under the age of five years: The difficulty of diagnosis. *Clin Orthop* 1993;296:218–224.

Seven patients under the age of five with an osteoid osteoma are reviewed. Most were misdiagnosed, because other concomitant signs and symptoms attracted more attention and led to unnecessary invasive procedures. Pain and gait disturbance were the most frequent presentations. In five of seven cases, initial radiographs were not conclusive. Bone scan and CT are additional helpful studies.

Kneisl JS, Simon MA: Medical management compared with operative treatment for osteoid-osteoma. *J Bone Joint Surg* 1992;74A:179–185.

Twenty four patients with osteoid osteoma were evaluated. Twelve patients treated initially with an operation had complete relief of pain. Twelve patients were treated initially with medical management consisting of nonsteroidal anti-inflammatory agents; of these, nine were successfully managed medically, and three subsequently requested surgical intervention, which gave complete symptom relief.

Komiya S, Minamitani K, Sasaguri Y, et al: Simple bone cyst: Treatment by trepanation and studies on bone resorptive factors in cyst fluid with a theory of its pathogenesis. *Clin Orthop* 1993;287:204–211.

Eleven patients with simple bone cysts were treated with saline perfusion with a two-trocar technique followed by trepanation, and all patients had good or excellent results. Bone resorptive factors were found in the cyst fluid.

Lee DH, Malawer MM: Staging and treatment of primary and persistent (recurrent) osteoid osteoma: Evaluation of intraoperative nuclear scanning, tetracycline fluorescence, and tomography. *Clin Orthop* 1992;281:229–238.

Fourteen patients were treated surgically for osteoid osteoma using the technique of IONS (intraoperative nuclear scanning), with 13 of the 14 cured with one surgical procedure.

Ruggieri P, Sim FH, Bond JR, et al: Malignancies in fibrous dysplasia. *Cancer* 1994:73:1411–1424.

Eight cases of sarcoma were found in 1,122 cases of fibrous dysplasia in a retrospective review of cases at the Mayo Clinic. Thirteen (46%) had received radiation therapy before the sarcoma developed. Although malignancy in fibrous dysplasia is rare, prognosis is poor.

Schmale GA, Conrad EU III, Raskind WH: The natural history of hereditary multiple exostoses. *J Bone Joint Surg* 1994;76A:986–992.

A retrospective review of patients and family members from a database of hereditary multiple exostoses in the state of Washington was carried out, including 113 affected individuals. Penetrance of the autosomal dominant gene was noted to be 96%. Thirty-nine percent of subjects had forearm deformities, 10% had limb-length inequalities, and 8% had knee deformity. Malignant transformation to chondrosarcoma had been detected in 1 (0.9%) patient.

Sessa S, Sommelet D, Lascombes P, et al: Treatment of Langerhans-cell histiocytosis in children: Experience at the Children's Hospital of Nancy. *J Bone Joint Surg* 1994;76A:1513–1525.

This is a retrospective study of 40 children with Langerhans-cell histiocytosis. Despite varying treatment methodologies, good results were ultimately obtained in all 30 children with disease localized to the bone. Nine of the 30 did have a disease recurrence within 4 years of initial treatment, which was successfully managed. Two of ten patients with multifocal disease died. Because of the frequent tendency of osseous lesions to heal spontaneously, the role of the orthopaedic surgeon should remain limited to symptomatic or easily accessible lesions.

Ward WG, Eckardt JJ, Shayestehfar S, et al: Osteoid osteoma diagnosis and management with low morbidity. *Clin Orthop* 1993;291:229–235.

Fifteen patients with osteoid osteoma were treated with a burr-down technique, in which careful preoperative localization with CT scans allowed for removal of the lesion by a high-speed burr instead of the more traditional en bloc resection. When compared to en bloc resection, the burr-down technique was associated with less postoperative immobilization, earlier weightbearing, and an earlier return to activity.

Malignant Bone Tumors

Bechler JR, Robertson WW Jr, Meadows AT, et al: Osteosarcoma as a second malignant neoplasm in children. *J Bone Joint Surg* 1992;74A:1079–1083.

Nine patients were treated for osteosarcoma developing in a previously radiated site. There was only one long-term survivor. Plans for tumor therapy should take into account the risk of post-radiation sarcomas, which usually are fatal.

Frassica FJ, Frassica DA, Pritchard DJ, et al: Ewing sarcoma of the pelvis: Clinicopathological features and treatment. *J Bone Joint Surg* 1993;75A:1457–1465.

Twenty-seven patients with Ewing's sarcoma of the pelvis treated over a 16-year time period were reviewed. There were no long-term survivors among the six patients who presented with metastatic disease. For patients with localized disease at presentation, five year survival was 45%; although the groups were not randomized, there was a lower survival rate in those patients treated with radiation for local control compared to those treated with surgery.

Glasser DB, Lane JM, Huvos AG, et al: Survival, prognosis, and therapeutic response in osteogenic sarcoma: The Memorial Hospital experience. *Cancer* 1992;69:698–708.

Two hundred and seventy-nine patients with Stage II osteogenic sarcoma of the appendicular skeleton were studied retrospectively. Five- and 10-year disease-free survival was 70% and 69% respectively. Histologic response to chemotherapy was the most important predictor for survival. Local control may be more difficult to achieve in some locations, particularly the proximal femur.

Marina NM, Pratt CB, Rao BN, et al: Improved prognosis of children with osteosarcoma metastatic to the lung(s) at the time of diagnosis. *Cancer* 1992;70:2722–2727.

Thirty-one patients who had metastatic osteosarcoma to the lungs at the time of diagnosis at the St. Jude Children's Research Hospital were identified over a 29-year time period. While there were no survivors among patients treated prior to 1982, there was a 30% 4-year survival rate for those patients treated subsequently.

Maygarden SJ, Askin FB, Siegal GP, et al: Ewing sarcoma of bone in infants and toddlers: A clinicopathologic report from the Intergroup Ewing's Study. *Cancer* 1993;71:2109–2118.

Nineteen patients with Ewing's sarcoma, who were younger than 3 years of age at the time of diagnosis, were identified. Although there was an unusual preponderance of female patients in this group, overall survival rate was comparable to survival rates of older children.

Menendez LR, Fideler BM, Mirra J: Thallium–201 scanning for the evaluation of osteosarcoma and soft-tissue sarcoma: A study of the evaluation and predictability of the histological response to chemotherapy. *J Bone Joint Surg* 1993;75A:526–531.

Sixteen patients had sequential thallium scans prior to and after preoperative chemotherapy, and scan results were compared to degree of necrosis at resection. Nine of ten patients with reduced thallium uptake after chemotherapy had tumor necrosis of at least 95%, and six patients with unchanged thallium scans had necrosis less than 95%. The authors propose that thallium scintigraphy is useful in predicting histologic response of high-grade osteosarcomas and soft-tissue sarcomas to preoperative chemotherapy.

Okada K, Frassica FJ, Sim FH, et al: Parosteal osteosarcoma. A clinicopathological study. *J Bone Joint Surg* 1994;76A:366–378.

Records of 226 patients with parosteal osteosarcoma were reviewed. Clinical follow-up was available for 67 patients treated at the Mayo Clinic, and data from 159 patients identified from consultation files was included. Five- and 10-year survival were 91% and 80% respectively. Of the tumors, 16% had undergone dedifferentiation, and 46% had invasion of adjacent soft tissue. Incomplete resection was associated with an increased risk of local recurrence, and dedifferentiation markedly increased the risk of metastases.

Rogalsky RJ, Black GB, Reed MH: Orthopaedic manifestations of leukemia in children. *J Bone Joint Surg* 1986;68A:494–501.

Of 107 patients under the age of 18 who had leukemia, 44% had radiographic abnormalities, which included osteopenia, lytic lesions, metaphyseal bands, periosteal new bone, and sclerotic lesions. Because bone pain is a common presenting symptom, and radiographic abnormalities are variable, a high index of suspicion for leukemia must be maintained when evaluating children with bone lesions.

Rougraff BT, Simon MA, Kneisl JS, et al: Limb salvage compared with amputation for osteosarcoma of the distal end of the femur: A long-term oncological, functional, and quality-of-life study. *J Bone Joint Surg* 1994;76A:649–656.

The outcome of treatment of non-metastatic high-grade osteosarcoma in the distal femur including 227 patients from 27 institutions, was reviewed. The authors found no difference in long-term survival or quality of life between patients treated with limb salvage versus amputation. Patients treated with limb salvage had a higher rate of reoperation but a better functional outcome.

Ruggieri P, De Cristofaro R, Picci P, et al: Complications and surgical indications in 144 cases of nonmetastatic osteosarcoma of the extremities treated with neoadjuvant chemotherapy. *Clin Orthop* 1993;295:226–238.

One hundred and forty-four patients with osteosarcoma of the extremities were treated with combined surgery and neoadjuvant chemotherapy, with a disease-free 5-year survival rate of 79% for good chemotherapy responders and 72% for nonresponders. Complications were frequent but usually manageable, and were more common in the limb salvage group.

Smith LM, Cox RS, Donaldson SS: Second cancers in long-term survivors of Ewing's sarcoma. *Clin Orthop* 1992;274:275–281.

Two of 25 Ewing's survivors treated with chemotherapy and irradiation developed secondary malignancies (one osteosarcoma, one acute myelogenous leukemia) at a median follow-up period of 7.6 years.

Toni A, Neff JR, Sudanese A, et al: The role of surgical therapy in patients with nonmetastatic Ewing's Sarcoma of the limbs. *Clin Orthop* 1993;286:225–240.

This is a retrospective review of 131 nonrandomized patients with primary Ewing's sarcoma in extremity locations, who were treated with chemotherapy, as well as surgery, radiation, or both. Although chemotherapy and radiation protocols changed over the time period in which patients were evaluated, patients treated with surgery more often had disease-free survival than those managed by radiation therapy alone.

Yasko AW, Lane JM: Chemotherapy for bone and soft-tissue sarcomas of the extremities. *J Bone Joint Surg* 1991;73A:1263–1271.

The effectiveness of adjuvant and neoadjuvant chemotherapy in osteosarcoma, Ewing's sarcoma and childhood rhabdomyosarcoma is well established, and has led to significantly improved survival rates for these diseases.

Limb Salvage in the Skeletally Immature

Buck BE, Malinin TI: Human bone and tissue allografts: Preparation and safety. *Clin Orthop* 1994;303:8–17.

The desire to safeguard against disease spread with allografts has led to current improvements in bone banking, which include intensive donor screening, application of sensitive tests for HIV and hepatitis, and a high discard rate for questionable grafts after harvest.

Eckardt JJ, Safran MR, Eilber FR, et al: Expandable endoprosthetic reconstruction of the skeletally immature after malignant bone tumor resection. *Clin Orthop* 1993;297:188–202.

Twelve skeletally immature patients with primary malignant bone tumors underwent extremity reconstruction with cemented custom-expandable endoprostheses. Seven patients have undergone a total of 11 expansions, and two patients required revision. Despite a high rate of expansion mechanism failure, expandable prostheses offer an alternative to amputation or rotationplasty.

Enneking WF, Dunham W, Gebhardt MC, et al: A system for the functional evaluation of reconstructive procedures after surgical treatment of tumors of the musculoskeletal system. *Clin Orthop* 1993;286:241–246.

A field-tested functional evaluation system for patients undergoing surgery for the treatment of musculoskeletal tumors is presented in order to standardize the reporting of results among investigators. Various indicators are on a five-point scale, and emphasis is on pain, function, and emotional acceptance. Lower extremity parameters include gait, need for supports, and walking ability, while upper extremity considerations are hand positioning and lifting ability.

Gottsauner-Wolf F, Kotz R, Knahr K, et al: Rotationplasty for limb salvage in the treatment of malignant tumors at the knee: A follow-up study of seventy patients. *J Bone Joint Surg* 1991;73A:1365–1375.

Seventy patients who had rotationplasties performed for malignant tumors about the knee were reviewed, and all 48 survivors were examined. Complications included vascular occlusion (10%), wound healing problems (11%), and transient or permanent nerve palsy. Late complications included fractures (11%), infection, and delayed union. More than half of the patients did not have complications related to the procedure. Patient acceptance of the procedure and psychosocial adjustment was good.

Steenhoff JR, Daanen HA, Taminiau AH: Functional analysis of patients who have had a modified Van Ness rotationplasty. *J Bone Joint Surg* 1993;75A:1451–1456.

Electromyographic analysis of gait in eight patients who had undergone Van Ness rotationplasty showed that 68% and 71%, respectively, of the strength of the ankle dorsiflexors and plantarflexors was retained following rotationplasty. Extension torque is nearly as good as that of the quadriceps on the normal side.

Thompson RC Jr, Pickvance EA, Garry D: Fractures in large-segment allografts. *J Bone Joint Surg* 1993;75A: 1663–1673.

Sixteen of 35 large-segment allografts implanted following resection of tumors were fractured at an average of 26 months following surgery. Multivariate analysis showed an increased risk of fracture for patients with graft fixation devices that penetrated the cortices of the graft and who were on chemotherapy.

Malignant Soft-Tissue Tumors

Hays DM: Rhabdomyosarcoma. *Clin Orthop* 1993;289: 36–49.

This comprehensive review article outlines the tremendous improvement in survival rates with contemporary chemotherapy regimens for rhabdomyosarcoma, the most common soft tissue malignancy of childhood.

8

Myelomeningocele

Spina bifida is a general term used to describe a broad spectrum of defects that occur during formation of the neural tube. Other commonly used terms are myelodysplasia and spinal dysraphism. Spina bifida occulta, a localized defect in formation of the vertebral arch, is present in 10% of normal adult spines. It is generally asymptomatic with no abnormalities of the meninges or spinal cord. Spina bifida cystica describes defects in which the meninges and spinal cord are involved. Myelocele, meningocele, myelomeningocele, and rachischisis are the four defects that make up this group. Together, they account for 55% of all neural tube defects. Anencephaly accounts for another 35% to 45% of defects and encephaloceles, 7%. Because it is rare for children with anencephaly to survive beyond birth, the majority of children who will be seen by the orthopaedist will have one of the forms of spina bifida cystica or an encephalocele. Ninety percent of these children will have myelomeningocele (MMC). It is on this group of children that the rest of this review will focus.

Most defects are now thought to result from a primary failure of closure of the neural tube rather than a reopening of the tube after closure. It is believed that closure of the neural tube is initiated at four separate sites, with each site being controlled by a different gene. Neural tube defects appear to be multifactorial, with environmental factors interacting with polygenic predisposition. Maternal hyperthermia, administration of valproic acid, maternal insulin-dependent diabetes, and folate deficiency are examples of environmental factors that have been associated with myelodysplasia. Each of these has an association with a different type of neural tube defect. The incidence of neural tube defects in the United States has been estimated to be 1 in 1,000 live births, but this number has been decreasing over the last few decades. Screening programs using maternal alphafetoprotein, ultrasound, and amniocentesis for amniotic alphafetoprotein and cholinesterase can now detect virtually all fetuses with open spina bifida by 18 weeks gestation. Periconceptual administration of folate has been shown to be effective in reducing the incidence of neural tube defects in several studies.

Natural History

Life Span and Function

Children who are born with MMC and who do not receive treatment have a less than 10% survival rate to school age. Selective treatment of infants as suggested by Lorber in 1972 has given way to nonselective closure and shunting in most Western societies. With nonselective early closure of the sac and shunting of the hydrocephalus, the survival rate at 25 years is 52%. Early deaths are generally due to central nervous system (CNS) infection or cardiorespiratory problems. The main causes of late death have been hydrocephalus, CNS infections, and renal failure. Better methods of managing these complications over the last 15 years is likely to improve long-term survival.

Adults with MMC can lead very full lives. Many will marry, have children, and be able to hold productive jobs. A survey of adults with spina bifida showed that two thirds listed themselves as independent, however, only 25% reported having a job. Thirty-nine percent were married or lived alone. Sixty-one percent lived with friends, family, or had chore services to assist them. Twenty-seven percent of women had had children. Recent emphasis on educational mainstreaming and intellectual development may alter these employment and functional statistics over time. Studies of adults with acquired and congenital paralytic conditions have shown that communication skills, self-help skills, and mobility are important factors in achieving independence. Ambulation ranks low in importance as a skill necessary for independent living.

Ambulation

There is no true natural history study of ambulatory function for children with MMC. All reported long-term series involve children who have undergone multiple interventions to enhance walking ability. Despite this, there are several consistent findings among these series. A high percentage of children with all levels of dysfunction will be able to achieve some functional ambulation by age 5 with the use of orthoses. The level of neurologic dysfunction is the best predictor of long-term ambulatory status. Few, if any, children with thoracic or high lumbar level involvement will be community ambulators as adults. Children who do not achieve ambulation by age 5 to 6 are unlikely to gain this ability with further efforts. Ambulatory function in children with midlumbar and sacral level involvement declines with long-term follow-up. Seventy-five percent of those with L3-L4 level involvement will be community ambulators at 15 to 20 years, but as few as 20% may still be community ambulators by 25 years. Of patients with sacral level lesions, 90% to 100% will be community ambulators at 15 years, but up to 30% of these patients may lose this ability by 30 years. The implication is that MMC is not a static disease, but is one in which there may be a slow, but relentless, deterioration of function over time. It is against this backdrop that orthopaedic surgeons must view their considerations for intervention.

Nonorthopaedic Considerations Before Treatment

There are many physical and societal factors that can greatly influence surgical outcome in patients with spina bifida. These factors make assessment of the effects of orthopaedic procedures extremely difficult to measure. No prospective controlled study of any surgical procedure in MMC has ever been performed. This makes the treatment of patients with MMC highly individualized. The surgeon must therefore consider many factors before undertaking surgical intervention. Orthopaedic training is generally not sufficient to assess many of these variables, which is why multidisciplinary teams exist in many centers for the care of patients with MMC.

Central Nervous System and Cognition

Of patients with MMC, 70% to 85% will have hydrocephalus and require shunting of cerebrospinal fluid (CSF). Of these, 70% to 80% will have IQs above 80 and 20% to 30% will be mentally disabled with IQs below 80. The verbal skills of these children can be quite good, but their perceptual scores will be low resulting in a social verbal child with poor performance in cognitive function and limited ability to participate in rehabilitation programs. Children who do not require shunting will have normal intelligence. CSF shunt technology has improved greatly in recent years, but the devices are still prone to malfunction. Most shunts work through a gravity flow system. In younger children and in postoperative patients, shunt malfunction may occur secondary to being in a recumbent position. Acute malfunction in the younger child will generally manifest with signs of increased intracranial pressure, but in the older child more subtle signs such as increased irritability, decreased attention span, headaches, worsening motor function, or progressive scoliosis may be present.

Three other major CNS problems may develop in children with MMC. The first is a hydromyelia (syringomyelia) of the spinal cord. Hydromyelic cavities have been found in up to 54% of the spinal cords of patients with MMC. The presumed mechanism is that fluid from an increasing hydrocephalus enters the central canal via the fourth ventricle. The fluid causes pressure and dilatation, with gradual expansion of the canal. In children with a functioning shunt, the mechanism is thought to involve a secondary block of the aqueduct. The child may manifest with increasing spasticity, weakness of the upper extremities, back pain, or worsening spinal deformity. Treatment recommendations have varied between centers. They include: ventriculoperitoneal shunt placement or revision, posterior fossa decompression with or without plugging of the obex, and direct shunting of the cavity.

The second CNS problem of concern is Arnold-Chiari malformations. These are displacements of the hind brain into the foramen magnum. There are three recognized types. In type I, the cerebellum is displaced, but the brainstem is spared. Headaches, lower extremity spasticity, and upper extremity pain may be the presenting symptoms in adolescence. In type II, the brainstem is displaced, and hydrocephalus is common. Apneic episodes, difficulty with feeding, and progressive respiratory insufficiency may occur in infancy. It has been estimated that up to 90% of children with MMC will have this malformation. Type III malformations involve an encephalocele at the craniocervical junction. Management of Chiari malformations is controversial. Occipital decompression has been advocated, but improvement in neurologic function has not been predictable.

The third major CNS finding in children with MMC is that of tethered spinal cord. Neural tube defects communicate with the overlying ectoderm at birth, resulting in a tether that prevents the normal migration cephalad of the spinal cord in the spinal canal during development. Thus, all children with MMC have a tethered cord at birth. With closure of the defect in the early perinatal period, the spinal cord is allowed to fall back within the canal, but rapidly scars to the overlying tissues. Virtually all children with MMC can be demonstrated with MRI to have a "tethered spinal cord," but neurologic changes or symptoms from the tethering occur in only 15% to 20% of patients. Progressive scoliosis, increasing spasticity, progressive weakness, back pain, hip pain, worsening foot deformity, and alterations in bowel and bladder function have all been associated with the presence of a tethered spinal cord. The exact mechanism by which the tethering causes symptoms is as yet unknown. Animal studies have shown that traction on cat spinal cords creates an increased susceptibility to hypoxia and extrinsic compression suggesting that repetitive movement stress on an adherent spinal cord leads to a reduction in circulation and neurologic deterioration. Unfortunately, the deterioration is often insidious and return of function after release of the cord is unpredictable. Serial somatosensory-evoked potential (SSEP) changes have been shown to correlate with neurologic changes and have been suggested as a means by which to detect evolving changes early and prevent serious loss of motor function. This method may hold some promise for future investigational studies.

Latex Allergy and Anesthesia Considerations

Much attention has recently been focused on latex reactions in children with MMC. The spectrum of reactions reported has ranged from urticaria and bronchospasm to anaphylactic shock and death. This hypersensitivity is IgE mediated. Both skin testing and use of a radioallergosorbent (RAST) test have been used to screen patients. In adult controls, the incidence of latex sensitivity is 1%; in operating room personnel it is 7.5%. Using the RAST test, the incidence of latex allergy in children with MMC has been found to range from 18% to 40%. It was found in one series to be 89% sensitive for patients who were known to have a history of hypersensitivity, but missed the one patient who did experience perioperative anaphylaxis. In another series, which used skin tests, 65% of the patients were positive. Most importantly, half of patients whose skin test was positive had no history of prior reaction to latex products. Proponents of the skin test point out that the RAST test is less sensitive than skin testing in the diagnosis of life-threatening anaphylactic states. Most recently, there has been testing of an IgE assay which uses flow cytometry and quantifies the level of IgE to latex. This method has been shown to be highly sensitive and specific. The factors that lead to a high rate of sensitivity to latex in the MMC population are unknown. Multiple exposures in early life from numerous surgical procedures and latex catheters have been postulated to be a major factor in developing a latex allergy. The risk factors that will trigger a systemic anaphylactic response in a child with a documented sensitivity are unknown. It is currently recommended that patients with MMC who are to undergo surgical procedures should be screened for latex allergy. For patients who are found to be positive, the most important precaution appears to be to provide a latex-free environment at the time of surgery. There are widely varying opinions regarding the need for premedication of children prior to surgery. Some authors have recommended the administration of histamine blocking agents and steroids prior to surgery, but to date there is no evidence to suggest that this is beneficial.

Malignant hyperthermia has been reported in patients with MMC. The paucity of reports indicates a weak association of the two conditions. Management is as with malignant hyperthermia in other conditions.

Urologic Considerations

Urologic dysfunction is common in children with MMC. Incomplete emptying due to bladder spasticity or flaccidity predisposes these children to recurrent urinary tract infections. Vesicoureteral reflux is common, leading to hydronephrosis and progressive renal deterioration. The use of urinary diversion, intermittent catheterization, and suppressive antibiotics has decreased the percent of patients with renal dysfunction from 75% to 30%.

Infection Risks

It has been speculated that spastic and paralytic bladder dysfunction resulting in recurrent urinary tract infections leads to a higher postsurgical infection rate in children with MMC. Blood-borne bacteria are presumed to seed surgical wounds and implanted devices, but to date no consistent commonality of organisms in the urine, blood, and wound infection has been established. One study of spinal fusions did note a decrease in the rate of infectious complications if prophylactic antibiotics, based on preoperative urine cultures, were given. Infection rates of 3% to 25% have been reported following spinal fusion. One series of tibial osteotomies combined with subtalar extra-articular arthrodesis reported a 20% infection rate for the tibial osteotomies. The relative importance of other factors, such as poor skin in the area of sac closure, insensate skin, and nutrition, has not been well studied, but these are presumed to be significant risk factors for infectious complications.

Fractures

Pathologic fractures of the long bones are common in patients with MMC. Local swelling, erythema, and mild elevations in temperature and white blood cell (WBC) count are common and may lead to confusion with infection. The etiology of fractures in MMC is obscure. From 70% to 90% of fractures are associated with the use of cast immobilization following surgery. Up to 85% of fractures occur in the first 8 to 9 years of life, when the majority of surgery upon the extremities is performed. The overall incidence has been reported to be 10% to 30% of all patients, with a direct correlation of frequency to level of involvement. In one series, reported in 1989, it was noted that 41% of thoracic level patients, 36% of upper lumbar level patients, 10% of lower lumbar level patients, and only 3% of sacral level patients would have a fracture. Recent studies have begun to explore a possible link between renal dysfunction, alterations in calcium and phosphorus homeostasis, and pathologic fractures in patients with MMC.

Half of the fractures occur around the knee, and 10% involve the growth plate. Diaphyseal and metaphyseal fractures will heal readily, but physeal fractures have been associated with significant healing problems. Clusters of fractures secondary to immobilization of an initial injury have been reported. Because of the good healing potential of these injuries, most authors advise against surgical stabilization, but prolonged immobilization in a cast is also felt to be detrimental because of the increased risk of further fractures. Compromises that involve short-term cast or splint immobilization followed by early return to ambulation in braces have been suggested.

Upper Extremity Function

Early gait training in many children with MMC involves the use of walkers, crutches, or other upper extremity assistive devices. Abnormalities in upper extremity function have been documented in 60% to 70% of patients with MMC. Risk factors for abnormal function include lumbar or thoracic level involvement, upper extremity spasticity, and need for more than three shunt revisions.

Orthopaedic Treatment

The primary goal of treatment in MMC is to improve function. The presence of unbalanced hip dislocation, pelvic obliquity, severe scoliosis, or severe lower extremity deformity may be cosmetically objectionable to the surgeon or family, but careful inspection of the functional deficit to the child must be performed before recommending treatment. Application of "rules" derived from treatment of other patient populations can be deleterious to the child with MMC.

Foot Deformities

The incidence of foot deformities in children with MMC ranges from 60% to 90%. Clubfoot occurs in 20% to 50%, equinus deformities in 25%, and calcaneus deformity in 9% to 30% of patients in reported series. Early series had postulated that foot deformity in MMC, like polio, was secondary to paralytic muscle imbalance. More recent reports, however, have shown that muscle imbalance alone does not explain the majority of foot deformities seen in these patients. Muscle spasticity has been associated with 50% of calcaneus and 17% of equinus deformities. Habitually assumed posture of the feet, intrauterine positioning, and subclinical spasticity have been proposed as etiologies for foot deformities, but all are speculative.

The goal of surgical intervention is to provide a braceable or shoeable foot that will accept and transfer weight effectively with minimal risk of decubiti. It has generally been assumed that a plantigrade foot is desirable, but a recent series has shown that plantigrade rigid feet may have a significant risk of skin breakdown compared to feet that are nonplantigrade and supple. Recurrent decubiti and resultant amputations have been implicated in the loss of ambulatory function over time in patients with low level MMC.

Clubfoot

If a clubfoot deformity occurs, it is generally present at birth. This deformity is recognized as being very rigid in children with MMC as compared to the idiopathic form of clubfoot. Successful nonsurgical treatment has been reported by only one group, with short-term follow-up. Surgical treatment has been superior to splinting or casting in all other series at achieving a plantigrade foot. Smith and Duckworth, however, had a high percentage of poor results in long-term follow-up of a group of patients treated with Turco type releases as reported in 1976. Similar results were reported by Dias in 1982. Incomplete correction, recurrence of deformity, and wound-healing problems have led to revisions in as many as 20% to 30% of patients. There have been no recent series reporting the results of surgical correction of this deformity in the MMC population. Small series of patients with resistant or recurrent deformity have been treated by talectomy, supramalleolar tibial osteotomy, or cuboid and talus decancellization procedures, with good clinical results. Force-plate studies of feet following talectomy indicate that it is rare that weightbearing forces are uniformly distributed over the plantar surface. High force concentration, found in up to 80% of feet, may predispose these patients to future decubiti formation.

Valgus Deformity

Valgus deformity of the foot can present as an isolated deformity in the young child or may be associated with external tibial torsion and ankle valgus in the older child. In both situations, skin breakdown can occur over the prominent talar head. Soft-tissue correction and subtalar extra-articular arthrodesis have been commonly recommended for treatment of the foot deformity if ankle valgus is not also present. Recently, promising results have been reported for calcaneal neck lengthening as an alternative to arthrodesis. A variety of methods have been tried for correction of the tibial torsion and ankle valgus. Supramalleolar osteotomy, medial tibial physeal stapling, and fibular-Achilles tenodesis have been reported to be successful in obtaining correction of ankle valgus. The mechanism by which fibular-Achilles tenodesis may improve ankle tilt is unknown. Improvements in valgus are generally modest, with a wide range in the series reported by Stevens. Abnormalities in tibial rotation are not addressed by this procedure. A report of combined tibial osteotomy with extra-articular subtalar arthrodesis noted a 25% recurrence rate requiring reoperation and a 10% delayed union rate for the tibial osteotomy.

Calcaneus Deformity

This deformity is thought to arise because of unopposed action of the tibialis anterior. It has been found most often in children with involvement at a low lumbar (L4) level. Several recent series have described improvement of heel ulceration, radiographic position of the calcaneus, and position of the foot after posterior transfer of the tibialis anterior through the interosseous membrane into the calcaneus. Follow-up has been only 6 to 8 years, with an average age at surgery of 4 to 7 years. Better results were seen in the series that required grade 4 strength of the tibialis anterior prior to transfer than in the series that did not measure muscle strength prior to surgery. No significant changes in level of bracing or ambulatory function have been noted. Problems with valgus deformity requiring surgical correction have been noted with follow-up. Equinus deformity after transfer of a spastic muscle has also been reported. The optimal age for this procedure is yet unknown. Several series suggest that age greater than 4 is better as one can better evaluate muscle strength and voluntary control in the older child.

Knee Problems

Knee flexion contractures are common in patients with MMC. It does not appear that muscle imbalance or spasticity alone explains the development of this deformity. In a natural history study of patients who had not undergone knee surgery, it was found that all babies with MMC have a knee flexion contracture of 10° at birth. This flexion decreased to an average of 5° by 9 months. Progressive flexion deformities then developed in patients with L3 or higher involvement. The average flexion contracture in adult patients was 30° in thoracic level patients, 20° in L1-L3 level patients, 5° to 10° in L4-L5 level patients, and 0° in sacral level patients. The standard deviation was quite broad for high level patients and very narrow for sacral level patients. The amount of physical therapy given, the use of long leg braces, and the presence of knee flexor spasticity did not appear to influence the degree of contracture in long-term follow-up. Nonambulatory patients were found to have higher degrees of knee flexion deformity, but it could not be determined which came first. Thoracic level patients who were kept in ambulation programs and "sat" late had an average knee flexion deformity of 8° as adults, but still were not able to ambulate due to the level of their involvement.

Concern about long-term knee problems in MMC has recently been raised. A 20- to 40-year follow-up of community ambulatory patients showed that 22% had knee pain or knee pain with instability related to activities. All were low lumbar or sacral level patients and the majority had an abductor lurch, stance phase internal rotation of the femur, and stance phase external rotation of the tibia. Lateral compartment degenerative changes were seen on radiographs of some patients. Flexion contractures alone were not found to correlate with knee pain or instability. No mention was made of the status of shunts or the spinal cord in these patients and the possibility of a CNS cause for their pain was not excluded. It was suggested that the position of the limb in stance led to significant valgus stress at the knee and contributed to the knee discomfort.

Correction of flexion and rotational deformities about the knee to achieve a braceable position can be difficult. Capsular contractures are frequent and often must be released. Hamstring releases or lengthenings can weaken the child enough to inhibit rather than aid ambulation. The use of osteotomies has been recommended to avoid this, but no comparative studies exist to show improved outcomes of one procedure over another.

Hip Deformities

Hip instability in children with MMC has been a controversial subject since Sharrard in 1964 recommended posterior transfer of the iliopsoas tendon to better balance muscle forces about the hip and thus prevent dislocation. A recent series found the incidence of hip dislocation was 28% for patients with thoracic level involvement, 30% for children with involvement at the L1-L2 level, 36% for L3, 22% for L4, 7% for L5, and only 1% for sacral level involvement. Children with L3 or lower involvement were found to dislocate by age 3 to 4 years, with few developing dislocation after this age. On the other hand, children with thoracic level involvement continued to develop dislocations well after 10 years of age. These children were also found to have significantly greater hip flexion contractures than children with mid-lumbar involvement. These findings of progressively worsening deformities in children without clinically evident muscle imbalance led the authors to conclude that muscle imbalance was not a factor in the development of hip instability. In another series, it was found that hip instability (subluxation or dislocation) was present in 86% of patients with L3 level involvement and 45% of those with L4 involvement. Only one hip that

was stable at the age of 1 subsequently dislocated over a 10-year follow-up.

There are now many published studies which have found that the presence of hip dislocation does not affect ambulation, bracing requirements, seating, progression of scoliosis, or lead to hip pain in patients with MMC. Two recent studies have added to this body of literature. High costs, a high redislocation rate, difficulty with sitting secondary to iatrogenic hip stiffness, loss of ambulatory function secondary to surgical complications, and little measurable benefit were noted by these authors for those patients who underwent surgical intervention for hip abnormalities.

Spine Deformities

Prevalence

Spinal deformities are common in children with MMC. Congenital scoliosis, scoliosis without vertebral anomalies, and kyphotic deformities will be seen in this population. The incidence of congenital scoliosis is estimated at 1% to 15% of patients. Kyphotic deformities, reported in 5% to 20% of patients, are virtually always limited to patients with thoracic level involvement. Estimates for significant kyphus deformities developing in this group of patients have run as high as 60%. The prevalence of the more typical neuromuscular scoliotic deformities has been found to be directly related to the level of involvement. A recent series found that 69% of all children with MMC had a spinal curvature of more than 10°. Ninety-four per cent of thoracic level patients had more than 10° of scoliosis compared to 20% of sacral level patients. Only 39% of patients were found to have curves greater than 30°. The majority of these patients had thoracic or high lumbar level involvement. Similar findings were reported by Shurtleff and associates in 1976. In that study, 80% to 90% of patients with L2 or higher involvement were expected to develop spinal curvature exceeding 30°, while only 9% of sacral level and 23% of L3-L5 level patients would develop deformity of that magnitude.

Scoliosis

Natural History There is little doubt that scoliotic deformities in MMC can become very severe. Reported series of surgically treated cases have included many patients with radiographic deformity greater than 100°. Several studies have shown that curve progression occurs in these children, but the extent of progression expected and factors that will lead to "significant" progression are not well documented. Curve magnitude, Risser sign, menarchal status, and bone age have not been linked to the likelihood of curve progression in this population as they have in idiopathic scoliosis. Etiologies for progressive spinal deformity in children with MMC remain speculative. Worsening hydrocephalus, tethered spinal cord, and hydromyelia have all been implicated and found in patients with worsening deformity. Correction of these associated findings has been linked to a temporary arrest of curve progression in some patients, but a true cause-and-effect relationship has yet to be proven. Level of paralysis appears to be the most significant predictor of progression. Two series reported that one fourth to one third of their patients developed curves greater than 60°. The majority of these patients had high level involvement. For patients with mid-lumbar or lumbosacral involvement, the likelihood of progression to large deformities appears to be much less.

The morbidity of severe spinal deformity in patients with MMC is poorly documented. Torso imbalance requiring the use of the arms for support, seating problems, ischial decubitus secondary to pelvic obliquity, difficult ambulation, pulmonary compromise, functional impairment of internal organs, progressive deformity, and problems in the management of urinary diversion appliances have been cited as indications for surgical intervention in several series. None of these series details how the severity of the problem was assessed or related to the spinal deformity or how surgical intervention improved the problem that was cited as the reason for treatment. Despite these limitations, there is a consensus that functional problems may be linked to spinal deformity on a case-by-case basis and that correction of the deformity may lead to improvement for the patient. A more controversial question is whether or not progressive spinal deformity in patients with MMC leads to pulmonary compromise. Studies of deterioration in lung volumes with curve progression in patients with idiopathic scoliosis are often cited. No similar longitudinal study has been performed in patients with MMC. Patients with severe spinal deformity are generally those with a high level of paralysis, and the natural history of changes in pulmonary function in the absence of spinal deformity for these patients is not known. Long-term survival studies do not cite pulmonary compromise as a common cause of death. One recent series claimed improvements in vital capacity and increased forced expiratory volume in approximately 50% of their patients who had undergone spinal stabilization. The average gain for the entire series was modest and several patients showed deterioration of pulmonary function postoperatively. At this time, it must be concluded that insufficient evidence exists to use pulmonary compromise as an indication for surgical stabilization of severe spinal deformity in the majority of these patients.

Brace Treatment   Because natural history studies of curve progression are lacking in MMC, it is difficult to assess the affect of brace management. Most authors have suggested that orthotic management is at best a "temporizing measure" that will delay, but not stop, curve progression. The Milwaukee brace, underarm thoracolumbo-sacral orthosis (TLSO) designs, and suspension jackets modified for use with a wheelchair have all been used for flexible deformities in children with MMC. Guidelines for the amount of time spent in brace are variable and range from daytime use in the wheelchair to 23 hours per day. Problems with pressure sores and worsening pulmonary status secondary to constriction by the brace have been reported.

Surgical Treatment   Historically, pseudarthrosis and infection rates following surgical treatment of scoliotic deformities in patients with MMC have been very high. Pseudarthrosis rates of 40% to 75% and infection rates of 20% to 40% have been reported using Harrington instrumentation and isolated anterior or posterior fusion. The addition of two-stage procedures combining anterior and posterior fusion with some form of instrumentation has decreased pseudarthrosis rates to less than 20%. The routine use of prophylactic antibiotics has decreased infection rates to 0 to 8%. Perioperative deaths are uncommon in recent published series. Reports of aborted cases due to intraoperative hypotension are present in several series and may represent latex sensitivity reactions.

Up to 57% of ambulatory patients with MMC will lose some of their ambulatory capacity following spinal arthrodesis to the pelvis. Fusion to the pelvis requiring restriction of ambulatory activities for 3 to 6 months may contribute to the loss of function. Increases in hip flexion contractures are seen in up to 50% of patients postoperatively. It has also been noted that many patients undergo surgery at an age when natural history studies would predict a loss of ambulatory potential independent of treatment of the spinal deformity.

Kyphosis

Natural History   Children with MMC can have a congenital or developmental kyphotic spinal deformity. The majority of children with this deformity will have high lumbar or thoracic level involvement. Of these children, 10% will have a kyphotic deformity greater than 65° at birth, but the number rises to one third of children by adolescence. The location of the deformity is typically the thoracolumbar or lumbar spine. Children with deformities greater than 80° at birth will inevitably progress. Most will exceed 120° by the third year of life, and progression to greater than 170° has been documented. A compensatory thoracic lordosis is generally not present at birth, but develops rapidly once a sitting posture is assumed. The natural history of smaller deformities is not well known. It is generally believed that progression will occur, but data on the rate and extent of this progression has not been published.

As with scoliotic deformities, the long-term morbidity of kyphotic deformities is not well documented. Recurrent skin ulceration over the gibbus deformity, poor seating balance, problems with management of urinary diversions, the poor cosmetic appearance of the back, and respiratory distress caused by crowding of the abdominal contents are all cited as indications for surgical intervention. The incidence of these problems among all patients with kyphotic deformities is not known. To date, no evidence has been presented that pulmonary compromise occurs as a result of this deformity. Improvements in skin ulceration problems by resection of the kyphus deformity have been docu-

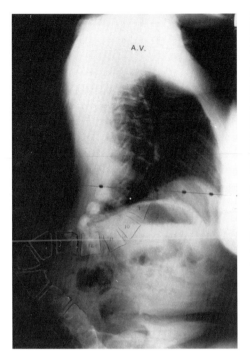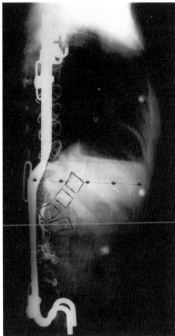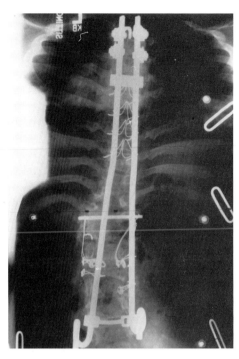

Fig. 1 An adolescent female with spina bifida and severe progressive lumbar kyphosis. **Left,** Kyphotic deformity. **Center,** Resection of kyphus and fixation with Dunn-McCarthy rods. The rods lie anterior to the sacral ala. **Right,** Postoperative anteroposterior radiograph demonstrating excellent frontal plane alignment.

mented. Quantification of improvements in the other listed indications has not been reported.

Treatment Orthotic management of kyphotic deformity in children with MMC has not been shown to be effective in controlling progression. Many authors have reported results for surgical treatment of this deformity. A recent series reporting an average 11-year follow-up of kyphectomy and arthrodesis found that there was loss of correction over time to less than 50% improvement of the original deformity. Figure-of-eight wiring was used for fixation in this series. Several patients had a deformity at follow-up that was worse than the preoperative abnormality. Other series using segmental fixation extended to the sacrum have shown, in short-term follow-up, correction of the kyphosis from a range between 100° and 130° down to a range between 7° and 45° (with little loss of correction). Two newer methods of fixation to the pelvis have included passage of a Luque rod through the S1 foramina to the anterior side of the sacrum and the Dunn-McCarthy rod which is pre-bent and also lies anterior to the sacral ala (Fig. 1). These methods have proven particularly useful in the management of kyphotic deformities.

Pseudarthrosis rates following kyphectomy have been reported as 25% to 40% in older series. Recent series report this problem in only 0 to 10% of cases in which segmental fixation is used. Similarly, infection rates of 20% to 25% have declined to 8% to 10%. Perioperative deaths have been reported in 0 to 10% of patients. Intraoperative death has been associated with ligation of the spinal cord leading to an acute elevation of intracranial pressure.

Miscellaneous Spinal Deformity

As previously mentioned, many children with MMC will be found to have Chiari II malformations. Occipital decompression has been used by many centers to treat this abnormality when swallowing or respiratory problems develop. The role of occipital decompression may be controversial, but a recent series found that 95% of children who underwent this procedure and had suboccipital cervical laminectomy that extended below C2 developed instability of the upper cervical spine (Fig. 2). The long-term prognosis of these children was not detailed and the authors did not recommend prophylactic arthrodesis of the spine at the time of decompression. This was partly due to the medical instability of many of the patients undergoing decompression. If progressive instability developed, the recommendation was to perform anterior interbody fusion. No data were presented to support this recommendation over a posterior fusion.

Bracing and Ambulation

As previously mentioned, the level of neurologic lesion has been found to be the best predictor of long-term ambula-

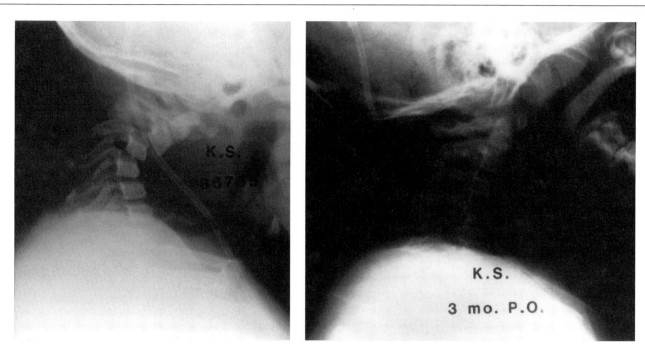

Fig. 2   **Left,** Cervical kyphosis after occipital decompression. **Right,** Following posterior fusion.

tory ability in children with MMC. Unfortunately, the classic neurosegmental pattern described by Sharrard in 1964 is seldom seen during the evaluation of muscle strength in patients with MMC. Variations in the patterns of muscle strength occur often. Large differences in ambulatory status have been noted in children with similar neurosegmental lesions. Previous reports have emphasized the importance of the quadriceps, hip abductors, and knee flexors for ambulation. A recent review of muscle strength testing and ambulatory outcomes in MMC patients suggests that specific patterns of lower extremity strength are more predictive of ultimate walking ability than testing of isolated muscle groups. In this study, patients with iliopsoas strength grade 3 or less ultimately relied upon wheelchairs for the majority of their mobility. Patients with grade 4 to 5 iliopsoas and quadriceps function and antigravity gluteal strength achieved community ambulatory ability without need for a wheelchair. The presence of grade 4 to 5 gluteal strength and grade 4 to 5 ankle dorsiflexion predicted independent ambulation without any aids or braces. Muscle testing was not reliable in children younger than 3 years of age.

Application of orthoses and gait training programs are widely used for patients with mid-lumbar, low lumbar, and sacral level involvement. More controversial is the use of bracing systems in children with thoracic and high lumbar level lesions. The high level of paralysis necessitates control of the trunk and limbs relative to each other to achieve ambulation. This has resulted in several bracing systems that combine knee-ankle-foot orthoses (KAFOs) with a

linked pelvic component. These systems are heavy and expensive. The cost of a reciprocating gait orthosis has been estimated at $3,500 to $5,000, with annual maintenance costs of $400 to $500. Natural history studies suggest that long-term ambulation is unlikely in these patients. The explanation for this is found by looking at the energy cost of ambulation in paraplegic patients. A report of 151 patients with traumatic paraplegia compared the energy cost of normal walking with ambulation in bilateral KAFOs, a crutch-assisted reciprocal gait without KAFOs, and the use of a wheelchair. Patients who used KAFOs and walked with a swing-through gait pattern had a velocity one third that of normal ambulation, a rate of oxygen consumption 38% greater, an oxygen cost of walking a set distance five times greater, and a velocity one third that of normal ambulation. Patients able to use a crutch-assisted reciprocal gait fared slightly better, but still had a rate of oxygen uptake 20% greater than normal. Smaller studies of patients with paraplegia secondary to MMC have reported similar findings. Normal adults walk at a rate of oxygen consumption that is 30% of maximum aerobic capacity and can do this indefinitely. Once the rate of oxygen uptake exceeds 50% of maximal aerobic capacity, anaerobic metabolism commences and endurance time decreases rapidly as the intensity of work increases. Unless a paraplegic patient maintains peak physical conditioning, swing-through ambulation rapidly pushes them above the 50% anaerobic threshold, making prolonged ambulation too costly to continue.

The benefits of bracing and short-term ambulation in

these patients is uncertain. A comparative study between two highly regarded programs with differing philosophies has been performed. Patients matched for age, sex, level of involvement, and intelligence had been involved in a walking program at one institution and had been prescribed a wheelchair early in life at the other center. No major differences were seen with regard to activities of daily living, function of the hands, or development of obesity. Deterioration of walking ability over time was seen in the patients enrolled in a walking program. Patients who walked early were found to average one fracture over 12 to 20 years versus an average of two fractures in the wheelchair group. Fewer pressure sores were seen in the ambulatory group. Patients who walked early were judged to be more independent and better able to transfer than the early wheelchair group. Ambulatory patients spent an average of 15 days in the hospital due to orthopaedic procedures versus an average of seven hospital days for the wheelchair patients.

Annotated Bibliography

General Articles

Beaty JH, Canale ST: Orthopaedic aspects of myelomeningocele. *J Bone Joint Surg* 1990;72A:626–630.

This is a concensus report by nine prominent orthopaedic surgeons experienced in the management of patients with MMC. It highlights much of the current thinking in the management of children with MMC and is well referenced.

Czeizel AE, Dudas I: Prevention of the first occurrence of neural-tube defects by periconceptional vitamin supplementation. *N Engl J Med* 1992;327:1832–1835.

In this randomized, controlled trial, women planning to become pregnant were either given a daily single multivitamin supplement containing folic acid or a trace-element supplement for one month before conception and until at least the date of the second missed menstrual period. There were approximately 2,100 women in each group. There were six cases of neural tube defects in the trace-element group and none in the folic acid group. The difference was statistically significant.

Van Allen MI, Kalousek DK, Chernoff GF, et al: Evidence for multi-site closure of the neural tube in humans. *Am J Med Genet* 1993;47:723–743.

This is a comprehensive review of experimental and clinical studies looking at the etiology of neural tube defects. The authors conclude that neural tube closure has several initiation sites and that this helps to explain the wide spectrum of spinal dysraphisms that are seen clinically. The clinical significance of this is that risk for subsequent children having the abnormality differs depending on the site of the defect, and that the response of these abnormalities to prenatal treatment (such as folate) will vary.

Natural History

Brinker MR, Rosenfeld SR, Feiwell E, et al: Myelomeningocele at the sacral level: Long-term outcomes in adults. *J Bone Joint Surg* 1994;76A:1293–1300.

This long-term study of sacral level patients followed at an experienced institution shows that at an average follow-up of 29 years up to one third of patients lost community ambulatory ability. An average of ten procedures per patient had been performed. The authors speculate that CNS deterioration due to tethered cord, hydromyelia, and Arnold-Chiari malformation led to the decline in most patients.

Dunne KB, Gingher N, Olsen LM, et al: *A Survey of the Medical and Functional Status of Members of the Adult Network of the Spina Bifida Association of America.* University of Washington, 1986. Thesis.

This survey of 263 adults aged 20 to 89 years with spina bifida asked questions regarding their age, motor level, shunt function, ambulatory status, independence, education, employment, continence, fertility, psychological health, decubiti, and renal function. Thirty-nine percent were married or lived alone. Sixty-one percent lived with friends, family, or had chore services to assist them. Twenty-five percent were employed. Sixty-seven percent were receiving social security insurance or social security disability insurance payments.

Hunt GM, Poulton A: Open spina bifida: A complete cohort reviewed 25 years after closure. *Dev Med Child Neurol* 1995;37:19–29.

This is a review of 117 children with spina bifida treated with early closure and CNS shunting with followup of 25 years. All patients were accounted for. The mortality rate was 44%, with the majority of deaths occurring in the first 5 years of life and being caused by renal failure, CNS infections, and cardiorespiratory insufficiency. Initial neurologic dysfunction was predictive of ultimate disability. Those with a sensory level L5 or below had no deterioration of function. Those with a sensory level L3 or L4 showed gradual deterioration of function over time. No patients with a sensory level above L3 maintained ambulatory ability. Treatment had no discernable effect on ultimate disability.

Nonorthopaedic Considerations

Anderson TE, Drummond DS, Breed AL, et al: Malignant hyperthermia in myelomeningocele: A previously unreported association. *J Pediatr Orthop* 1981;1:401–403.

This is a report of three patients with malignant hyperthermia and MMC in a total clinic population of 200 children. None of the patients were related. The likelihood of this number of cases in a population of this size is very unlikely and leads the authors to conclude that there may be an association.

Boor R, Schwarz M, Reitter B, et al: Tethered cord after spina bifida aperta: A longitudinal study of somatosensory evoked potentials. *Childs Nerv Syst* 1993;9:328–330.

This small study looks at serial SSEP data in 25 ambulatory patients with MMC. All had MRI findings of a tethered spinal cord. Declining posterior tibial nerve SSEPs were seen in 15 patients, and 14 were noted to have clinical signs of a tethered cord. Repeat MRI showed a hydromyelia in six patients. The SSEP improved in eight of the ten patients who underwent untethering. Five of the eight were improved clinically. Two remained stable and one deteriorated.

Breningstall GN, Marker SM, Tubman DE: Hydrosyringomyelia and diastematomyelia detected by MRI in myelomeningocele. *Pediatr Neurol* 1992;8:267–271.

MRI studies were performed on 45 patients with MMC out of a clinic population of 49 patients. Twenty-four (54%) had a hydromyelia and two had a diastematomyelia. All patients were felt to be asymptomatic prior to the MRI.

Emans JB: Allergy to latex in patients who have myelodysplasia: Relevance for the orthopaedic surgeon. *J Bone Joint Surg* 1992;74A:1103–1109.

This is a comprehensive review of our understanding of latex allergy in patients with MMC. Testing methods, prevention methods, and surveillance of populations at risk are discussed and referenced.

Lock TR, Aronson DD: Fractures in patients who have myelomeningocele. *J Bone Joint Surg* 1989;71A:1153–1157.

This is a review of existing literature and the authors' own experience with pathologic fractures in their 186 patients with MMC. The frequency of fractures increased with higher levels of involvement. Overall, 20% of their patients had fractures. Most followed surgical immobilization. Physeal fractures were prone to nonunion and growth arrest. Diaphyseal and metaphyseal fractures healed uneventfully.

Tosi LL, Slater JE, Shaer C, et al: Latex allergy in spina bifida patients: Prevalence and surgical implications. *J Pediatr Orthop* 1993;13:709–712.

Ninety three patients at D.C. Children's Hospital were tested for latex allergy with the RAST test. Thirty-five patients (38%) tested positive. Only nine patients had a clinical history of reaction. Only one of these patients was not detected by RAST testing, but it was the one patient who had a documented anaphylactic reaction to latex.

Yassin MS, Sanyurah S, Lierl MB, et al: Evaluation of latex allergy in patients with meningomyelocele. *Ann Allergy* 1992;69:207–211.

This is a prospective review of 76 patients with MMC who were skin tested for latex allergy. Sixty-five percent were positive. Of these, half had no clinical history of reaction. None of the skin test negative patients had a history of latex reaction.

Foot Deformities

Broughton NS, Graham G, Menelaus MB: The high incidence of foot deformity in patients with high-level spina bifida. *J Bone Joint Surg* 1994;76B:548–550.

This review of 124 consecutive children with MMC above the L3 level found deformity in 89% of all feet. Fifty-one percent had equinus deformities, 19% had a clubfoot deformity, and 28% had a calcaneus deformity. Muscle spasticity of the tibialis anterior, peroneus tertius, or toe extensors was associated with 50% of the calcaneus deformities. Spasticity of the gastrocnemius was found in 17% of the equinus deformities. The authors conclude that muscle imbalance is not the etiology of foot deformities in many children with MMC.

Fernandez-Feliberti R, Fernandez SA, Colon C, et al: Transfer of the tibialis anterior for calcaneus deformity in myelodysplasia. *J Bone Joint Surg* 1992;74A:1038–1041.

Fifteen patients (22 feet) had a transfer of the tibialis anterior tendon to the calcaneus. All were L4 or L5 level MMC. Seven other patients had been lost to follow-up. No selection criteria other than the development of progressive calcaneus deformity were used. Patients younger than 5 years old at the time of surgery were found to be less likely to need additional procedures and had the best correction of the deformity.

Georgiadis GM, Aronson DD: Posterior transfer of the anterior tibial tendon in children who have a myelomeningocele. *J Bone Joint Surg* 1990;72A:392–398.

Twenty of 26 children who had undergone a transfer of the tibialis anterior tendon to the calcaneus were reviewed at an average of 6 years postoperative. Of 39 feet, 37 were plantigrade at review. Grade 4 muscle strength was a prerequisite for the surgery. In 14 feet, the transfer was nonfunctional at review, but 12 of 14 had a good clinical result. Brace needs and ambulatory ability were not significantly altered. Valgus deformity developed in 25% of operated feet.

Maynard MJ, Weiner LS, Burke SW: Neuropathic foot ulceration in patients with myelodysplasia. *J Pediatr Orthop* 1992;12:786–788.

The authors reviewed 36 patients at an average follow-up of 14 years. All were ambulatory. The incidence of decubitus formation in flexible plantigrade feet was 0%; in flexible nonplantigrade feet, 25%; in rigid plantigrade feet, 36%; and in rigid nonplantigrade feet, 100%. Many of the rigid feet had undergone arthrodesis. Arthrodesis in a nonplantigrade position may increase the risk of decubitus formation.

Mosca VS: Calcaneal lengthening for valgus deformity of the hindfoot: Results in children who had severe, symptomatic flatfoot and skewfoot. *J Bone Joint Surg* 1995;77A:500–512.

This review of 20 patients with valgus hindfoot deformities treated by calcaneal neck lengthening with interposition of tricortical bone graft showed good correction of the deformity and relief of symptoms. Talonavicular joint plication, Achilles tendon lengthening, and cuneiform or distal tibial osteotomies were added in many of the patients. Nine patients had MMC. The procedure was combined with a corrective tibial osteotomy in eight of 20 feet for patients with MMC. Subtalar motion was preserved.

Sherk HH, Marchinski LJ, Clancy M, et al: Ground reaction forces on the plantar surface of the foot after talectomy in the myelomeningocele. *J Pediatr Orthop* 1989;9:269–275.

Nineteen patients with MMC and severe foot deformities had undergone talectomy and were seen at an average follow-up of 12 years. Force-plate and photoelastic sheets were used to examine the pattern of distribution of forces on the plantar aspect of the feet. Only 20% of the feet had a normal distribution of forces. In the remaining feet, there were high peaks of pressure at various locations. Four patients subsequently developed decubiti in areas of high forces.

Stevens PM, Toomey E: Fibular-Achilles tenodesis for paralytic ankle valgus. *J Pediatr Orthop* 1988;8:169–175.

The authors review 26 extremities in 18 patients who underwent fibular-Achilles tenodesis for ankle valgus. Four also had a Grice procedure. Improvement in talar tilt was reported in

80% of patients. Improvements in fibular length were seen in 17 of 26 ankles.

Knee Problems

Williams JJ, Graham GP, Dunne KB, et al: Late knee problems in myelomeningocele. *J Pediatr Orthop* 1993;13:701–703.

A long-term review of 72 community ambulators was done. Sixteen patients (24%) had activity-related knee pain, knee pain with instability, or instability alone. Thirteen of these patients had a characteristic gait in which there was an abductor lurch with stance phase internal rotation of the femur and external rotation of the tibia. Degenerative changes were seen in some, but not all knees. Spinal cord problems were not excluded. Patients with flexion contractures alone were not found to be symptomatic.

Wright JG, Menelaus MB, Broughton NS, et al: Natural history of knee contractures in myelomeningocele. *J Pediatr Orthop* 1991;11:725–730.

Pooled data from 850 patients entered into a spina bifida data base were used to plot the course of nonsurgically treated knee flexion deformities. At 1 year of age, 257 patients were available. At age 15, only 70 patients were available. Higher degrees of knee flexion contracture were seen in patients with L3 or higher involvement, with very little deformity in sacral level patients. More severe contractures were also seen in nonambulatory patients, but the contractures could not be cited as the cause of nonambulatory status. The use of physical therapy, orthotics, and the presence of knee flexor spasticity was not associated with the degree of flexion contracture.

Hip Deformities

Broughton NS, Menelaus MB, Cole WG, et al: The natural history of hip deformity in myelomeningocele. *J Bone Joint Surg* 1993;75B:760–763.

The authors analyzed the development of hip deformity in children with MMC and found that the highest rates of hip dislocation and flexion contracture were in children with thoracic level involvement. Muscle imbalance was not clinically present in these children. Children with L3 or lower involvement tended to develop hip dislocations by age 3 or 4 if they were going to. Children with thoracic level involvement continued to develop dislocations well past 10 years of age.

Fraser RK, Hoffman EB, Sparks LT, et al: The unstable hip and mid-lumbar myelomeningocele. *J Bone Joint Surg* 1992;74B:143–146.

Fifty-five patients with L3 or L4 level MMC were reviewed for ambulatory ability and hip instability. Twenty-four patients had documentation of their hip status from birth to dislocation. Instability (subluxation or dislocation) developed in 86% of hips in L3 level children and 45% of hips in L4 level children. Only one patient with a stable hip at 1 year of age subsequently developed hip dislocation. Hip instability had no bearing on ultimate ambulatory ability. Only 32% of hips that were surgically treated for instability achieved stability.

Spine Deformities

Aronson DD, Kahn RH, Canady A, et al: Instability of the cervical spine after decompression in patients who have Arnold-Chiari malformation. *J Bone Joint Surg* 1991;73A:898–906.

This review of 40 patients with MMC showed that 19 of the 20 who had posterior occipital decompression of a type II Arnold-Chiari malformation and cervical laminectomy developed instability on lateral flexion extension radiographs. Of the 20 who had not undergone surgery, none had instability. Prophylactic fusion at the time of decompression was not recommended for patients who were medically unstable.

Carstens C, Paul K, Niethard FU, et al: Effect of scoliosis surgery on pulmonary function in patients with myelomeningocele. *J Bone Joint Surg* 1991;73A:459–464.

In this small series of 13 patients with MMC who had spinal stabilization, eight patients had improvement in vital capacity and six had increased forced expiratory volume after surgery. Patients with larger preoperative curves and with high levels of paralysis seemed to have the most improvement.

Lintner SA, Lindseth RE: Kyphotic deformity in patients who have a myelomeningocele: Operative treatment and long-term follow-up. *J Bone Joint Surg* 1994;76A:1301–1307.

At an average of 11 years follow-up, 39 patients were reviewed following surgical treatment of kyphotic spine deformities. The technique of fixation was figure-of-eight wiring around the pedicle remnants. Postoperative bracing for up to a year was used. There was a loss of correction over time. Ultimately, less than 50% correction resulted. Several patients had deformities worse in followup than they had preoperatively. Infectious and pseudoarthrosis complications were low. One perioperative death occurred.

Muller EB, Nordwall A: Prevalence of scoliosis in children with myelomeningocele in western Sweden. *Spine* 1992;17:1097–1102.

This review of 131 patients with MMC found that 69% had a scoliotic deformity greater than 10°. Thirty-nine percent had a curve greater than 30°. The prevalence of scoliosis was strongly correlated to level of involvement, with deformity in 94% of thoracic level patients and only 20% of sacral level patients. The prevalence did not increase above age 9.

Muller EB, Nordwall A, von Wendt L: Influence of surgical treatment of scoliosis in children with spina bifida on ambulation and motoric skills. *Acta Paediatr* 1992;81:173–176.

Fourteen children with MMC who had undergone spinal arthrodesis to the pelvis were assessed for ambulation ability after surgery. Fifty-seven per cent lost some of their preoperative ambulatory ability. No effect was seen on the patient's ability to perform activities of daily living.

Ward WT, Wenger DR, Roach JW: Surgical correction of myelomeningocele scoliosis: A critical appraisal of various spinal instrumentation systems. *J Pediatr Orthop* 1989;9:262–268.

Thirty-eight patients with MMC underwent surgical management by a variety of techniques over an 18-year period. Patients who had a single stage anterior or posterior procedure with or without instrumentation had a pseudarthrosis rate of 50%. Patients who underwent a variety of two-stage procedures using instrumentation had pseudarthrosis rates of 0 to 17%. Hardware failures were common; infectious complications were rare. Wound necrosis was, however, seen in 25% of patients.

Warner WC Jr, Fackler CD: Comparison of two instrumentation techniques in treatment of lumbar kyphosis in myelodysplasia. *J Pediatr Orthop* 1993; 13:704–708.

This review of 33 patients compares 21 who had Harrington compression instrumentation with 12 who had Luque instrumentation and fixation to the pelvis using a modified Dunn technique with placement of the rod through the S1 foramina. Of the patients with Harrington instrumentation, 38% had pseudarthroses versus none in the Luque group. The rate of infection in the Harrington group was 24% versus 8% in the Luque group.

Bracing and Ambulation

Duffy CM, Hill AE, Cosgrove AP, et al: Three dimensional gait analysis in spina bifida. *J Pediatr Orthop,* in press.

The authors of this study evaluate ambulation of 30 children with low lumbar or sacral level spina bifida. Analysis was performed using a Vicon system. Pelvic obliquity and rotation, hip abduction in stance, and persistent knee flexion in stance were the most significant abnormalities noted. Characteristic patterns of abnormalities were identified depending on the level of involvement. Tendon transfers about the hip (Sharrard) or ankle did not appear to alter the gait patterns of operated patients.

Guidera KJ, Smith S, Raney E, et al: Use of the reciprocating gait orthosis in myelodysplasia. *J Pediatr Orthop* 1993;13:341–348.

This is a review of a Shriners Hospital experience with the reciprocating gait orthosis (RGO) with a maximum follow-up of 5 years. The average cost of an RGO was $5,000. Eleven of 21 patients were no longer using their orthosis at follow-up. Only four patients were community ambulators in their RGO. The average time of use was 25 months. All patients reported some problems with use of the brace. Twelve families had a negative

impression of the orthosis after usage. An average of three repairs a year were necessary for maintenance. Parental and child motivation, good upper extremity strength, absence of obesity, and absence of significant scoliosis were the most important factors for prolonged brace usage.

Mazur JM, Shurtleff D, Menelaus M, et al: Orthopaedic management of high-level spina bifida: Early walking compared with early use of a wheelchair. *J Bone Joint Surg* 1989;71A:56–61.

This study compares similar patient groups with high level MMC from two institutions. Patients from Melbourne were enrolled in ambulation programs while the Seattle patients were prescribed wheelchairs early. Follow-up was at 12 to 20 years of age. Deterioration of ambulatory ability was seen in the ambulatory group. No differences in ability to perform activities of daily living, hand function, or obesity were seen. Ambulatory patients had an average of one fracture over 12 to 20 years versus two fractures in the wheelchair group. Decubiti were more common in the wheelchair group. Ambulatory patients had an average of 15 hospital days versus 7 days for the wheelchair group. Ambulatory patients were judged to be more independent and be better at transfers than the wheelchair group.

Waters RL, Lunsford BR: Energy cost of paraplegic locomotion. *J Bone Joint Surg* 1985;67A:1245–1250.

An energy cost analysis was performed for 151 patients with traumatic paraplegia. One hundred twenty four were evaluated in their wheelchair. Sixty-seven were studied while ambulating. For patients who used bilateral KAFOs for ambulation, a swing-through gait was preferred. Velocity was 66% slower, rate of oxygen consumption 40% higher, and oxygen cost per meter walked 5 times higher than normal walking. In contrast, use of a wheelchair resulted in a velocity that was comparable to, rate of oxygen consumption equal to, and oxygen cost per meter equal to, normal walking.

9

Arthrogryposis

The term "arthrogryposis" is commonly used to describe multiple congenital contractures. Derived from Greek terminology, arthrogryposis means "hooked or curved joints." This syndrome complex is characterized by multiple joint contractures, poorly developed and contracted muscles, limb deformities, and intact sensation. Stern coined the term arthrogryposis multiplex congenita in 1923. Neither term represents a specific diagnosis, because there are well over 150 conditions that can lead to the presence of multiple congenital contractures (Outline 1). The multiple heterogeneous etiologies of this syndrome have led to considerable confusion and great difficulty in determining effects of treatment. Arthrogryposis is a term often used to describe any number of common orthopaedic conditions that result in multiple congenital contractures, such as myelomeningocele, congenital muscular dystrophy, Larsen syndrome, Möbius syndrome, and skeletal dysplasias. These conditions have different etiologies, prognoses, and treatments.

Etiology

The etiology of most forms of arthrogryposis is unknown. Common to all conditions causing congenital contractures, however, is limited intrauterine movement. Persistent immobility as a result of neuropathic, myopathic, connective tissue, and mechanical processes leads to joint contractures and subsequent abnormal joint development. Neuropathic changes, resulting from abnormalities of the central and peripheral nervous system, are responsible for 90% of all cases of arthrogryposis. Myopathic processes, such as dystrophies or myopathies and abnormalities associated with connective tissues, can also lead to decreased joint motion and contractures. Finally, mechanical factors, such as oligohydramnios, amniotic bands, or structural uterine abnormalities, can cause limitations in fetal motion. The role of environmental factors, teratogens, intrauterine infections, and other multifactorial processes in the development of arthrogryposis is unknown. It is estimated that the syndrome occurs in one of 3,000 live births.

Pathology

In most forms of arthrogryposis, the affected muscle tissue is grossly atrophic, lightly pigmented, and, in some cases, completely replaced by fibro-fatty tissue. Histologic examination of muscle tissue varies according to the etiology. The more common neurogenic processes lead to changes in fiber type predominance and disproportion, amyoplasia, hypoplasia, and denervation atrophy. Magnetic resonance imaging (MRI) will often reveal spinal cord atrophy consistent with a reduction in the number of anterior horn cells. Electromyography may reveal neuropathic or myopathic changes, again depending upon the etiology. Serum enzymes and chromosome studies should be performed, although they will be normal in most cases.

The initial evaluation of children with arthrogryposis requires a multidisciplinary approach. In addition to the previously noted tests, it is important for the child to be seen and evaluated by a pediatrician, neurologist, geneticist, physical therapist, occupational therapist, and social worker, in addition to the orthopaedic surgeon. A genetic evaluation is important, because several of the arthrogrypotic disorders are inherited.

Despite the large heterogeneous group of disorders described by the term arthrogryposis, orthopaedic surgeons are most likely to be confronted with children affected by amyoplasia, a specific arthrogrypotic disorder. The etiology of amyoplasia is not understood, but the condition refers to what orthopaedic surgeons commonly refer to as the "classic" form of arthrogryposis. Like other arthrogrypotic conditions, amyoplasia is characterized by multiple symmetric contractures of the upper and lower extremities (Fig. 1). Approximately 40% of patients with arthrogryposis are specifically diagnosed with amyoplasia. Most orthopaedic surgeons recognize this group of patients as having normal intelligence, intact sensation, and symmetric contractures. The contractures involve adduction/internal rotation of the shoulders, fixed extension of the elbows, volar and ulnar contractions at the wrist, thumb-in-palm deformities, flexed but relatively rigid interphalangeal joint contractures, flexion-abduction and external rotation at the hip, fixed flexion or extension of the knees, and severe rigid talipes equinovarus (clubfoot) deformities. Hip dislocations are common. Associated abnormalities include occasional elbow flexion contractures, pronation of the forearm, soft-tissue dimpling of the skin, loss of flexion creases, digital hypoplasia, and scoliosis. Nonmusculoskeletal findings include an inconsistent capillary hemangioma over the forehead, micrognathia, and loss of the characteristic whorl patterns typically seen on the distal end of the digits. In general, the skin is tense and glossy or waxy, with limited subcutaneous tissue. Webbing may be present at the elbow and knee. The side-to-side asymmetry of this condition is often striking, with distal deformities being the most severe.

Laboratory testing in amyoplasia is of limited benefit. Electromyography is nondiagnostic. Nerve conduction

Outline 1. Characteristics of types of arthrogryposis

Primarily limb involvement

Absence of dermal ridges	Coalitions (eg, fusion of tarsals or carpals)	Nievergelt-Pearlman syndrome
Absence of distal interphalangeal creases	Contractures, continuous muscle discharge	Poland syndrome
Amniotic bands	Distal arthrogryposis	Radioulnar synostosis
Amyoplasia	Humeroradial synostosis	Symphalangism
Antecubital webbing	Impaired pronation, supination of forearm	Symphalangism/brachydactyly
Camptodactyly	(familial)	Tel Hashomer camptodactyly
Clasped thumbs, congenital	Liedenberg syndrome	Trismus pseudocamptodactyly

Limb involvement plus other body areas

Camptomelic dysplasia	Metaphyseal dysostosis	Pseudothalidomide syndrome (Robert
Conradi–Hünermann (chondrodysplasia	Metatropic dysplasia	syndrome)
punctata)	Möbius syndrome	Puertic syndrome
Contractural arachnodactyly	Multiple pterygium syndrome	Sacral agenesis
Craniocarpotarsal dystrophy (whistling face,	Nail-patella syndrome (hereditary osteo-	Schwartz-Jampel syndrome
Freeman-Sheldon)	onychodysplasia)	Spondyloepiphyseal dysplasia congenita
Diastrophic dysplasia	Nemaline myopathy	Sturge-Weber syndrome
Focal femoral dysplasia	Neurofibromatosis	Tuberous sclerosis
Hand muscle wasting and sensorineural	Oculodentodigital dysplasia	Vertebral defects, imperforate anus,
deafness	Ophthalmomandibulomelic dysplasia	tracheoesophageal fistula, and radial
Holt-Oram syndrome	Oral cranial digital syndrome	and renal dysplasia (VATER)
Kniest syndrome	Osteogenesis imperfecta (Type I)	Weaver syndrome
Kuskokwim syndrome	Otopalatodigital syndrome	Winchester syndrome
Larsen dysplasia	Pfeiffer syndrome	X-trapezoidocephaly, midfacial hypoplasia,
Leprechaunism	Popliteal pterygium	cartilage abnormalities
Megalocornea with multiple skeletal	Prader-Willi habitus, osteoporosis, hand	
anomalies	contractures	

Limb plus CNS involvement

Adducted thumbs	Miller-Dieker syndrome (lissencephaly)	46,XXY/48,XXXY
Cerebro-oculo-facio-skeletal syndrome	Multiple pterygium, lethal	49,XXXXX and 49,XXXXY
Cloudy corneas, diaphragmatic defects,	Myotonic dystrophy, severe, congenital	Trisomy 4p
distal limb deformities	Neu Luxova syndrome	Trisomy 8/trisomy 8 mosaicism
Craniofacial/brain anomalies/intrauterine	Neuromuscular disease of larynx	Trisomy 9
growth retardation	Nezelof's syndrome	Trisomy 9q
Cryptochidism, chest deformity, contractures	Osteogenesis imperfecta (Type II)	Trisomy 10q
Faciocardiomelic syndrome	Pena-Shokeir phenotype (ankylosis, facial	Trisomy 10p
Fetal alcohol syndrome	anomalies and pulmonary hypoplasia)	Trisomy 11q
FG syndrome	Popliteal pterygium with facial clefts	Trisomy 13
Marden-Walker syndrome	Potter syndrome	Partial trisomy 14p
Meningomyelocele	Pseudotrisomy 18	Trisomy 15
Mietens-Weber syndrome	Zellweger syndrome (cerebrohepatorenal)	Trisomy 18

(Reproduced with permission from Hall JG: Arthrogryposis. *Am Fam Physician* 1989;39:113–119.)

studies, serum enzymes, and chromosome studies are normal.

Parents often ask about the recurrence risk of arthrogryposis when planning for additional children. Depending on the diagnosis, this risk may be anywhere from 0 to 50%. Because of this variability, genetic counseling is essential. When no specific diagnosis can be made, the risk for recurrence in subsequent children is 5%.

Prognosis

The majority of children with arthrogryposis, and certainly those with amyoplasia, have a relatively good prognosis and should be treated as such. It is not unreasonable to expect that such children should be able to ambulate and function independently. Children with arthrogryposis

who have significant mental retardation or identifiable chromosomal abnormalities have a much less favorable prognosis, both in terms of longevity and function. Survival during the first year may be compromised by respiratory insufficiency and weakness.

Management

Management of the child with arthrogryposis begins at birth. A multidisciplinary team is most useful, because the care of these patients is often too complex for one or two professionals to manage without assistance. Genetic and neuromuscular studies are initiated soon after birth. The earliest orthopaedic treatment is likely to involve the treatment of birth fractures. Twenty-five percent of infants with multiple congenital contractures sustain birth fractures.

long bones, in particular, are likely to produce only short-lived improvement because in many individuals the deformity will recur prior to skeletal maturity.

Management of Foot and Ankle Deformities

Perhaps the most common single orthopaedic deformity affecting children with arthrogryposis is a rigid form of talipes equinovarus (clubfoot). Like other deformities, the rigid clubfoot is static and nonprogressive. Unlike idiopathic clubfeet, however, nonsurgical treatment of the arthrogrypotic clubfoot is rarely successful. Manipulation and serial casting often leads to some correction, but rarely enough to avoid the need for surgery. Surgical treatment should be delayed until the child is approximately 1 year of age because of the high risk of recurrence. Surgery usually consists of an extensive posteromedial release or talectomy. Because of the extensive rigidity and marked fibrosis, recurrence rates of up to 46% have been reported following extensive posteromedial release. Talectomy or decancellization of the talus can be considered if posteromedial release does not allow for full correction of the foot deformity or if a recurrence develops. While primary talectomy for arthrogrypotic clubfoot deformities may seem aggressive, one study showed better results, decreased recurrence rates, fewer procedures per foot, and better maintenance of ambulatory status for children who underwent primary talectomies when compared to a group of children treated with extensive posteromedial releases. Following either posteromedial release or talectomy, orthotic management with an ankle/foot orthosis is necessary to maintain correction.

In an attempt to deal with the rigid soft-tissue contractures associated with arthrogrypotic clubfeet, soft-tissue expanders have been used around the ankle. Although several case reports have suggested that this is a useful technique, the single study reporting more than one case noted success for only two of the seven foot deformities reported. The authors concluded that soft-tissue expanders have limited usefulness in the surgical treatment of equinovarus foot deformities in patients with arthrogryposis. Triple arthrodesis remains a viable option for patients older than 10 years of age who have rigid clubfoot deformities.

Management of Knee Deformities

Most patients with arthrogryposis have flexion contractures at the knee, sometimes in excess of 90°. Extension contractures also occur but are less common. Other deformites include patellar elongation, flattening of the femoral condyles, and joint incongruity. Initial treatment should involve aggressive physical therapy with passive range-of-motion exercises. Active motion usually does not improve, because there is marked weakness of both hamstring and quadriceps. Ambulation is possible with residual knee flexion contractures of as much as 15° to 20°.

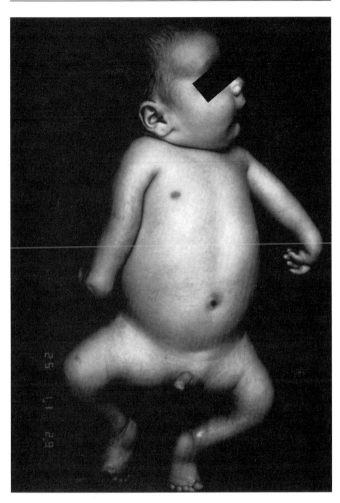

Fig. 1 Photograph of an infant with arthrogryposis. The contractures are consistent with amyoplasia.

Long-term orthopaedic treatment for children with arthrogryposis is directed at obtaining maximum function. Function is never sacrificed for the sake of cosmesis. Because of the large number of variable disorders leading to arthrogryposis, no single treatment plan can serve as a template for all patients with arthrogryposis. Despite this, several principles can generally be applied. Long-term goals must be realistic. Independent ambulation or self-mobility, self-care, and the potential for eventual employment are reasonable goals. Physical and occupational therapy are useful for improving and maintaining range of motion. In general, these modalities should always be used prior to the consideration of the surgery for any deformity. Long-term orthotic management is necessary to maintain correction. The risk of developing a recurrent deformity is inversely proportional to age. As such, very little surgery should be done during the first year of life. Osteotomies of

Hamstring lengthening, posterior capsulotomy, and distal femoral shortening may be necessary for contractures of greater than 20° to 30°. Extension producing osteotomy of the distal femur also can be performed to correct rigid knee flexion deformities. Internal fixation is necessary to avoid displacement of the osteotomy and injury to the popliteal neurovascular structure. Recurrent flexion contractures may develop if the osteotomy is done before adolescence.

When extensive soft-tissue webbing is associated with knee flexion contractures it may be necessary to consider the use of a circular frame external fixator with slow, gradual distraction to obtain knee extension prior to soft-tissue releases. External fixator treatment of flexion contractures and popliteal webbing, such as in the pterygium syndromes, is always accompanied by a rapid recurrence following fixator removal if formal soft-tissue procedures are not also performed. Soft-tissue procedures may involve Z-plasty lenthening of the skin, skin grafting, or flap coverage of the popliteal space.

Although the less common extension contractures are initially helpful for ambulation, problems arise at the end of the first decade when sitting and tying shoes become difficult because of the extended position. Untreated extension contractures are also associated with a high incidence of late degenerative arthritis. Treatment of extension contractures at the knee involves extensive anterior Z-plasty lengthening of the quadriceps followed by aggressive range of motion exercises. Postoperative casting should be avoided as this leads to stiffness. The goal of all lower extremity surgery is to obtain plantigrade feet, knee extension, and hip extension prior to the age of 2 years so as to permit ambulation if the child's condition allows.

Management of the Hip Joint

The characteristic deformities of the hip in infants with arthrogryposis are flexion, abduction, and external rotation. Unilateral or bilateral dislocations are common. Contractures cause more functional problems than dislocations. Bilateral dislocations with satisfactory motion are best left untreated. The dislocations themselves do not interfere with functional ambulation. Likewise, pain is an uncommon sequela of hip dislocations in this patient population. Passive stretching exercises can be done to improve or maintain motion.

Contractures about the hip joint should be corrected with soft-tissue procedures, osteotomies when the child nears skeletal maturity, or a combination of these two techniques. Unilateral dislocations of the hip should be treated because of the high incidence of associated pelvic obliquity, leg length discrepancy, and scoliosis. Closed procedures are almost never successful and the necessary prolonged period of cast immobilization results in stiffness. Open reduction, combined with soft-tissue release and proximal femoral shortening, is usually performed between 6 and 12 months of age. Medial-approach open reduction at an early age (between 3 and 6 months) has recently been shown to be effective.

Management of Spinal Deformities

Between 20% and 35% of patients with arthrogryposis develop scoliosis. Spinal deformities are usually developmental and are not associated with vertebral malformations. Nonsurgical brace treatment is recommended for patients with scoliosis of between 20° and 40°. Thoracolumbar and lumbar curves are most common.

When curve progression to greater than 40° or 50° occurs, spinal fusion with instrumentation should be considered. Fusion to the pelvis is recommended if lumbosacral obliquity exceeds 15°. Because some of these individuals use their lumbosacral spine for mobility, care should be taken to fuse only those segments necessary to obtain a balanced spine.

Upper Extremity Management

Management of the upper extremity in children with arthrogryposis is directed at improving hand function. Feeding, toileting, and assisting with ambulation are all important goals. As with the lower extremity, a passive stretching program is the initial step in upper extremity management. Surgery can be considered to correct some of the deformities. Internal rotation contractures at the shoulder can be treated with proximal humeral osteotomies. Elbow extension contractures can be treated with posterior capsulotomy and triceps tendon lengthening. Active elbow flexion can be established in most patients with 90° of passive elbow motion. Both anterior transfer of the triceps and pectoralis transfers have been described for restoration of active flexion. Shoulder and elbow procedures should be carried out only if the child has functional use of the hand.

The common volar flexion/ulnar deviation wrist deformity is accepted when the hand is stiff and the fingers lack active function. For those patients having some active digital flexion, soft tissue release of the tight volar structures, tendon transfer of the wrist flexors to the dorsum of the wrist, proximal row carpectomy, or a combination of these procedures can be considered. Failure to adequately balance the wrist flexors and extensors will lead to a recurrence. Finger deformities are best treated with therapy to obtain and maintain finger mobility. Surgery has not been particularly useful in assisting with finger function. Thumb-in-palm deformities can be adequately managed by releasing the adductor pollicis and performing a Z-plasty of the first webspace.

It is important to emphasize that all treatment for the child with arthrogryposis must be directed at improving or maintaining function. Despite having what initially appear to be severe deformities, these children often show surprising dexterity, resourcefulness, and function. This compensatory ability often makes surgical intervention unnecessary.

Annotated Bibliography

Pathology

Banker BQ: Arthrogryposis multiplex congenita: Spectrum of pathologic changes. *Hum Pathol* 1986; 17:656–672.

This classic article describes the pathologic features of muscle and spinal cord found in 96 infants and children with arthrogryposis. The specific muscle changes observed included primary myopathic alterations, fiber type predominance and disproportion, hypoplasia, aplasia, and denervation atrophy. The author concludes that a pathogenic feature common to all these conditions appears to be the occurrence of severe weakness early during intrauterine life, permitting the immobilization of joints at various stages of development.

Fedrizzi E, Botteon G, Inverno M, et al: Neurogenic arthrogryposis multiplex congenita: Clinical and MRI findings. *Pediatr Neurol* 1993;9:343–348.

Eleven children with neurogenic arthrogryposis were studied clinically, electromyographically, and with muscle biopsies. Evidence of anterior horn cell involvement was noted in all patients. Fifty percent of the patients also showed impaired cerebral function. MRI scans revealed spinal cord atrophy in 50% of the patients studied. The etiology of these changes, however, remains unclear.

Sarwark JF, MacEwen GD, Scott CI Jr: Current concepts review: Amyoplasia (A common form of arthrogryposis). *J Bone Joint Surg* 1990;72A:465–469.

This review article describes in significant detail the characteristics, known etiology, and treatment of amyoplasia, the most common form of arthrogryposis. Amyoplasia is perhaps best described as the "classic" form of arthrogryposis, common to pediatric orthopaedic clinics. This is the first article describing amyoplasia in the orthopaedic literature. Twenty-three excellent references are included.

Prognosis

Hall JG: Arthrogryposis. *Am Fam Physician* 1989;39: 113–119.

This review article is a well-written, easy-to-read summary of arthrogryposis from the perspective of a geneticist. Emphasis is placed on the possible etiologies, the extensive differential diagnosis, the risk of recurrence, and the generally favorable prognosis.

Management

Bassett GS, Mazur KU, Sloan GM: Soft-tissue expander failure in severe equinovarus foot deformity. *J Pediatr Orthop* 1993;13:744–748.

This retrospective study of seven feet with severe equinovarus foot deformities reveals that only two feet were successfully treated with soft-tissue expanders. Complications, including ischemia, infection, and sepsis, resulted in failure for five of the seven affected feet. Although isolated case reports have supported the use of this technique, the authors conclude that soft-tissue expanders have limited usefulness in the surgical treatment of equinovarus foot deformities.

Guidera KJ, Kortright L, Barber V, et al: Radiographic changes in arthrogrypotic knees. *Skeletal Radiol* 1991; 20:193–195.

The authors retrospectively reviewed the radiographs of 62 patients with arthrogryposis. Slightly more than 50% showed changes consistent with long-standing clinical deformities, including patellar elongation, malposition, flattening of the femoral condyles, joint incongruity, tibial plateau irregularities, tibial and femoral fractures, fibular hypoplasia, soft-tissue thickening, valgus deformity, and dislocation. Based on this review, the authors recommend early surgical treatment of the arthrogrypotic knee to prevent these chronic changes.

Mennen U: Early corrective surgery of the wrist and elbow in arthrogryposis multiplex congenita. *J Hand Surg* 1993;18B:304–307.

The authors describe treatment of 47 arthrogrypotic upper extremities in children treated surgically between 3 and 6 months of age. The early one-stage corrective procedure involves proximal row carpectomy, tendon transfers, and triceps-to-radius transfer for elbow flexion. Active motion of 49°, 27°, and 65° was noted at 2-year follow-up for the elbow, wrist, and metatarsophalangeal joints respectively. This occurred in the absence of intensive physiotherapy. Unfortunately, the necessity for early surgical intervention does not allow adequate time to study the child's preoperative upper extremity function or adaptive potential.

Segal LS, Mann DC, Feiwell E, et al: Equinovarus deformity in arthrogryposis and myelomeningocele: Evaluation of primary talectomy. *Foot Ankle* 1989;10: 12–16.

This retrospective study of 16 children with arthrogryposis (30 feet) and 16 myelodysplastic children (26 feet) compares primary talectomy with extensive posteromedial release. The authors conclude that primary talectomy led to better results, decreased recurrence rates, fewer procedures per foot, and better maintenance of ambulatory status compared to those children treated with extensive posteromedial release.

Shapiro F, Specht L: The diagnosis and orthopaedic treatment of childhood spinal muscular atrophy, peripheral neuropathy, Friedreich Ataxia, and arthrogryposis. *J Bone Joint Surg* 1993;75A:1699–1714.

This is the most recent review article in the literature dealing with arthrogryposis and several other neurologic conditions. The article emphasizes the confusion created by orthopaedists, geneticists, and neurologists, each of whom tend to recognize and concentrate on different aspects of the arthrogryposis syndrome. The article contains an excellent bibliography citing 92 references.

Sodergard J, Ryoppy S: The knee in arthrogryposis multiplex congenita. *J Pediatr Orthop* 1990;10:177–182.

This retrospective review of 30 patients with knee deformities due to arthrogryposis suggests that extension contractures are more successfully treated than flexion contractures. Despite this, surgical treatment of flexion contractures does seem to be justified because in this series all patients so treated were functional walkers. Shortening of the femur was often necessary.

Of 17 patients with extension contractures, 11 had good primary results compared to only three good results in the group with flexion contractures. The risk for degenerative arthritis was 27% overall but was significantly greater among patients with extension contractures.

Solund K, Sonne-Holm S, Kjolbye JE: Talectomy for equinovarus deformity in arthrogryposis: A 13 (2–20) year review of 17 feet. *Acta Orthop Scand* 1991;62:372–374.

This is a retrospective study of 17 arthrogrypotic feet with severe equinovarus deformities treated with talectomy. Fourteen of 17 feet were felt to be satisfactory at follow-up. Five feet required further surgical treatment. The authors recommend talectomy for the treatment of primary or recurrent equinovarus foot deformity in children with arthrogryposis.

Staheli LT, Chew DE, Elliott JS, et al: Management of hip dislocations in children with arthrogryposis. *J Pediatr Orthop* 1987;7:681–685.

These authors reviewed 18 hip dislocations in 14 children. The range of motion was much better when the medial approach was used instead of the anterolateral approach. The range of motion was also greater in children with bilateral dislocations when the medial approach was used when compared to closed reductions. There were no redislocations and only one case of osteonecrosis.

Because of their good results, these authors recommend an early (3 to 6 months of age) medial open reduction of the dislocated arthrogrypotic hip, whether unilateral or bilateral.

Szöke G, Staheli LT, Jaffe K, et al: Medial-approach open reduction of hip dislocation in amyoplasia-type arthrogryposis. *J Pediatr Orthop* 1996;16:127–130.

This study provides follow-up of the previous Staheli article and reports a high success rate following medial-approach open reduction for hip dislocations in amyoplasia-type arthrogryposis. Eighty percent achieved good results, and 12%, fair results. Only one of 25 hips redislocated and four had transient evidence of AVN.

Thompson GH, Bilenker RM: Comprehensive management of arthrogryposis multiplex congenita. *Clin Orthop* 1985;194:6–14.

This classic review paper discusses the comprehensive management of arthrogryposis including the need for a multispecialty team. Emphasis is placed on communication with the parents. An outline of general management principles is also presented. Perhaps most importantly, this is the lead in a series of 15 excellent articles on arthrogryposis covering 124 pages in the same issue.

10

Osteogenesis Imperfecta

Introduction

Osteogenesis imperfecta (OI) is a genetically and phenotypically diverse group of inherited connective tissue disorders. Manifestations of the syndrome have great variability and include generalized osteoporosis, dentinogenesis imperfecta, blue sclerae, hearing loss, short stature, easy bruising, excessive sweating, joint laxity, and cardiopulmonary abnormalities. Osteoporosis, present to some extent in all patients with OI, is responsible for the hallmark feature of this disease, a tendency for fractures to occur with minimal inciting trauma.

The earliest described case suggestive of OI was that of a mythical Danish prince, Ivan Benløs, who was carried into battle on a shield due to his brittle bones. Eckman in his doctoral thesis in 1788 described a family with inherited bone fragility. It was not until 1849 that Vrolik used the term osteogenesis imperfecta to describe a newborn with multiple fractures. Other historical terms for this disease include osteopsathyrosis idiopathica, Lobstein's disease, fetal rickets, and hereditary fibrous osteodysplasia.

There is no preferential distribution of OI by gender, race, or ethnic origin. The incidence of OI, diagnosed by fractures at birth, ranges from one per 20,000 births to one per 50,000 births. Less severe forms of OI, which may not be diagnosed at birth, have a reported incidence of four to five cases per 100,000 births. Based on these statistics OI, in all its various forms, probably affects about one individual per 10,000.

Classification

In 1906, Looser proposed a classification of OI based on the chronologic appearance of fractures. Patients with numerous fractures at birth exhibited the congenita form of the disease while those in whom fractures occurred after the perinatal period exhibited the tarda form of the disease. In 1949, Seedorff subclassified the tarda form into tarda gravis and tarda levis based on whether the first fracture occurred before or after the first year of life. In 1979, Sillence proposed a clinical, radiographic, and genetic classification that divided OI into four main types (Table 1). Although this remains the most universally accepted classification scheme in use today, many patients with OI do not fit readily into any of the Sillence types as defined. The ultimate classification will presumably be based on the location and nature of the various molecular abnormalities responsible for the clinical spectrum present in this disease.

The most severe form of OI in the Sillence classification is the type II phenotype. Perinatal fatality is the rule, although some infants may survive for months to a few years with optimized neonatal care. These infants are extremely fragile, with vaginal delivery often resulting in intracranial hemorrhage or multiple fractures. Those who survive delivery will eventually succumb to death from pneumonia or respiratory insufficiency secondary to decreased thoracic size. Originally described as a recessive condition, recent biochemical data suggest that most type II cases represent new dominant mutations.

The Sillence type III category represents a rare autosomal recessive form of the disease. These patients are characterized by severe bone fragility and often sustain in utero fractures. Progressive bone deformity and bowing with extreme short stature and triangular facies are present in this group of patients (Fig. 1). There is some phenotypic overlap in mild type II patients and those with type III disease. It is this type III group of patients that will often require multiple orthopaedic procedures, such as intramedullary rodding, in order to decrease the incidence of fractures, prevent deformity, and improve rehabilitation potential.

Sillence type I and IV patients represent the milder forms of OI, with type I being the most mild. Both are inherited in an autosomal dominant pattern and both are divided into A and B subtypes based on the absence or presence of dentinogenesis imperfecta. There are usually multiple affected family members in the pedigree. Type I patients will exhibit blue sclera and 30% to 60% will also have presenile hearing loss, which may be the most significant long-term handicap in this patient group. Fractures are usually associated with moderate trauma and occur after walking age. Type IV patients have normal sclerae and more severe osseous abnormalities. Bowing of the bones is often present even in patients with infrequent fractures. The fracture rate in this group decreases around puberty. Type IV patients do not have presenile hearing loss but are often of short stature.

Pathogenesis

Histologic and biochemical analyses of the various types of OI have shown that quantitative and/or qualitative defects in the formation of type I collagen are fundamentally responsible for the disease and its manifestations. Type I collagen is the principal protein found in bone, dentin, sclera, and ligaments. Therefore, these are the tissues that are primarily affected in patients with OI.

Table 1. Sillence classification of osteogenesis imperfecta

Type	Genetics	Description
I	Autosomal dominant	Mildest form of OI Mild-to-moderate bone fragility without deformity Associated with blue sclerae, early hearing loss, easy bruising May have mild to moderate short stature Type IA: Dentinogenesis imperfecta absent Type IB: Dentinogenesis imperfecta present
II	Autosomal dominant or recessive	Perinatal lethal Extreme fragility connective tissue, multiple in utero fractures, usually intrauterine growth retardation Soft, large cranium Micromelia, long bones crumpled and bowed, ribs beaded
III	Autosomal recessive	Progressive deforming phenotype Severe fragility of bones, usually have in utero fractures Severe osteoporosis Relative macrocephaly with triangular facies Fractures heal with deformity and bowing Associated with white sclerae and extreme short stature, scoliosis
IV	Autosomal dominant	Skeletal fragility and osteoporosis more severe than type I Associated with bowing of long bones; light sclerae, with or without moderate short stature, with or without moderate joint hyperextensibility Type IVA: Dentinogenesis imperfecta absent Type IVB: Dentinogenesis imperfecta present

(Reproduced with permission from Marini JC: Osteogenesis imperfecta: Comprehensive management. *Adv Pediatr* 1988;35:391–426.)

The synthesis of collagen is extraordinarily complex. Each type I collagen molecule consists of two α1(I) and one α2(I) polypeptide chains. Each chain has its own gene located on different chromosomes. Transcription of the gene produces an exact messenger RNA copy (pre-mRNA) from which mRNA is produced. Translation of mRNA produces pre-pro α chains which are processed to pro α1(I) and pro α2(I) chains, which then form type I procollagen molecules. Repeating triplet sequences of glycine-X-Y form the major central part of each chain, which enables the three α chains to wind into a triple helix, essential for the normal structure and function of collagen. Enzymatic modifications result in the final procollagen molecule, which is secreted from the cell. The amino- and carboxy-terminal extensions are enzymatically removed to yield the collagen molecule, which then becomes cross-linked with other collagen molecules to form the characteristic quarter stagger array.

Recent dramatic advances in OI research have resulted in the localization and characterization of mutations responsible for the various forms of the disease. Type I collagen deficiencies as well as mutant type I collagen have been found (Table 2). It is hoped that a biochemical classification of this disease will be the fruit of these research efforts, with eventual insights into strategies to control tissue expression of type I collagen genes.

Differential Diagnosis

Except for mild elevations in the serum levels of alkaline phosphatase, there are no specific laboratory abnormalities in patients with OI. Therefore, the diagnosis is usually made based on the characteristic clinical and radiographic features.

The clinical features have been outlined above (Table 1). Radiographically, there are several findings that reflect the severity of osseous involvement. In patients with mild forms of the disease, generalized osteoporosis, with thin cortices, is evident. Flaring of the metaphyseal regions is indicative of impaired bone modeling. Fractures in various stages of healing, as well as bowing of long bones, may be present. Scoliosis and kyphosis with biconcave vertebrae may also develop.

The radiographic findings in newborns with severe congenital forms are striking. Bones are short and wide with thin cortices. Numerous fractures in all stages of healing will be present and angular deformities from malunions will occur (Fig. 2). Popcorn calcifications in the metaphyseal and epiphyseal regions have been described. Skull radiographs demonstrate wormian bones, which are a salient feature of OI. Spine films reveal marked osteoporosis, biconcave vertebral bodies, and eventually, scoliosis and kyphosis.

Differential diagnosis according to age is summarized in Table 3. In the majority of cases, the combination of a detailed family history, clinical features, and skeletal survey will enable the physician to make the correct diagnosis. Several recent reports have documented the difficulty in differentiating a child with OI from a case of nonaccidental trauma. In the unusual instance where routine diagnostic criteria are inconclusive, dermal punch biopsies can be performed. The synthesis and structure of type I collagen produced by the cultured fibroblasts obtained from biopsy

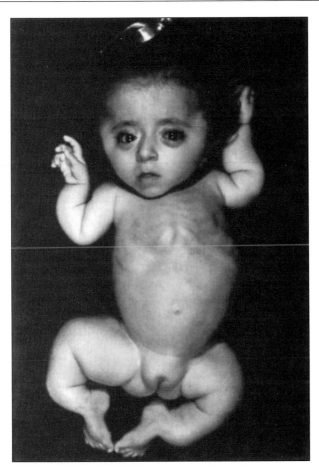

Fig. 1 Phenotypic appearance of patient with type III osteogenesis imperfecta. Triangular facies, thoracic deformity, and bowing of long bones are evident. (Reproduced with permission from Gertner JM, Root L: Osteogenesis imperfecta. *Orthop Clin North Am* 1990;21: 151–162.)

Table 2. Biochemical classification of osteogenesis imperfecta

Tissue Collagen	Clinical type of OI
Type I collagen deficiency alone	
50%	OI-IA and OI-IB (mild)
20%	OI-II (lethal perinatal)
0%	Lethal in utero
Type I collagen deficiency plus mutant	OI-II (lethal perinatal)
type I collagen	OI-IV (moderate severity)

(Reproduced with permission from Cole WG: Etiology and pathogenesis of heritable connective tissue diseases. *J Pediatr Orthop* 1993;13:392–403.)

Patient Management

Systemic Management

Several systemic treatment modalities have been tried in patients with OI in an attempt to enhance the strength and stability of the skeleton. Unfortunately, to date no known systemic drug therapy has proved effective in a controlled clinical trial. Medications tried have included calcium, vitamin C, vitamin D, fluoride, calcitonin, diphosphonates, gonadal hormones, magnesium oxides and APD ([3-amino-1-hydroxypropylidene]-1,1-biphosphonate). Research in this area continues; however, no currently known agent is able to modify the structure and composition of type I collagen fibers.

Orthopaedic Management

The orthopaedic surgeon has a primary role to play in the management of patients with OI. Orthopaedic treatment consists of physical therapy, casts and orthotics, and surgical stabilization of long bones and spinal deformities.

The active involvement of a physical therapist in order to maximize the age-appropriate activities and skills of the child is an important component of a successful treatment plan. Beginning in the neonatal period, proper positioning and handling must be taught to parents and caregivers. Hydrotherapy is a relatively safe form of exercise and allows active motion of all extremities. It also aids in the development of head and trunk control and strengthens extremity musculature. Improved muscle strength will increase the stresses on bone, which will in turn strengthen the bone. With the assistance of an involved physical therapy team, muscle and bone strengthening, standing, and even ambulation are desirable and attainable goals for many patients with OI.

Orthotics are another important adjunct to the management of these patients. Orthotic use starts with custom-molded seating to align the head, spine, pelvis, and lower extremities in young patients. Patients with standing and walking potential should be fitted with lightweight lower extremity braces to prevent bowing of long bones. Patients with already significant lower extremity deformities may require surgical realignment prior to brace fitting. Braces should be lightweight and total contact in design with joint hinges. The extent of the braces will depend on the

can then be analyzed. This process typically takes 3 to 4 weeks.

Noninvasive prenatal diagnosis of OI has received much attention in the literature. A recent review documented the efficacy of ultrasonography in those fetuses with type II and severe type III OI disease. Detection can reliably be achieved with ultrasound at 17 to 20 weeks of gestation. More invasive methods, such as chorionic villus sampling, can be used for families with the milder dominant forms of OI and for the severe forms of OI in which the biochemical or molecular defect in type I collagen is known. This information can then be used by the families for planning or by the physicians in order to anticipate the method of delivery of the fetus.

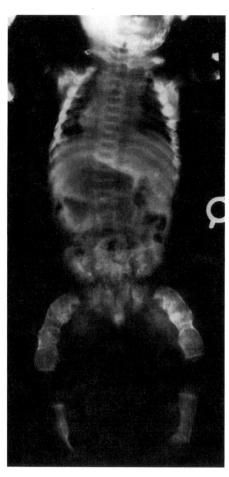

Fig. 2 Radiograph of patient with type II osteogenesis imperfecta. Multiple fractures are present. Femurs are short and wide with thin cortices. (Reproduced with permission from Zaleske DJ, Doppelt SH, Mankin HJ: Metabolic and endocrine abnormalities of the immature skeleton, in Morrissy RT (ed): *Lovell and Winter's Pediatric Orthopaedics,* ed 3. Philadelphia, PA, JB Lippincott, 1990, pp 203–262.)

Table 3. Differential diagnosis of OI by age

Age	Diagnostic Possibilities
At birth	Hypophosphatasia
	Achrondrogenesis
	Thanatophoric dwarfism
	Asphyxiating thoracic dystrophy
	Achondroplasia
	Chondroectodermal dysplasia
Infancy	"Battered baby"
	Scurvy
	Congenital syphilis
	Infantile cortical hyperostosis (Caffey's disease)
	Immobilization osteoporosis (spina bifida)
	Pyknodysostosis
	Osteopetrosis
Childhood and adolescence	Idiopathic juvenile osteoporosis
	Fibrous dysplasia
	Sarcoma (hyperplastic callus)
Adult life	Postmenopausal osteoporosis

(Reproduced with permission from Smith R, Francis MJO, Houghton GR (eds): *The Brittle Bone Syndrome: Osteogenesis Imperfecta.* London, England, Butterworth-Heineman, 1983.)

severity of bone involvement. Bracing does not replace the need for muscle strengthening and range-of-motion activities in these patients. The use of a vacuum pant orthosis to prevent recurrent fractures has been reported in a limited study (four patients). A decrease in the number of fractures as well as an increased bone density was documented in one patient who was studied sequentially. Pneumatic trouser splints can also be used but can irritate the skin, exacerbate sweating, and cause arterial compromise if overinflated.

Acute fractures can usually be treated with closed reduction and cast immobilization, and this treatment may also provide an opportunity to realign a previously deformed bone to a straighter position. Immobilization should be limited to 3 to 4 weeks for upper extremity frac-

tures and up to 6 weeks for lower extremity fractures. Splints that allow for joint motion may then be used if further fracture consolidation is needed. Nonunions do occur with increased frequency in this population. In a study of 12 nonunions in an OI population, nine underwent surgery, and eight of the nine subsequently healed after excision of the nonunion, nailing, and bone grafting. The primary causes of the nonunions were inadequate immobilization of a fracture and recurrent fracture through an area of progressive bowing. The vicious cycle of prolonged immobilization, disuse osteoporosis, and repeat fractures can significantly impair the rehabilitation process and is frustrating to caregivers.

The most popular and successful surgical method for treating the long-bone deformities in patients with OI was pioneered by Sofield and Millar. Their technique consists of multiple osteotomies with realignment of the fragments and intramedullary nail fixation. Bailey and Dubow refined this procedure through the use of a telescoping intramedullary nail that was fixed within the epiphyses at the proximal and distal ends of the involved bone. The proposed advantage of the telescoping nail technique is that with growth of the bone the nail has the ability to elongate and thus continue to allow the entire length of the bone to remain stabilized and aligned. With static intramedullary nails growth can result in loss of stabilization and eventual deformity or fracture distal or proximal to the rod.

Several recent reports have discussed the merits of intramedullary stabilization and have compared elongating versus nonelongating nail systems. A study of 20 patients with OI undergoing stabilization of long bones reported the overall complication rate with the Bailey-Dubow (B-D) nail to be 72% compared to 50% for the nonelongating nail. Reoperation rates were similar in both groups. The median time interval from the primary operation to reoperation was 3.0 years for the B-D nail and 2.0 years for the static nails. In another report of 29 patients who underwent 108 intramedullary roddings, the B-D group again had a higher complication rate but a lower reoperation and replacement rate. Of their B-D rod complications, 34% were related to proximal T-piece problems. The authors recommend the following steps to avoid these problems: (1) crimping of the proximal T-piece sleeve after insertion of the T-piece to prevent disassembly; (2) placing the T-piece below subchondral bone but not deep enough to result in migration into the medullary canal; and (3) after insertion, rotating the T-piece 90° to prevent backing out. In a study on intramedullary stabilization using a closed or semiclosed technique combined with manual osteoclasis, many of the patients in the series were first operated on when younger than 2 years of age. Because this closed technique avoids extensive surgical exposure of bone, it is possible to stabilize all four lower extremity long bones at one surgical sitting. These severely involved patients were able to progress from a rehabilitation standpoint following this early surgery as the number of fractures decreased and the children were easier to care for.

It is clear that surgical stabilization of deformed bones, even in the severely involved type III patient, results in improved alignment, decreased incidence of fractures, ease of handling, and improved rehabilitation potential. The choice of elongating versus nonelongating rods as well as the choice between the traditional open osteotomy technique versus the closed percutaneous technique is based on surgeons' preference and experience. In the very young patient with significant deformity of all four lower extremity long bones, the closed technique with nonelongating rods offers the advantages of minimizing surgical time and blood loss. In patients older than 5 years of age, a more lasting correction can usually be achieved by using the telescoping rods inserted in the standard open fashion. This often requires staging of bilateral procedures to minimize blood loss. The surgical technique is demanding and a high complication rate is associated with this patient population. Realistic goals and expectations on the part of the family, surgeon, and rehabilitation team are crucial.

Spinal deformity consisting of scoliosis and kyphosis is a relatively common finding in patients with OI. The reported incidence ranges from 40% to 80%, depending on the particular study. Factors that are associated with the development of spine deformities are severity of disease, age of patient, history of long bone fractures, and ambulatory status. The etiology is probably multifactorial but weak bone combined with ligamentous laxity are thought to be the primary factors. Natural history studies have indicated that the incidence and severity of scoliosis increases with age. Approximately 25% of patients between the ages of 1 and 5 have scoliosis, and in older patients the incidence increases to 75%. When curves do occur, they tend to be progressive even past skeletal maturity.

The management of spinal deformities in this population can be divided into observation, bracing, and surgery. By observation, it is meant that patients with OI must be followed closely from an early age for the development and progression of scoliosis and must also continue to be monitored as adults.

The role of bracing in the management of spinal deformities in this population has been questionable. The combination of pre-existing chest wall deformities, fragile ribs, and deformed vertebral bodies severely impairs the ability of a brace to transmit effective forces to the spine. The pressure exerted by a spinal orthosis can result in worsening of chest and rib deformities in these patients. In many cases bracing is instituted too late or is discontinued because of some brace-related complication. In summary, bracing is generally unsuccessful in controlling curve progression and, in fact, often worsens the chest and rib deformities present in the child with OI. Whether there is any role for brace wear in the patient with milder disease and curves of lower magnitude has yet to be determined.

Surgical indications in children with OI are variable and must be tailored to the individual patient. Children with mild OI can be treated with posterior spinal fusions and instrumentation, remembering that segmental instrumentation may be needed and that hook cutout can occur. Children with severe OI are very difficult to instrument, often sustain excessive blood loss, and are clearly prone to increased operative risks, often without benefit. In a recent series of children with OI and spinal deformity, only those children with maintenance of vertebral contours had their curve progression halted by arthrodesis. The more severely involved children had variable results from surgery.

A less common area of spinal involvement is at the craniocervical junction. In a report on the neurologic complications of OI, a significant incidence of basilar invagination was found in patients with the more severe forms of the disease. Three of their eight patients presented with neurologic signs due to brainstem compression. In those patients with neurologic signs and documented basilar invagination, decompression and spinal stabilization is recommended.

Hypertrophic callus formation following a fracture or surgical intervention is a well described occurrence in patients with OI. Although it is thought to be an abnormal response to trauma, its exact pathophysiology is unclear. Clinical features include massive swelling, dilated superficial veins, and tense skin. The condition most commonly occurs in the femur. It is often accompanied by fever, weight loss, malaise and anorexia. Laboratory studies reveal leukocytosis, and elevations in the erythrocyte sedimentation rate (ESR) and alkaline phosphatase level. High output cardiac failure has been described in association with this condition. Radiographs reveal massive callus formation. Recognition of this condition and differentiation from osteogenic sarcoma is of paramount importance and may require open biopsy. Treatment is for the most part symptomatic and consists of splinting and restriction of motion. Despite the long-term risks of low dose radiation therapy in this age population, it has been used with some success in this unusual condition.

Nonorthopaedic Management

From an anesthesia standpoint, patients with OI are at high risk for a variety of reasons. Restricted neck and jaw mobility, pulmonary function abnormalities due to thoracic cage distortion, dentinogenesis imperfecta and valvular heart disease are present in many of these patients. In addition, anesthesia-induced hyperthermia has been observed. Although the findings of fever, tachycardia, hypoxia, acidosis, and elevated creatine phosphokinase (CPK) that occur under anesthesia in some patients are similar to malignant hyperthermia, it is now believed that patients with OI are not at an increased risk of developing true malignant hyperthermia (MH). Rather OI patients are prone to a hypermetabolic state which can mimic MH. Although routine use of prophylactic dantrolene is not justified, certain drugs should be avoided. These include succinylcholine, which can cause fractures due to muscle fasciculations, and anticholinergics, which can exacerbate hyperthermia.

Hearing loss is present in many patients with OI. In type I patients, this may represent their most significant handicap and is reported to occur in 25% to 60% of this patient group. Audiologic abnormalities predate clinically significant hearing loss, which occurs in the third decade of life. The loss can result from conductive abnormalities or, less commonly, sensorineural deficits. Two lesions responsible for the conductive hearing loss are functional ossicular discontinuity and a thick, crumbly, lightly fixed stapes footplate. Surgical treatment consisting of stapedectomy can give satisfactory long-term results in patients whose severe hearing loss is not responsive to treatment with a hearing aid.

Dentinogenesis imperfecta, due to a deficiency of dentin, is present in patients with type IB, type IVB and in some patients with type III disease. The enamel is unaffected. The primary dentition is generally more severely involved than the permanent dentition. The teeth appear grayish, bluish, or brown and opalescent. They break easily, are prone to caries, and fillings do not hold well. These children should be seen by their dentist every 3 to 6 months. Artificial crowns to preserve tooth structure and new dental restorative materials for milder cases are the available treatment options.

Annotated Bibliography

Pathogenesis

Cole WG: Etiology and pathogenesis of heritable connective tissue diseases. *J Pediatr Orthop* 1993;13: 392–403.

This is a review of the current state of knowledge regarding collagen mutations in OI, as well as Ehlers-Danlos syndrome and spondyloepiphyseal dysplasia. Future directions in OI research are discussed.

Differential Diagnosis

Cohn DH, Byers PH: Clinical screening for collagen defects in connective tissue diseases. *Clin Perinatol* 1990; 17:793–809.

The authors review the biochemical defects present in OI and in other collagen disorders. They discuss methods of prenatal diagnosis of OI, including ultrasound, amniocentesis, and chorionic villus biopsy.

Smith R, Francis MJO, Houghton GR (eds): *The Brittle Bone Syndrome: Osteogenesis Imperfecta.* London, England, Butterworth-Heineman, 1983.

This entire textbook is devoted to OI. The chapter on differential diagnosis (from which Table 3 is taken) is particularly helpful.

Thompson EM: Non-invasive prenatal diagnosis of osteogenesis imperfecta. *Am J Med Genet* 1993;45:201–206.

The authors review the role of ultrasonography in the prenatal diagnosis of OI. The article includes the ultrasonic findings suggestive of the diagnosis and discusses which forms of OI can be reliably diagnosed by ultrasound and which forms may be missed by this imaging method.

Patient Management

Binder H, Conway A, Hason S, et al: Comprehensive rehabilitation of the child with osteogenesis imperfecta. *Am J Med Genet* 1993;45:265–269.

The authors report on their experience with a comprehensive rehabilitation protocol consisting of positioning, exercises, and bracing in children with OI. They conclude that a rehabilitation program is beneficial for most children with OI.

Charnas LR, Marini JC: Communicating hydrocephalus, basilar invagination, and other neurologic features in osteogenesis imperfecta. *Neurology* 1993;43:2603–2608.

Seventy-six patients with OI were evaluated regarding the frequency and spectrum of neurologic features associated with their disease. Seventeen patients had communicating hydrocephalus. Eight patients had basilar invagination; three of these had evidence of brainstem compression. Skull fractures and seizure disorders were also found. Neurologic evaluation is recommended in patients with OI.

Gamble JG, Rinsky LA, Strudwick J, et al: Non-union of fractures in children who have osteogenesis imperfecta. *J Bone Joint Surg* 1988;70A:439–443.

Twelve nonunions in 10 patients with OI were identified. In nine cases, surgical treatment was undertaken, consisting of excision of the nonunion, intramedullary nailing, and bone grafting. Healing occurred in eight of these nine cases.

Occurrence of nonunion was associated with repeated fractures at a progressively deforming site.

Gamble JG, Strudwick WJ, Rinsky LA, et al: Complications of intramedullary rods in osteogenesis imperfecta: Bailey-Dubow rods versus nonelongating rods. *J Pediatr Orthop* 1988;8:645–649.

A retrospective review of the authors' experience with Bailey-Dubow rods and nonelongating rods is presented. The complication rate was higher in the Bailey-Dubow group but the reoperation rate was lower. The authors recommend use of the Bailey-Dubow rod and offer several helpful hints to avoid complications.

Hanscom DA, Winter RB, Lutter L, et al: Osteogenesis imperfecta: Radiographic classification, natural history, and treatment of spinal deformities. *J Bone Joint Surg* 1992;74A:598–616.

Six well-defined groups of patients with OI were established based on radiographic appearance of long bones, pelvis, and vertebral body shape. Scoliosis was progressive in patients in groups B, C, D, and E. Bracing was not thought to be an effective method of treatment. Thirteen patients underwent surgical treatment. Five of these patients had mild group A disease and good results. In the remaining eight patients, whose disease was more severe, the results were variable.

Letts M, Monson R, Weber K: The prevention of recurrent fractures of the lower extremities in severe osteogenesis imperfecta using vacuum pants: A preliminary report in four patients. *J Pediatr Orthop* 1988;8:454–457.

The authors describe a vacuum pants orthotic system, which allows for comfortable standing in those patients with multiple fractures and they include a description of the fabrication technique.

Lubicky JP: The spine in osteogenesis imperfecta, in Weinstein SL (ed): *The Pediatric Spine: Principles and Practice.* New York, NY, Raven Press, 1994, pp 943–958.

This complete and up-to-date review of the topic includes a discussion of spinal deformity treatment, craniocervical and cervical abnormalities, and anesthetic considerations.

McHale KA, Tenuta JJ, Tosi LL, et al: Percutaneous intramedullary fixation of long bone deformity in severe osteogenesis imperfecta. *Clin Orthop* 1994;305:242–248.

Seven patients with severe OI and unbraceable deformities underwent 25 long-bone percutaneous intramedullary rod fixation procedures. The patients ranged in age from 8 months to 35 months. Early stable fixation was achieved. The authors describe their surgical technique.

Porat S, Heller E, Seidman DS, et al: Functional results of operation in osteogenesis imperfecta: Elongating and nonelongating rods. *J Pediatr Orthop* 1991;11:200–203.

Twenty patients with OI underwent intramedullary rodding of long bones. Thirty-two Bailey-Dubow rods and 24 nonelongating rods were placed. The B-D nail had a higher complication rate (72%) than the nonelongating nail (50%). The reoperation rates were similar. The longevity of the primary operation was slightly longer (3.0 years vs 2.0 years for the B-D nail). The authors conclude that surgical intervention improves or maintains the gait capacity in these children, and that the choice of nail should be based on surgeons' preference.

Stockley I, Bell MJ, Sharrard WJ: The role of expanding intramedullary rods in osteogenesis imperfecta. *J Bone Joint Surg* 1989;71B:422–427.

Eighty-three expanding intramedullary rods were used in 24 children with OI. Thirty-four additional operations were required for revision of rods or correction of deformity. Despite the complications, the expandable rods improved ambulation, reduced the frequency of fractures, and prevented deformity.

II
Spine

George S. Bassett, MD
Section Editor

11

Idiopathic Scoliosis: Etiology and Evaluation

Epidemiology

Idiopathic scoliosis, the most common type of scoliosis, is a distinct entity, which has no known etiology and is characterized by a lateral curvature of the spine with rotation. Scoliosis should be considered idiopathic only after other causes have been excluded.

The reported prevalence of idiopathic scoliosis in the general population is influenced by the study method employed and the minimum Cobb angle used to define true scoliosis. Some of the early studies of prevalence were based on a review of chest radiographs, which had been taken to examine for pulmonary tuberculosis. Most of the information in recent studies was derived from patients identified through school screening programs, a method that introduces uncertainty regarding the status of those individuals who were not selected for radiographs. When a Cobb angle of 10° is used as the minimum angulation to define scoliosis, the prevalence reported in most studies is in the range of 1.9% to 3%. The prevalence drops to 0.3% for curves greater than 20°. There is an overall female predominance, which increases substantially for larger curves. For curves between 11° and 20°, the female-to-male ratio has been reported as 1.4 to 1. This ratio increases to more than 5 to 1 for curves greater than 20° and for those requiring treatment.

Patients who have idiopathic scoliosis are frequently divided into three groups, based on the age of onset. The infantile group includes those whose scoliosis appeared between birth and age 3. Juvenile onset is between the ages of 4 and 10, although some define the upper limit as the beginning of adolescence. Adolescent onset, the most common type, develops after the age of 10 years. The infantile form affects more males than females and has associated features, such as plagiocephaly and developmental hip dysplasia, that distinguish it from other forms of idiopathic scoliosis. This type of scoliosis is almost completely absent from North America. Another distinguishing feature of infantile scoliosis is the clinical course, which is usually either spontaneous resolution or significant progression. Juvenile onset scoliosis is often difficult to distinguish from the adolescent type. A factor that obscures the demarcation between adolescent and juvenile scoliosis is the difficulty of precisely determining the age of onset for adolescents with already established curves at initial presentation. As is also true for the adolescent group, females with the juvenile form outnumber the males.

Etiology

The role of genetics in idiopathic scoliosis has been debated. There have been numerous published reports of scoliosis in twins, but these have not been helpful in elucidating inheritance patterns. Based on information derived from familial studies, sex-linked dominant, autosomal dominant, and multifactorial inheritance have all been postulated. It has been established that if one parent has idiopathic scoliosis, it increases the risk for the couple's children. The reported magnitude of this risk has varied widely, with females at considerably higher risk than males. Approximately 30% of the time, the family history is positive for scoliosis. A family history of scoliosis is not helpful for determining curve magnitude or risk of progression. Although the mode of genetic transmission has not been unequivocally established, some form of either autosomal dominant or multifactorial inheritance has the most support in the literature. Because both adolescent and infantile idiopathic scoliosis have been observed in the same family, a genetic link between these conditions has been suggested.

The roles played by hormones and alterations of growth patterns in the etiology of scoliosis have been questioned. It is likely that hormonal function influences scoliosis, but it is not the sole etiologic factor. There have been conflicting reports regarding serum levels of growth-stimulating hormone and other hormones. Clinical studies have shown that individuals with idiopathic scoliosis are taller than matched control subjects. Growth is known to be associated with the progression of existing deformities; but growth, which in normal circumstances is symmetrical, does not explain the initiation of the deformity.

Growth, in conjunction with existing short segment thoracic lordosis or hypokyphosis, has been proposed as a biomechanical explanation for the development and progression of idiopathic scoliosis. The premise of this assertion, that the apical segment is lordotic in all cases of idiopathic scoliosis, has been questioned. This type of analysis does not take into consideration the anatomic complexity of the spinal column or the role of the multiple dynamic forces acting on the spinal motion segments. Advanced imaging techniques, used to reconstruct the three-dimensional anatomic deformity, have been unsuccessful in predicting curve progression. It is accepted that biomechanical forces play a role in the progression of large curves. The contribution of biomechanical forces to the etiology and early progression of idiopathic scoliosis remains unresolved.

Alterations in connective tissue have been noted when comparing the convexity and concavity of curves. The differences in collagen type and intervertebral disk proteoglycan content is believed to be a result, rather than a cause of scoliosis. A similar question has been raised regarding convex-concave differences in muscle fiber type. Platelets have been examined because of their structural and functional similarities to muscle. The fact that platelets are not attached to the deformed spine makes it less likely that alterations are caused by the scoliosis. Observed abnormalities in platelet function are significant, because they may be an indication of a more general alteration in cellular function. This concept is of particular importance in its relation to muscle activity. A recent study demonstrated elevated platelet calmodulin levels in patients with progressive idiopathic scoliosis. Calmodulin, a calcium-binding receptor, is involved in the regulation of both skeletal muscle and platelet contractile systems. A longitudinal study was recommended to determine the clinical usefulness of calmodulin for the prediction of curve progression.

Much of the investigation into the etiology of idiopathic scoliosis has focused on the equilibrium system. Studies have demonstrated variations in vestibular, ocular, and proprioceptive functions. Vibratory response, a sensitive indicator of posterior column function, has also been found to be abnormal. The role of the brain stem in the equilibrium system is to integrate the afferent input. Anatomic asymmetry in the brain stem has been reported in idiopathic scoliosis patients studied by magnetic resonance imaging (MRI). Attempts to relate handedness to curve direction have been unsuccessful. Despite the existence of conflicting reports, abnormal function involving some aspect of the equilibrium system currently is the most widely supported theory for the etiology of idiopathic scoliosis.

In summary, the results of research efforts to uncover the etiology of idiopathic scoliosis have been inconclusive. Among the reasons for continuing research in this area is that the information derived may be valuable in the clinical management of this condition. Out of necessity, current treatment modalities are directed toward controlling the manifestations of scoliosis. Treatment derived with an understanding of the etiology can be directed toward the cause, leading to more effective intervention. In addition, clinical decision making will be further facilitated if insight can be gained into the prediction of curve progression.

Patient Evaluation

History and Physical Examination

The diagnosis of idiopathic scoliosis is made by excluding other conditions known to cause scoliosis. Obtaining a complete history is an essential component in this process.

It is important to note the severity, duration, and character of any back pain. Radicular pain, abnormal sensation, weakness, incontinence, and balance or coordination problems can be indications of neurologic involvement. Information pertaining to the patient's level of skeletal maturity can be valuable when attempting to predict remaining growth, a crucial factor for determining the probability of curve progression.

When examining patients, physical features and body proportions are frequently clues to the existence of conditions known to be associated with scoliosis. The position of the trunk and the sagittal plane contours should be noted. Rotational malalignments are best determined with the forward bending test. The patient is asked to bend forward, placing the palms together, letting the upper extremities hang in a dependent position. The examiner sights tangentially along the spine from the seated position, checking for any rotation or paraspinal asymmetry. The forward bending test also provides an opportunity to assess mobility of the spine. The level of the pelvis is frequently an indication of relative leg lengths. Discrepancies in lower extremity circumference and deformities of the feet are sometimes observed in association with intraspinal pathology. The neurologic examination must be thorough. Significant intraspinal pathology, such as syringomyelia and spinal cord tumors, can be associated with subtle neurologic abnormalities. The abdominal reflex has received much attention as an early indicator of spinal cord pathology.

Objective Measurement of Body Shape

There have been many attempts to quantify the body surface changes observed in idiopathic scoliosis. One of the goals has been to develop a technique that could be used to identify scoliosis, to monitor curve progression, and to provide information to be used for treatment decisions, without the use of radiographs. These efforts have not only been hampered by the difficulty in reproducibly measuring body surfaces, but also by the complexity of spinal deformities. In most cases, natural history data and treatment decisions are based on Cobb angles taken from standard upright frontal radiographs. Because the Cobb angle is obtained from a single plane radiographic image, it does not always accurately demonstrate the severity of the three-dimensional spine deformity. In addition, the Cobb angle fails to account for vertebral rotation, a major factor determining the magnitude of body surface changes.

A variety of methodologies are available to measure and document back contours. The simplest documentation of the rib deformity involves direct measurement of the prominence with a level and ruler. Other sophisticated techniques have evolved, such as Moire Topography, Raster-Stereophotography, and the Integrated Shape Imaging System (ISIS), which use computer analysis of digitized topographic information. Correlation of these techniques with radiographic measurements of Cobb angle has been variable.

The Scoliometer™ is a specially designed inclinometer used to measure the angle of trunk rotation. The goal of this device is to provide a simple, yet effective method of identifying patients who need further evaluation and treatment of their scoliosis. As the patient bends forward with hands clasped, the device is gently placed on the surface of the back, perpendicular to the long axis of the body and centered over the apex of the maximum deformity. The angle of trunk rotation is read directly off the device. In cases of multiple deformities, each should be measured independently. In order to identify the maximum rotation for each deformity, it may be necessary to vary the amount of forward flexion.

The initial study on the Scoliometer™ reported data from 1,065 patients referred from screening programs. The trunk rotation (from the Scoliometer reading) was correlated with the radiographically determined Cobb angle. Patients with Cobb angles less than 20° and trunk rotation greater than or equal to 5° were considered false positives. False negatives were defined as Cobb angles greater than or equal to 20° and trunk rotation less than 5°. False positives were found to be high, representing 36% of the total; while false negatives represented only 1.2%. The mean trunk rotation for patients with a 20° Cobb angle was 7°. The angle of trunk rotation correlated well with the magnitude of the curve as radiographically measured by the Cobb angle.

The false positive results from scoliosis screening programs have been a topic of much concern recently. In a follow-up study by the same author, it was recommended that patients with trunk rotation of 7° be referred for further evaluation. Seven degrees would result in an estimated referral rate of 3% of the individuals screened. The false-negative rate, which is 12% if the goal is to identify curves with 20° Cobb angles, drops to 8% for a Cobb angle of 25°. The Scoliometer™ has gained widespread acceptance because it is an inexpensive, noninvasive tool that can be used for obtaining objective measurements during scoliosis screening of large populations.

Radiography

Anteroposterior (AP) or posteroanterior (PA) upright radiographs have been the standard for objective measurement of spine deformities. The radiograph should be done on a 36-inch cassette, which allows adequate space to include the entire thoracic and lumbar spine on a single view. For standing radiographs, known leg length discrepancies should be equalized with a lift.

Lateral radiographs are needed in cases in which the physical findings indicate significant sagittal plane alterations, when the patient is symptomatic, and when there is suspicion of spondylolisthesis. Obtaining a lateral radiograph of every patient at the time of initial presentation is unnecessary. Additional views can be added when warranted by clinical concerns. Radiographs that are truly lateral to the scoliotic section of the spine frequently demonstrate lordosis of the apical segment.

Bending radiographs assess the flexibility of the deformity and are best performed with the patient in the supine position. These views, which are needed preoperatively for the selection of instrumentation levels, are also used when there is a need to determine flexibility, as is the case with certain types of bracing.

The Cobb technique is considered the standard for measuring scoliosis on radiographs. A recent study evaluating the Cobb technique found interobserver variability averaging 7.2° when the endpoints were not selected. The intraobserver variability under similar circumstances averaged 4.9°. When the endpoints were preselected, the observed variability improved, indicating the importance of consistent endpoint selection when evaluating serial radiographs. Another study found that a 10° measurement difference between radiographs taken at different times was necessary in order to be 95% confident that a true change in the scoliosis had occurred. A diurnal variation has also been observed. In a study of 19 patients, an average increase of 5° was noted on afternoon radiographs when compared with those obtained in the morning of the same day. This increase was determined to be statistically significant.

Vertebral rotation has been graded according to the system of Nash and Moe. This system assigns grades of 0 to 4, based on asymmetry of the pedicles as they appear on the radiograph. In grade 0, there is no asymmetry. In grade 4, the convex pedicle has rotated past the midline toward the concave side. Rotation may also be measured with a Perdriolle torsionmeter. In a laboratory study, measurement with this device has been shown to have a satisfactory correlation with known amounts of rotation. A variety of measurements have been described to document the presence of significant spinal decompensation or trunk shift.

Ossification of the iliac apophysis radiographically begins laterally and then extends medially, eventually fusing to the ilium. Grading according to the system of Risser involves dividing this excursion into four segments. Ossification of the lateral one fourth is Risser 1, one half is Risser 2, and three fourths is Risser 3. Complete excursion of the ossification without fusion is Risser 4. Risser 5 denotes fusion of the ossified apophysis to the ilium. Complete excursion of the ossification requires approximately 1 year. The average time from complete ossification to fusion with the ilium is 2 years.

Published reports have indicated that, for most females, Risser 4 corresponds with the completion of spinal growth. A recent study has questioned this association, after performing a careful statistical analysis of the literature assessing the use of the Risser sign as an indication of skeletal age. The authors concluded that chronologic age may be more accurate than the Risser sign for determining skeletal age. The Risser sign is considered a less reliable indicator in males, because growth of the trunk is frequently observed after Risser 4. As the iliac wings are frequently included on the full-length spine radiographs, use of the Risser sign makes it unnecessary to take separate hand radiographs for the assessment of skeletal maturity.

The number of radiographs required to monitor scoliosis until the completion of growth has led to concerns regarding radiation exposure. Most of the patients followed on a regular basis are adolescent females, and there is particular concern about the carcinogenic effect of radiation on breast tissue. In a retrospective study of women previously seen for idiopathic scoliosis, a higher than normal rate of breast cancer was reported. The 973 subjects for whom there was usable information had an average follow-up of 25.6 years. There was an average of 41.5 radiographs per patient. Eleven cases of breast cancer were identified, (six cases expected in this sample size). None were detected within 15 years of the initial examination. The ratio of observed cases to expected cases was greater after 30 years for those with more than 30 years of follow-up. This ratio also increased as the estimated dose of radiation and number of radiographs increased. It is important to realize that this study involved patients treated before the development of techniques designed to limit the exposure of breast tissue to radiation. The average estimated breast radiation was 12.8 rads. The use of newer techniques, and the reduction in the number of radiographs taken while following patients, have dramatically reduced breast tissue radiation.

The PA radiographic projection significantly decreases breast and thyroid exposure to radiation. The risk associated with the increased marrow radiation resulting from PA exposures has been debated. When the AP projection is used, breast shielding must be employed. High speed radiographic films, intensifying screens, beam collimation, modification of radiographic technique, and filters are also used to decrease radiation exposure. Other techniques of radiation reduction, such as digital radiography, are being investigated.

Further reduction in radiation exposure can be achieved by reducing the number of radiographs taken. Avoidance of technical errors will decrease the number of studies repeated because of poor quality or incorrect patient positioning. Better objective criteria for obtaining radiographs at the time of initial presentation are needed. Among the important factors to consider are the magnitude of the body surface changes, skeletal maturity, and the existence of symptoms. The radiographic views should be limited to those that are likely to yield information pertinent to the care of the patient. The optimal frequency of follow-up radiographs should be determined by the likelihood of curve progression and the influence of progression on treatment recommendations.

Magnetic Resonance Imaging

The role of MRI in the evaluation of scoliosis patients is evolving. Syringomyelia, Arnold-Chiari malformation, hydromyelia, spinal cord tumor, tethered spinal cord, diastematomyelia, and intraspinal lipoma have all been identified in scoliosis patients previously presumed idiopathic. Identifying these conditions is important, because in some instances effective treatment is available. Treatment not only directly addresses the identified problem, but also may have a beneficial effect on the course of the scoliosis. Chiari malformation and hydromyelia have been among the more common abnormalities found on MRI of scoliosis patients (Fig. 1). A prospective study of 11 patients younger than 16 years of age, who had scoliosis and Chiari malformations, reported on the course of scoliosis following surgical decompression of the Chiari malformation. The follow-up ranged from 20 to 68 months, with a mean of 35 months. The scoliosis improved in eight, stabilized in one, and increased in two patients. All patients younger than 10 years of age had improvement in their curves. Even when no effective treatment is available, the information gained from the MRI can still be of value in patient management. Curves with a known etiology should not necessarily be expected to mimic the course of idiopathic scoliosis.

It is frequently suggested that all patients with atypical scoliosis be referred for MRI. The problem arises in defining what actually is classified as atypical. It is generally agreed that the typical patient with scoliosis is asymptomatic, female, neurologically normal, adolescent at the time of presentation, and has a right thoracic curve that follows one of several defined typical curve patterns. Neurologic deficit, left thoracic curve, male patient, onset before adolescence, unusually rapid curve progression, lower extremity deformity, and the presence of symptoms have all been proposed as indications for an MRI. In many of the reports describing MRI abnormalities in association with these conditions, the patients studied were those selected from a larger population of scoliosis patients, which makes it difficult to discern the actual incidence of abnormalities associated with these atypical presentations. In a prospective study, 26 consecutive scoliosis patients younger than age 11 were evaluated by MRI. Intraspinal abnormalities were identified in five of the 26 patients. Abnormalities included: Chiari I malformation with hydromyelia, syringomyelia, intramedullary tumor, and terminal lipoma (Fig. 1).

To date, the primary disadvantage of routine MRI is the cost. Even in selected groups of patients, many of the studies are normal. Although the studies are noninvasive, many of the young children require sedation to keep them immobile during the long scanning sequences. The MRI is very sensitive and frequently demonstrates subtle changes. Questions then arise as to the relationship between these findings and the scoliosis. As a result, the potential for unnecessary treatment exists. The scoliotic deformity can make MRI technically demanding. Close collaboration with the involved radiologist, with clear communication of the study goals, is essential. It is important for the images to extend from the brainstem to the lumbar spine. Proper image sequences and orientation are necessary to limit the occurrence of technically inadequate studies.

Despite some limitations, MRI has made a substantial contribution to the treatment and understanding of scoliosis. The high frequency of MRI abnormalities in preadolescent patients increases skepticism on whether

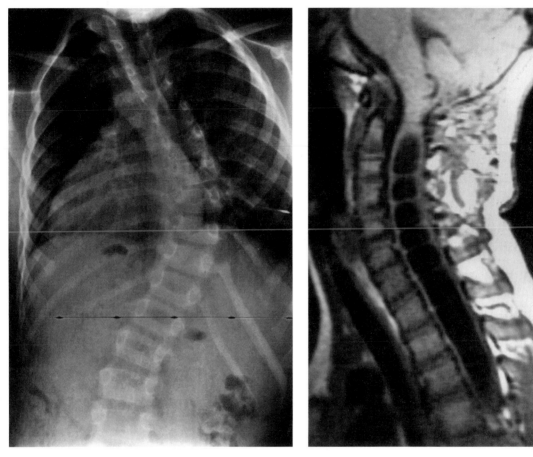

Fig. 1   Left, Spine radiograph of a 10-year-old male with scoliosis. **Right,** MRI of the same patient showing hydromyelia of the spinal cord. The patient was also found to have a Chiari I malformation.

juvenile idiopathic scoliosis is really a distinct diagnosis. Although the precise indications for an MRI are still undefined, it is important to remember when evaluating patients that scoliosis may be the only apparent manifestation of an intraspinal abnormality. Patients who have neurologic abnormalities, even stable ones, or those with features that are felt to be inconsistent with idiopathic scoliosis, should be considered for further study.

Computed Tomography/Myelogram

Computed tomography (CT) is not routinely indicated. When there is a need for better definition of the skeletal anatomy, CT, combined with two- or three-dimensional reconstructions can be of value. Myelography and CT myelography have been replaced by MRI for most indications. There are instances when spinal canal evaluation is indicated postoperatively in patients with stainless steel hardware. Because the hardware limits the effectiveness of the MRI, myelography combined with CT is preferred in these situations.

Scoliosis Screening

The goal of a screening program is to identify any unrecognized disease or defect. The screening test is not intended to be diagnostic, but rather is a method of identifying those patients most likely to be affected by the condition in question. Those found positive by screening are to be referred for diagnosis and, if necessary, treatment of the condition.

School screening for scoliosis has been endorsed by the American Academy of Orthopaedic Surgeons (AAOS) and the Scoliosis Research Society. The AAOS position paper on school screening recommends screening for girls at ages 11 and 13; and for boys, at age 13 or 14. A 1989 publication reported the results of a survey dealing with school screening for spine deformity in North America. Screening was required by law in 15 states, and five states had administrative regulations related to screening. Some form of screening was being conducted in all 50 states and the District of Columbia. The inclinometer was the most commonly used apparatus for screening. Several screening programs began in Canada during the 1970s; but, at the time of the survey, only two provinces were conducting some kind of organized screening. The British Orthopedic Association and the British Scoliosis Society advised against scoliosis screening in a 1983 statement. In a 1993 published statement, the U.S. Preventive Services Task Force concluded that there is insufficient evidence to recommend for or against routine screening for scoliosis.

The World Health Organization has defined principles for a successful screening program. It is helpful to use some of these basic screening guidelines as a framework for exploring in greater depth the controversy that has surrounded these programs.

First, the condition being screened for should be an important problem. The prevalence of scoliosis has been reported to be in the range of 1.9% to 3%. The prevalence of a spinal curve greater than 30° is 0.3%, which indicates that only a small proportion of curves progress. Although the prevalence is low, the reported complications of idiopathic scoliosis have been used to justify the need for school screening. There is controversy regarding the incidence of back pain and related disability in adult scoliosis patients. There are cosmetic and emotional concerns, but these are difficult to measure. Cardiopulmonary problems are associated with only the most severe cases, which constitute a small fraction of the total number of individuals with scoliosis.

Second, the natural history should be understood. Studies that define the natural history of scoliosis in skeletally immature patients allow determination of the probability of curve progression based on several factors. There is no way to determine accurately the prognosis for curve progression in an individual patient. Inability to precisely predict curve progression may result in management dilemmas once the scoliosis is identified. The incomplete knowledge of the natural history has hindered the evaluation of nonsurgical treatment.

Third, there should be a suitable screening test, acceptable to the population being screened. Scoliosis screening tests are based on the identification of body asymmetry. The forward bending test, with or without objective measurement of rotation, is a component of most screening programs. This type of screening is generally well tolerated and easily administered. The specificity and sensitivity are substantially influenced by the guidelines used to determine a positive test. The desire to decrease the false-positive rate, thereby increasing the specificity, has led to the recommendation to raise the angle of trunk inclination necessary for referral from 5° to 7°. The positive predictive value (the probability that scoliosis exists if the test is abnormal) has varied in published reports. Some of the inconsistency is attributed to the minimum Cobb angle used to define true scoliosis. The positive predictive value is lower if a larger minimum angle is used. A potential harmful effect of screening relates to incorrectly labeling people with the diagnosis of scoliosis. Assigning a diagnosis of scoliosis, when in fact there is either no curve or the curve is so small that it is inconsequential, can have a negative impact on employment and future insurance coverage.

Fourth, once the disease is identified, there should be an accepted treatment available. A goal of screening is to allow early identification and nonsurgical treatment, thereby limiting the number of curves requiring surgery. Curves that do require surgery can be identified earlier, which will improve the outcome. The assumption is made that, unless screening is implemented, many asymptomatic people will go unrecognized until very late in the course. The validity of this assumption is questioned, because the number of cases and stage of scoliosis identified without screening have not been well documented. A treatment rate of 2.75 per thousand individuals screened has been reported. A 1981 Swedish study reported a decrease in the number of surgically treated patients due to early detection and awareness of the condition. In a 1993 publication from Sweden, an improvement in outcome following brace treatment (less surgery) was noted after the implementation of screening. This improvement was attributed to the younger skeletal age and smaller curves at the time of initial diagnosis, a result of the screening program. A study from Minnesota, published in 1982, reported a decrease in the number of patients requiring surgery after the development of a comprehensive screening program. The average curve treated surgically decreased from 60° to 42° over the 8 years of the study.

Finally, the program should be cost effective. To establish cost effectiveness, the cost of late diagnosis and related problems must be compared with the cost of the program. Some of the program costs are difficult to determine. It has been shown that the screening itself can be done inexpensively. The study from Minnesota reported the direct screening cost to be 6.6 cents for each student screened. Indirect costs include physician referrals, follow-up visits, treatment, and radiographs. Although the costs associated with follow-up and treatment of positive cases has been estimated, these figures are an inaccurate indication of the actual costs resulting from screening programs.

The reported rate of referral from screening programs has ranged from 3.4% to greater than 30%. Much of this variability is a reflection of the screening method employed and the guidelines for referral. Contrasting these referral rates with the prevalence of scoliosis, the potentially large expense from false positives becomes apparent. In addition, as progression is unpredictable, many cases of true scoliosis have had unnecessary follow-up or treatment, creating another expense that is difficult to evaluate.

In summary, the debate regarding the value of scoliosis screening has not been resolved. The effectiveness of treatment, as it relates to a screening program, assumes that those identified by screening will receive subsequent care. The consistency of this follow up has been questioned. As more information regarding the natural history and effectiveness of nonsurgical treatment becomes available, a more objective evaluation of the issues will be possible.

Annotated Bibliography

Etiology

Geissele ME, Kransdorf MJ, Geyer CA, et al: Magnetic resonance imaging of the brain stem in adolescent idiopathic scoliosis. *Spine* 1991;16:761–763.

MRI was used to study the brain stems of 27 patients with idiopathic scoliosis. The studies obtained were compared to a control group of nonscoliotic patients. The control group comprised 25 females and two males. Brainstem asymmetry was found in seven of the study group patients, and in only one of the 11 controls. The findings of this study add support to the hypothesis of a central nervous system contribution to the etiology of idiopathic scoliosis.

Kindsfater K, Lowe T, Lawellin D, et al: Levels of platelet calmodulin for the prediction of progression and severity of adolescent idiopathic scoliosis. *J Bone Joint Surg* 1994; 76A:1186–1192.

Platelet calmodulin levels were measured in 17 idiopathic scoliosis patients and 10 controls. Calmodulin is a calcium binding receptor protein involved in the regulation of the skeletal muscle and platelet contractile systems. Progressive curves were defined as those which had increased more than 10° in the previous 12 months; and those curves greater than 30°, with 5° of progression in the previous 12 months. Significantly higher levels of platelet calmodulin were found in the patients with progressive curves. A longitudinal study was recommended to determine the clinical usefulness of calmodulin for the prediction of curve progression.

McInnes E, Hill DL, Raso VJ, et al: Vibratory response in adolescents who have idiopathic scoliosis. *J Bone Joint Surg* 1991;73A:1208–1212.

Vibratory thresholds of 14 scoliosis patients were tested with the PVD Bio-Thesiometer and compared with 23 controls. An initial test on four subjects showed that, of the four sites tested, only the first metatarsophalangeal (MTP) joint yielded reproducible results. Vibratory thresholds at the first MTP joint were significantly higher in controls. There was no left to right difference noted for either group. The authors concluded that the lack of a left-right difference makes it unlikely that a posterior column defect is the cause of idiopathic scoliosis.

Patient Evaluation

Beauchamp M, Labelle H, Grimard G, et al: Diurnal variation of Cobb angle measurement in adolescent idiopathic scoliosis. *Spine* 1993;18:1581–1583.

Measurements of the spinal curves of 19 females with idiopathic scoliosis were conducted to investigate the daily variation in curve magnitude. A standing AP radiograph was taken at 8:00 am and was repeated at 4:00 pm on the same day. The mean morning Cobb angle was found to be 60°, with a range of 42° to 91°. In the afternoon, the mean was found to be 65°, with a range of 47° to 87°. Comparison of the measurements taken in the morning and afternoon revealed a statistically significant increase of 5° in the afternoon.

Carman DL, Browne RH, Birch JG: Measurement of scoliosis and kyphosis radiographs: Intraobserver and interobserver variation. *J Bone Joint Surg* 1990;72A:328–333.

Four orthopaedists and one physical therapist measured eight scoliosis and 20 kyphosis radiographs to assess measurement variability. The mean value of the intraobserver variability was 3.8°. Tolerance limits were used to determine that a measurement difference of 10° was necessary to be 95% confident that a true change in the scoliosis had occurred.

Hoffman DA, Lonstein JE, Morin MM, et al: Breast cancer in women with scoliosis exposed to multiple diagnostic x-rays. *J Nat Cancer Inst* 1989;81:1307–1312.

The risk of breast cancer was retrospectively determined for 1,030 women who had been seen for idiopathic scoliosis. There were 973 subjects with usable information. The average follow-up was 25.6 years. There were 11 cases of breast cancer identified, compared with six expected from the population. The risk increased with the number of spinal radiographs and the estimated dose of radiation to the breast. The increased risk was greater after 30 years of follow-up.

Kalmar JA, Jones JP, Merritt CR: Low-dose radiography of scoliosis in children: A comparison of methods. *Spine* 1994;19:818–823.

The quality of 1,582 radiographic images of children with scoliosis was evaluated using a low dose computed radiography system. The diagnostic quality images obtained were made with radiation doses 5% or less than those needed for conventional film screen systems. A major shortcoming of this processing system is the costly hardware.

Lewonowski K, King JD, Nelson MD: Routine use of magnetic resonance imaging in idiopathic scoliosis patients less than eleven years of age. *Spine* 1992;17 (suppl 6):S109–S116.

Twenty-six consecutive idiopathic scoliosis patients younger than 11 years of age underwent MRI to evaluate them for intraspinal pathology. The neurologic examination was normal in all patients. Spinal cord abnormalities were found in five patients. The abnormalities included: Chiari I malformation with hydromyelia, syringomyelia, intramedullary tumor, and terminal lipoma. The authors recommend routine MRI evaluation for all individuals younger than age 11 with presumed idiopathic scoliosis.

Little DG, Sussman MD: The Risser sign: A critical analysis. *J Pediatr Orthop* 1994;14:569–575.

The existing literature was assessed to evaluate the use of the Risser sign as an indication of skeletal age. Critical statistical analysis was used to assess the validity of the conclusions in the studies. The authors concluded that the literature does not support the use of the Risser sign as an accurate predictor of skeletal age or the end of curve progression. Risser 4 was not found to be a reliable indicator that spinal growth had been completed.

Morrissy RT, Goldsmith GS, Hall EC, et al: Measurement of the Cobb angle on radiographs of patients who have scoliosis: Evaluation of intrinsic error. *J Bone Joint Surg* 1990;72A:320–327.

Interobserver and intraobserver measurement variability was assessed for the measurement of scoliosis radiographs using the

Cobb technique. Fifty AP radiographs were measured by four orthopaedic surgeons. The interobserver variability was found to be 7.2°, decreasing to 6.3° when the endpoints were preselected. The intraobserver variability was 4.9° without endpoint selection. This study examined only intrinsic variability. Extrinsic factors, such as patient position and radiographic technique, could increase this variability in the clinical setting.

Muhonen MG, Menezes AH, Sawin PD, et al: Scoliosis in pediatric Chiari malformations without myelodysplasia. *J Neurosurg* 1992;77:69–77.

A prospective study was undertaken to better understand how the surgical manipulation of hindbrain herniation affected abnormal spinal curvature. Eleven patients younger than 16 years of age with Chiari malformation and scoliosis of at least 15° were studied. The mean curve angle at the time of original treatment was 29°. The most common presenting signs were myelopathy and weakness. Surgical intervention consisted of a posterior fossa decompression in all patients. The scoliosis improved in eight patients, stabilized in one, and progressed in two. Only one child required postoperative spinal fusion and instrumentation for progression of scoliosis.

Schwend RM, Hennrikus W, Hall JE, et al: Childhood scoliosis: Clinical indications for magnetic resonance imaging. *J Bone Joint Surg* 1995;77A:46–53.

MRI studies were reviewed for 95 patients who had idiopathic scoliosis. The average age at the time of imaging study was 13 years. The average curve was 41°. Fourteen patients were seen to have an intraspinal abnormality on the imaging study: 12 had a syrinx, one had a syrinx and an astrocytoma of the spinal cord, and one had dural ectasia. Five of the eight patients who were younger than 11 years old and who had a left thoracic curve had an intraspinal abnormality on the imaging study. Four of the intraspinal abnormalities in the 14 patients necessitated neurosurgical intervention.

Scoliosis Screening

Bunnell WP: An objective criterion for scoliosis screening. *J Bone Joint Surg* 1984;66A:1381–1387.

The angle of trunk inclination determined from an inclinometer and the Cobb angle were compared for 1,065 patients referred from screening programs. The mean trunk rotation for patients with a 20° Cobb angle was 7°. The angle of trunk rotation and the Cobb angle correlated well. Screening with this technique was found to have a high degree of sensitivity.

Bunnell WP: Outcome of spinal screening. *Spine* 1993; 18:1572–1580.

The trunk rotation angle of 1,000 physically mature high school students was measured with the scoliometer. The results were then compared with existing natural history information and a previous report relating Cobb angle to the angle of trunk rotation measured with the scoliometer. Trunk rotation of 3° or more was found in 80% of the students. The prevalence and severity of trunk rotation was the same for males and females. Using 5° of trunk rotation as the referral criterion would result in 12% referral rate. Referrals would decrease to 3% with a referral criterion of 7°. Costs and current trends in treatment were considered. The author recommends a trunk rotation angle of 7° or more as a guideline for referral.

Lonstein JE, Bjorklund S, Wanninger MH, et al: Voluntary school screening for scoliosis in Minnesota. *J Bone Joint Surg* 1982;64A:481–488.

Eight years of the scoliosis school screening program in Minnesota was retrospectively reviewed. The referral rate from the screening program was 3.4%. Scoliosis was found in 1.2% of those screened. The number of surgical cases and mean curve at the time of surgery declined over the period studied. The cost of the program was low. The authors concluded that the program was efficient and cost effective.

Montgomery F, Willner S: Screening for idiopathic scoliosis: Comparison of 90 cases shows less surgery by early diagnosis. *Acta Orthop Scand* 1993;64:456–458.

In a review of 90 cases from Sweden, outcome of brace treatment instituted during a period of time prior to school screening was compared with a period after screening. Eighty-nine of the patients were brace treated. The demand for surgery decreased from 45% to 10% after the institution of the screening. The decrease in the demand for surgery was attributed to the lower skeletal age and smaller curve at diagnosis, a result of the screening program.

US Preventive Services Task Force: Review article: Screening for adolescent idiopathic scoliosis. *JAMA* 1993;269:2667–2672.

A summary of the existing literature regarding screening for adolescent idiopathic scoliosis is presented by the U.S. Preventive Services Task Force. The authors found the evidence regarding the outcome of screening to be inconclusive. The task force was not able to make a recommendation either for or against screening. Further clinical research to demonstrate the effectiveness of school screening is advocated.

12

Idiopathic Scoliosis: Natural History and Nonsurgical Management

Natural History

Accurate natural history information is essential for determining the most appropriate management of patients and for evaluating the effectiveness of nonsurgical treatment. Access to large numbers of untreated patients is limited, which makes it difficult to complete long-term natural history studies. The influence of study design on the outcome should be considered when interpreting the results. Retrospective studies of the natural history have a tendency to focus on large curves and to underrepresent small to mild curves. Many of the early long-term follow-up studies included patients with scoliosis of mixed etiologies. The minimum curve size used to define scoliosis can influence observed rates of progression in the sample. In addition, the classification of a curve as progressive must take into account the variability of the measurement technique employed.

Idiopathic Scoliosis Prior to Skeletal Maturity

For curves presenting after infancy, the natural history before skeletal maturity differs greatly from that after the completion of growth. Relatively few studies have evaluated the natural history of curves prior to skeletal maturity. The probability of curve progression is the primary consideration in determining treatment indications for this group of patients. Several factors have been examined for their influence on curve progression prior to skeletal maturity.

Progression of scoliosis is known to be associated with growth. The exact mechanism by which this change occurs is still debated. Several studies have shown that curves at greatest risk for progression are those that present at an early age. Late onset curves, such as those detected after the onset of puberty, are less likely to have significant progression. In one study, patients diagnosed between the ages of 10 and 12 had an 88% risk of their curves progressing at least 5°; for those aged 12 to 15, the risk was 56%; and for those over 15 years, it was 29%. In another study, the overall frequency of curve progression at age 10 was 50%, and at age 13, it was 21%.

Determination of skeletal maturity is often helpful in the prediction of curve progression. The onset of puberty is associated with a rapid increase in spinal growth velocity. Menarche occurs after the peak velocity has already been reached. For females, the mean period between the onset of iliac ossification and Risser 4 is 1 year. Risser 4 is generally considered to be an indication of the end of spinal growth in females. For males, it is a less reliable indication, with iliac ossification occurring relatively earlier with respect to continuing growth. There is a much higher probability of curve progression for patients Risser 0 or 1, when compared with those Risser 2 to 5.

Although bone age can be helpful in identifying discrepancies between skeletal and chronological age, it can be misleading in the prediction of spinal growth. The timing of spinal and long bone growth differ. Spinal growth has been observed after documentation of skeletal maturity on wrist and hand radiographs.

Curves that are larger at the time of detection are also at greater risk for progression. In one study, the probability of progression for curves 20° or larger was more than twice that for smaller curves. In another study, the average nonprogressive curve was 15°, and the average progressive curve was 20°. Progression of 5° or more occurred in 78% of curves between 40° and 50°, compared with 52% of curves between 20° and 30°. Progression of 10° or more in these two groups averaged 67% and 30%, respectively.

Although a relationship between curve type and progression is acknowledged, comparison between studies is difficult because of discrepancies in the classification systems used. In general, thoracic curves present earlier and are more likely to progress than lumbar curves. Double curves progress more frequently than single curves. One study reported that, in double (thoracic and lumbar) curves that worsened, the thoracic curve progressed in 25%, the lumbar curve progressed in 43%, and both curves progressed in 32%.

The female-to-male ratio increases for larger curves, but there is conflicting information regarding the influence of gender on the probability of progression once a curve is identified. Scoliosis in males can develop later and progress longer than in females. Follow-up on male adolescents with idiopathic scoliosis is recommended until Risser 5. A study of patients identified in school screening reported that for curves of at least 11°, 15% of the females and 4% of the males had at least 5° of progression. Conversely, a higher likelihood of male progression has been reported in other studies. Finally, in other studies, no difference between genders was reported. This lack of consistency may be a reflection of the small number of males in most natural history studies.

Most studies show no correlation between family history and risk of progression. A study of the influence of parental age on scoliosis found that maternal age 27 years or older at the time of the patient's birth correlated with a larger eventual curve.

Thus, for young patients with scoliosis, the major factors that influence curve progression are skeletal maturity, curve magnitude, and curve type. In the clinical setting, combinations of these factors are useful in assessing the probability of progression. As an example, curves of 20° to 29° in patients Risser 0 or 1 have a 68% probability of curve progression of 5° or more. For the same curves, the risk of progression for patients Risser 2 to 4 is only 23%. Family history, spinal rotation, and gender generally are not helpful in predicting progression.

Idiopathic Scoliosis After Skeletal Maturity

In addition to curve progression, the probability of functional impairment is a concern in adults with idiopathic scoliosis. The effects of scoliosis during adulthood have a major impact on the management of this deformity in adolescence. Surgery is frequently offered to adolescent patients who are likely to experience progression during adulthood, in an effort to limit future disability. The following information is useful in counseling young patients on the probability of encountering problems related to their scoliosis.

Progression in adults tends to be much slower than that observed in adolescents. Curves less than 30° at skeletal maturity, regardless of the curve pattern, are unlikely to progress. However, 68% of curves greater than 50° at maturity will worsen progressively. Thoracic curves between 50° and 75° progress nearly a degree per year. Lumbar curves greater than 30° are likely to progress and may have translatory shifts. A fifth lumbar vertebra seated below the intercrest line is protective against translatory shifting. The observed progression of right lumbar curves is twice that observed for left lumbar curves.

Progression related to pregnancy has been reported in patients with unstable curves and in women who have multiple pregnancies before age 23. Most studies, however, indicate that there is little or no relationship between pregnancy and curve progression. Three hundred fifty-five skeletally mature idiopathic scoliosis patients were reviewed to examine the effects of pregnancy on curve progression. Patients were divided into two groups, based on whether or not they had been pregnant. In both groups, spinal curve progression of at least 10° was noted in 10% of the patients. No significant correlation was found between age at first pregnancy and curve progression. Pregnancy and delivery complications, including cesarean section, have been reported in proportions similar to the average for nonscoliotic patients. In general, it is believed that mild to moderate idiopathic scoliosis has no negative effect on pregnancy or delivery.

Cardiopulmonary compromise is uncommon and symptoms, if they appear, are usually late. Most adolescents with idiopathic scoliosis have normal or near-normal lung volume. Restrictive lung disease is the pulmonary impairment associated with scoliosis. During childhood, even those with a measured decrease in pulmonary function tend to be asymptomatic. Pulmonary symptoms and decreased vital capacity correlate positively with the severity of the thoracic curve. Marked diminution of pulmonary function in nonsmokers does not occur until the thoracic

curve approaches 100°. There is no correlation between lumbar or thoracolumbar curves and pulmonary impairment. A study of 79 adolescent idiopathic scoliosis patients, who had a mean curve of 45°, found a reduction in work capacity, unrelated to the nature or extent of spinal deformity. The authors concluded that physical activity should be encouraged for scoliosis patients, to maintain and improve peripheral muscle and cardiovascular conditioning. In a study that sought to identify risk factors for respiratory failure, only patients with vital capacity less than 45% of predicted, and a Cobb angle greater than 110°, were at risk for subsequent failure. This respiratory failure was believed to be the result of age-related diminution of pulmonary function in an already compromised individual. Hypokyphosis further contributes to a decrease in pulmonary function.

Early estimates of mortality associated with scoliosis described rates much higher than those predicted for the general population. These studies overestimated the death rate due to idiopathic scoliosis because they included patients with scoliosis of other etiologies. A more recent study from Sweden again demonstrated an increase in the mortality rate for a group of scoliosis patients. However, when the adolescent idiopathic scoliosis patients were examined separately, it was found that this group was not at increased risk when compared with the expected mortality rates in the general population. Although there are individual exceptions, as a group, patients with adolescent idiopathic scoliosis are not at increased risk for early death.

Many studies of back pain report a greater than 50% occurrence in the general population. In most studies, the incidence of back pain associated with scoliosis does not differ significantly from that observed in the normal population. Differences in the characteristics of back pain have been associated with scoliosis. Reports have described pain along the convexity and concavity of the curve, as well as paraspinal and interscapular pain. Patients with thoracic curves are less likely to experience back pain than are patients who have other types of curves. One study reported that the incidence of pain was associated with age and curve severity. Degenerative changes do not correlate with the severity of the curve or with back pain. As a group, the daily function of adult idiopathic scoliosis patients is similar to that of the general population.

Cosmetic concerns related to scoliosis are frequently expressed by patients, but are difficult to measure objectively. Patients claim to be more self-conscious during their teenage and early adult years than when older. One study showed a positive correlation between the degree of psychological handicap and clinical deformity, a finding that has been disputed by others. Severe psychological reactions to scoliosis requiring treatment are unlikely.

Nonsurgical Management

Most patients with an established diagnosis of adolescent idiopathic scoliosis do not require treatment. The percentage who do varies among published reports, and is influenced by the composition of the study population, minimum curve size used to define the scoliosis, and the length of follow-up. A major study, which looked at patients identified through school screening, reported that 6.8% of those with scoliosis required treatment. Nevertheless, periodic observation is necessary to monitor for curve progression.

Multiple factors must be considered when determining the ideal time interval between visits. Progression is not the sole concern; what the progression will mean in relation to the management of the patient must also be considered. Skeletal maturity is important, because the potential for further growth has a great influence on the risk of progression. More frequent follow-up will be required if curve progression results in a change in treatment. For example, an immature patient, who may need bracing if further progression occurs, may need to be reevaluated within 4 months. On the other hand, a much longer follow-up interval is suitable for someone with a small curve, for which more progression could be accepted without changing the management plan. Skeletally mature patients can be allowed a much longer interval between visits because progression, when it occurs, is at a much slower rate. Predetermined guidelines that apply to all cases have not been established. Decisions regarding the follow-up interval must be individualized, with careful consideration of the many pertinent factors.

The need for radiographs influences the follow-up interval. The ability to monitor patients according to body surface changes has been limited by the lack of correlation between these changes and the Cobb angle. Natural history data and thresholds for treatment are based on the Cobb angle. If accurate determination of the Cobb angle is critical to patient management, radiographs are a necessity. The number of radiographs should be minimized. Occasionally, it is possible to monitor body surface changes for smaller curves using a scoliometer. A radiograph is then requested if a significant change is noted.

The Milwaukee brace was first introduced as a method of postoperative immobilization. Its use was later extended to the nonsurgical management of scoliosis. As bracing evolved, there was a desire to produce better tolerated and, in some cases, less expensive braces. This resulted in the development of lower profile braces constructed without a suprastructure, such as the Boston, Wilmington, Miami, and Charleston. The concept of the Boston brace was to have a prefabricated design, which could be modified to fit the individual patient. The Wilmington brace was constructed from a thermoplastic material molded to a plaster positive mold from a cast of the patient. The Charleston bending brace, designed to conform to a side-bending patient, is for nighttime use.

Early Milwaukee braces had a mandibular support, which was found to cause dental problems, and was later replaced by a neck ring. Computer simulations have shown that lateral forces are primarily responsible for correction, with longitudinal traction playing a minor role.

Some of the correction has been attributed to the role of active muscle forces. In a study using electromyograms to assess muscle activity, the difference between braced and unbraced activity was not significant, leading to the conclusion that muscle forces were not a major factor contributing to brace correction of scoliosis. The reduction of lumbar lordosis resulting from bracing is also believed to contribute to curve correction.

The goal of brace treatment is to control curve progression. Suitable candidates for bracing must fit the profile of the patient at risk for progression. Natural history studies, and other studies evaluating the effects of bracing, have clarified the indications for brace treatment. Patients should be skeletally immature (Risser 0, 1, or 2), have a curve in the range of 20° to 40°, have a deformity that they consider cosmetically acceptable, and be willing to accept brace treatment. Patients classified as Risser 3 and 4 do not have enough growth remaining to make them suitable candidates for bracing. Even if progression has not been demonstrated, curves between 30° and 40° in immature patients should be braced upon presentation. Those between 20° and 30° can be observed. If curve progression of 5° or more occurs in this group, brace treatment should be initiated. Documenting progression will avoid unnecessary treatment. This decision to delay treatment must be individualized, especially for curves between 25° and 30°. Because brace treatment is effective in managing smaller curves, some authors advocate initiating bracing for curves of 25° or more, when the patient is Risser 0. Significant spinal decompensation, even if the curve magnitude is not large enough to meet the usual guidelines, is a relative indication for brace treatment. Most studies concur that bracing is ineffective in controlling larger curves, especially those greater than 45°. Low profile braces may be used for curves with the apex at T7 or below.

Bracing is contraindicated for patients who do not meet the described prerequisites. Thoracic lordosis and hypokyphosis are considered relative contraindications. Adolescents adamantly opposed to bracing, despite counseling on the issues, cannot realistically be expected to comply with bracing.

After the brace is fitted, an in-brace radiograph is compared with the initial radiograph. If adequate correction is not achieved, brace adjustments are needed to maximize correction. Studies have shown that curves that correct by 50% or more in the brace are more likely to have a positive response.

The optimal number of hours a brace should be worn each day is controversial. The standard recommendation in the past was for the brace to be worn full-time, which was defined as 23 hours per day. However, satisfactory outcomes were observed when patients partially complied with bracing, and this has been interpreted as an indication that part-time bracing would be as effective as full time. This issue remains unresolved. Exercise, initially considered an integral component of the bracing regimen, has since been shown to be ineffective. Patients in braces should be monitored periodically to assess for brace-

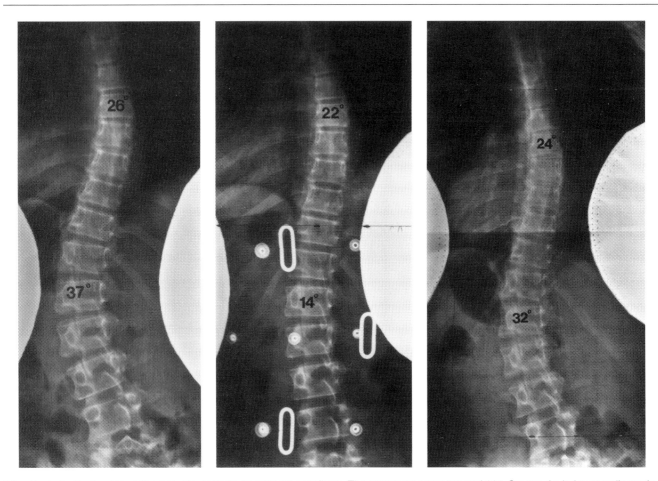

Fig. 1 **Left,** Pre-bracing radiograph of a patient with idiopathic scoliosis. The curves measure 37° and 26°. **Center,** An in-brace radiograph of the same patient, demonstrating correction of the curves to 22° and 14°. **Right,** A 5-year follow-up radiograph of the same patient. There has been some loss of the initial correction achieved in the brace, but the curves remain less than that observed on the pre-bracing radiograph.

related problems, growth, and clinical changes. It is generally unnecessary to radiograph patients at every visit. A 4- to 6-month interval has been mentioned as a reasonable frequency for follow-up visits, but the final determination should be made on an individual basis. Bracing should be continued until skeletal maturity (Risser 4) (Fig. 1). Weaning from the brace has been advocated, but the value of weaning prior to discontinuing bracing has not been established in the literature.

There have been numerous reports examining the efficacy of brace treatment. Despite evidence supporting this form of treatment, bracing remains quite controversial. Studies are often criticized for the lack of suitable control patients, short follow-up, and the composition of the study group. To be successful, bracing must positively alter the natural history of scoliosis. As noted, not all patients with scoliosis have curve progression. The sample population must be composed of patients truly at risk for progression, and it must be large enough to demonstrate that, as a

group, patients have had a course that differs from the natural history. Differences in sample composition, length of follow-up, and grouping of curve types are among the factors that make study comparisons difficult.

A recent long-term follow-up of 1,020 patients compared the outcome of patients treated with a Milwaukee brace with the natural history as defined in an earlier series from the same institution. Failure was defined as progression of 5° or more. For curves of 20° to 39°, the rate of failure was less than that observed in the natural history study. A Risser sign of 0 or 1, or a curve measuring 30° or more at the time bracing is initiated were factors that increased the likelihood of surgery being necessary. As is also true in other series, loss of the correction initially achieved in the brace occurred with follow-up.

In a 1990 retrospective review of 76 adolescent idiopathic scoliosis patients treated with a Wilmington brace for curves ranging from 20° to 39°, curve progression of 5° or more was observed in 28%. This compares favorably with published natural history data. There was a minimum follow-up of 5 years from the conclusion of bracing for those patients not treated surgically. The authors of this study conclude that the Wilmington brace appears to be an acceptable alternative to the Milwaukee brace for the nonsurgical treatment of adolescent scoliosis. In an earlier study, the Wilmington brace was also shown to improve pretreatment lateral trunk shift.

A study of 295 patients treated with a Boston brace found that young age and larger pretreatment curves increased the probability of surgery. Bracing for curves greater than 40° had a high rate of failure. A strong correlation between best in-brace correction and follow-up correction was observed. The results suggest that the Boston brace is beneficial. In a more recent study, 32 patients treated with a Boston brace were compared with 32 paired untreated patients from a separate institution. All patients were Risser 0. Follow-up terminated when patients were weaned from the brace. No statistically significant difference in curve progression was found between the two groups. The small number of patients and the short follow-up are weaknesses of this study.

An important recent prospective study supported by the Scoliosis Research Society compared adolescent patients with idiopathic scoliosis who were braced with untreated adolescents who also had idiopathic scoliosis. There were 129 observed and 111 braced patients. Forty-six patients were treated with electrical surface stimulation. The method of management was determined by the preference of the ten centers involved. Follow-up was incomplete for 14% of the patients. Failure was defined as progression of 6° or more observed on two consecutive radiographs. Bracing was found to have a significant beneficial effect on curve progression, even if all patients with incomplete follow-up were considered failures. As would be expected, there was no difference in curve progression between patients who were observed and those who received electrical stimulation. This study did not address the effect of nonsurgical treatment on the probability of surgery.

The Charleston brace is designed to bend the trunk toward the convexity of the curve being treated, thus correcting the deformity (Fig. 2). It is intended for nighttime use, which makes it less of a burden for patients. The results of treatment with this brace are preliminary. One study reported less than 5° of curve progression for 83% of the 139 patients treated with the brace. Patients included in this study were Risser 0, 1, or 2 and had curves between 25° and 49°. Double major curves are a special concern, because the side bending that corrects one curve could accentuate the curve in the opposite direction. The authors recommend accepting a minimum of 50% correction in the structural curve being addressed with the side bending, and no increase in the associated compensatory curve while in the brace. It is also advised that double major curves be examined closely, and that the patient be switched to another form of bracing if initial brace correction is not satisfactory.

Compliance with the prescribed bracing schedule is

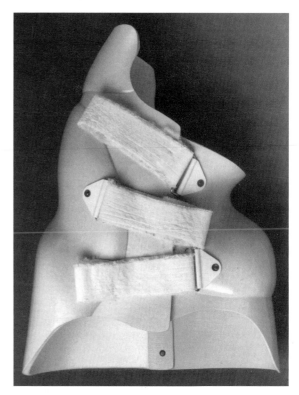

Fig. 2 A Charleston bending brace. This brace is generally recommended for use at night.

often difficult to assess when managing patients. One study evaluating brace compliance found that only 15% of the patients wore the brace at least 90% of the recommended time. For the entire group, the average wear was 65% of the recommended time. Grade school children had a higher rate of compliance than adolescents. A study utilizing a transducer to monitor compliance found that the time actually in the brace was much lower than that reported by the patients. In a study of the Boston brace, the results of those treated in a brace with a superstructure were compared with those treated in a brace without a superstructure. Contrary to expectations, there was no difference in compliance between the two groups.

In an assessment of the long-term functional and social impact of Milwaukee brace treatment, the braced and control groups were found to be similar. A lower frequency of low back pain was observed in those patients who had been treated with the brace. The decrease in patients' pulmonary function observed while a thoracolumbosacral orthosis was being worn returned to normal after removal of the brace. When measured in the brace, adaptive changes in breathing pattern have been observed after several months of bracing. Reduction in glomerular filtration rate (GFR), effective renal plasma flow (ERPF), and urinary sodium secretion have all been noted shortly after application of the Boston brace. It was postulated that these changes were the result of reduction in the transverse section area of the body caused by the brace. It is unlikely that there is long-term clinical significance of these observed changes in renal function. Other complications related to bracing include skin ulceration or hypersensitivity and exacerbation of lordosis.

Brace-related psychological changes are frequently mentioned as a concern. Patients able to adapt to bracing have been found to have measurable psychological differences from those who fail to adapt. Routine psychological counseling for brace users is not recommended.

Other nonsurgical treatments have included lateral electrical surface stimulation (LESS), which was introduced in 1977. This device sought to achieve active curve correction through intermittent transcutaneous muscle stimulation on the convex side. This alternative to bracing was designed for use at night. Although early reports on the results of patients treated with LESS were encouraging, numerous subsequent studies have shown that treatment with LESS results in a course that parallels the disease's natural history. This discrepancy in results has been attributed to the selection of patients at low risk for progression, and to short follow-up in the early studies. Surface stimulation is no longer considered an effective method for the management of scoliosis.

Implantable electrical stimulation has also been attempted. Here, too, the early studies by the originators reported successful treatment of patients. A subsequent study of the same patients, by investigators not involved in the design of the device, failed to demonstrate effectiveness. Physical therapy and manipulation have not been shown to alter the natural history of idiopathic scoliosis.

Annotated Bibliography

Natural History

Dhar S, Dangerfield PH, Dorgan JC, et al: Correlation between bone age and Risser's sign in adolescent idiopathic scoliosis. *Spine* 1993;18:14–19.

Status of iliac apophysis development was compared with bone age assessed by wrist and hand radiographs, using the Turner and Whitehouse II systems. The study sample consisted of 86 females with idiopathic scoliosis ranging in age from 10 to 18 years. A significant correlation between the two methods was noted.

Henderson MH Jr, Rieger MA, Miller F, et al: Influence of parental age on degree of curvature in idiopathic scoliosis. *J Bone Joint Surg* 1990;72A:910–913.

The curves of 177 adolescents with idiopathic scoliosis were measured to determine the effect of maternal age at the time of birth on curve severity. Follow-up was from the time of initial diagnoses until skeletal maturity (mean age of 18.2 years). Curves of adolescents whose mothers were 27 years of age or older at the time of the patient's birth (mean curves of 35.2°) were compared with curves of those whose mothers were younger than 27 years of age at that time (mean curves of 30.4°). Using an unpaired *t*-test to compare group means, a significant difference was found.

Howell FR, Mahood JK, Dickson RA: Growth beyond skeletal maturity. *Spine* 1992;17:437–440.

Growth after skeletal maturity was examined in a group of patients identified as having truncal asymmetry on a forward bending test. Scoliosis was defined as a Cobb angle of 10° or more. Skeletal maturity was determined from hand and wrist radiographs. Standing and sitting heights were measured using the Harpenden standiometer. Increases in sitting height were found after skeletal maturity in both scoliotic and nonscoliotic patients, indicating growth after skeletal maturity for both groups. The authors conclude that these findings may account for the progression of idiopathic scoliosis after skeletal maturity.

Karol LA, Johnston CE II, Browne RH, et al: Progression of the curve in boys who have idiopathic scoliosis. *J Bone Joint Surg* 1993;75A:1804–1810.

Curve progression was evaluated by retrospectively reviewing the initial and most recent radiographs of 210 male idiopathic scoliosis patients. Progression was defined as an increase in Cobb angle of 10° or more. Curves that were larger at the time of presentation were more likely to progress. Fifteen percent of the Risser 4 patients had curve progression. Based on these findings, follow-up to Risser 5 was recommended for males with idiopathic scoliosis.

Kearon C, Viviani GR, Killian KJ: Factors influencing work capacity in adolescent idiopathic thoracic scoliosis. *Am Rev Respir Dis* 1993;148:295–303.

A cross-sectional study of 79 adolescent idiopathic scoliosis patients with a mean curve of 45° was conducted to determine the influence of spinal deformity, pulmonary impairment, and muscular function on work capacity. The cardiorespiratory response to exercise and an incremental cycle test to measure work capacity were compared to those of normal subjects. Significant reduction in work capacity, unrelated to the nature and extent of spinal deformity ($p > 0.05$) was found in the idiopathic group. The authors conclude that disability exists in individuals with mild to moderate idiopathic scoliosis and suggest that physical activity be encouraged in these patients to maintain and improve peripheral muscle and cardiovascular conditioning.

Lonstein JE, Carlson JM: The prediction of curve progression in untreated idiopathic scoliosis during growth. *J Bone Joint Surg* 1984;66A:1061–1071.

Curve progression in 727 patients with idiopathic scoliosis was evaluated. Progression of 5° or more was observed in 23.2% of the patients. The risk of progression for curves of 20° to 29° in patients Risser 0 or 1 was 68%. Progression was found to be related to curve pattern, curve magnitude, age at presentation,

Risser sign, and menarchal status. A method of calculating a progression factor was described.

Pehrsson K, Bake B, Larsson S, et al: Lung function in adult idiopathic scoliosis: A 20-year follow-up. *Thorax* 1991;46:474–478.

Twenty-four of 45 idiopathic scoliosis patients previously studied in 1968 were re-examined in 1988 to assess changes in lung function and risk factors for respiratory failure. The age of the patients in the initial study ranged from 15 to 67 years. The range in the spinal curves was 10° to 190°. None of the patients in the follow-up group had been treated with a spinal fusion. As a group, only age-predicted changes were found. Respiratory failure occurred only in patients with spinal curves greater than 110° and vital capacities below 45% of predicted levels. No curve progression was observed in the patients with respiratory failure. The respiratory failure was believed to result from a decrease in function due to age, coupled with pre-existing pulmonary compromise.

Pehrsson K, Larsson S, Oden A, et al: Long term follow-up of patients with untreated scoliosis: A study of mortality, causes of death, and symptoms. *Spine* 1992;17:1091–1096.

The cause of death for 115 of the 130 consecutive patients who were seen for scoliosis between 1927 and 1937 was investigated in Sweden. Overall, the mortality rate of the group was found to be greater than that predicted by the Swedish statistics for mortality. The mortality rate for patients with adolescent idiopathic scoliosis was found to be the same as expected for the general population. A statistically significant increase in the mortality rate was identified for those patients with infantile and juvenile idiopathic scoliosis.

Rogala EJ, Drummond DS, Gurr J: Scoliosis: Incidence and natural history. A prospective epidemiological study. *J Bone Joint Surg* 1978;60A:173–176.

The incidence and natural history of scoliosis was determined by examining radiographs of individuals referred from school screening programs. The incidence of idiopathic scoliosis of 6° or greater in the 26,947 students was determined to be 4.5%. The female-to-male ratio for the entire group was 1.25 to 1, increasing to 5.4 to 1 for those with curves greater than 20°. For those with follow-up data, progression was found in 6.8%. Progression occurred in 15.4% of females with a curve of 10° or greater on initial radiograph.

Weinstein SL, Ponseti IV: Curve progression in idiopathic scoliosis. *J Bone Joint Surg* 1983;65A:447–455.

Curve progression was evaluated for 102 patients with idiopathic scoliosis followed for an average of 40.5 years. Progression after skeletal maturity was greatest for curves greater than 50°, especially thoracic curves. Curves less than 30° at skeletal maturity tended to be stable. Other factors influencing progression were described.

Nonsurgical Management

Bassett GS, Bunnell WP, MacEwen GD: Treatment of idiopathic scoliosis with the Wilmington brace: Results in patients with a twenty to thirty-nine-degree curve. *J Bone Joint Surg* 1986;68A:602–605.

The results of Wilmington Brace treatment for 79 patients with idiopathic scoliosis, Risser 0 or 1, and Cobb angle 20° to 39° were reported in this study. Curve progression of 5° or more was observed in 28%, an improvement when compared with the

existing natural history data. Eleven percent of patients were subsequently treated with a fusion. A gradual loss of initial in-brace correction was observed. The authors concluded that the Wilmington Brace altered the natural history of scoliosis for this group of patients.

Emans JB, Kaelin A, Bancel P, et al: The Boston bracing system for idiopathic scoliosis: Follow-up results in 295 patients. *Spine* 1986;11:792–801.

The use of the Boston brace for treatment of idiopathic scoliosis in 295 patients was retrospectively reviewed. The curves ranged from 20° to 59° and the mean pre-bracing age was 13.2 years. Patients were followed for at least 1 year after the completion of bracing. Progression of 5° or more was observed in 7%. Twelve percent of the patients were treated surgically. There was a strong correlation between in-brace correction and correction observed at follow-up. The larger pre-bracing curves were more likely to require surgery.

Goldberg CJ, Dowling FE, Hall JE, et al: A statistical comparison between natural history of idiopathic scoliosis and brace treatment in skeletally immature adolescent girls. *Spine* 1993;18:902–908.

This prospective study addresses the effectiveness of bracing for altering the natural history of idiopathic scoliosis. Thirty-two adolescent girls treated with a brace were compared with a matched control group from another medical center on the basis of curve size, curve type, and age at diagnosis. All participants in the study were classified as Risser 0 at the time of bracing. No statistically significant difference in curve progression was found between the two groups. All of the girls who had progression of 10° or more were premenarchal. The authors indicate that, although this study is not definitive, it does raise questions about the efficacy of bracing.

Lonstein JE, Winter RB: The Milwaukee brace for the treatment of adolescent idiopathic scoliosis: A review of one thousand and twenty patients. *J Bone Joint Surg* 1994;76A:1207–1221.

The course of 1,020 patients treated with a Milwaukee brace for idiopathic scoliosis was retrospectively reviewed. Curve progression was compared with the previously reported natural history of idiopathic scoliosis observed in a group of patients with comparable curves from the same institution. Factors influencing curve progression were analyzed. The authors conclude the Milwaukee brace altered the natural history, effectively controlling progression of 20° to 39° curves in this group of patients.

Nachemson AL, Peterson LE: Effectiveness of treatment with a brace in girls who have adolescent idiopathic scoliosis: A prospective, controlled study based on data from the Brace Study of the Scoliosis Research Society. *J Bone Joint Surg* 1995;77A:815–822.

This prospective study, involving 10 centers, compared patients with treated and untreated adolescent idiopathic scoliosis. There were 129 observed and 111 braced patients. Forty-six patients were treated with electrical stimulation. The method of management was determined by center preference. Follow-up was incomplete on 14% of the patients. Failure was defined as 6° or more of progression observed on two consecutive radiographs. Bracing was found to have a significant effect on curve progression, even if all patients with incomplete follow-up were considered failures. There was no difference in curve progression between the electrical stimulation and observation groups.

O'Donnell CS, Bunnell WP, Betz RR, et al: Electrical stimulation in the treatment of idiopathic scoliosis. *Clin Orthop* 1988;229:107–113.

The results of surface electrical stimulation for the treatment of 62 patents with idiopathic scoliosis were retrospectively reviewed. The patients were Risser 0, 1, or 2, with curves between 20° and 39°. The rate of failure was higher than the failure rated reported in orthotic studies. After comparing the results to the natural history previously reported, the authors concluded that electrical stimulation did not alter the natural history.

Piazza MR, Bassett GS: Curve progression after treatment with the Wilmington brace for idiopathic scoliosis. *J Pediatr Orthop* 1990;10:39–43.

The records and radiographs of 76 idiopathic scoliosis patients treated with a Wilmington brace were retrospectively reviewed. There was a minimum follow-up of 5 years from the conclusion of bracing for those patients not treated surgically. Pretreatment curves were between 20° and 39°. Twenty-nine percent had progression of 5° or more, which compared favorably with the reported natural history data. Sixteen patients (21%) experienced 5° to 16° of curve progression after bracing was discontinued. For nine of these 16 patients, the progression reflected a loss of correction that had been achieved with bracing. The authors conclude that the Wilmington brace appears to be an acceptable alternative to the Milwaukee brace for treatment of adolescent idiopathic scoliosis.

Price CT, Scott DS, Reed FE Jr, et al: Nighttime bracing for adolescent idiopathic scoliosis with the Charleston bending brace: Preliminary report. *Spine* 1990;15:1294–1299.

This preliminary study reports the outcome for 139 patients following treatment of adolescent idiopathic scoliosis with a Charleston bending brace. Brace wear was recommended for nighttime only. The curves ranged between 25° and 49°. All patients were either Risser 0, 1, or 2. Follow-up was a minimum of 1 year from the initiation of brace treatment. Eighty-three percent showed either improvement or less than 5° of increase in the curvature. Double major curves had the poorest response to brace treatment. The authors advocate close examination of double major curves, and a switch to another form of bracing if satisfactory correction is not achieved.

13

Idiopathic Scoliosis: Surgical Management

Surgical Indications

The surgical treatment of idiopathic scoliosis has undergone tremendous changes in the past 15 years, as newer techniques of instrumentation, monitoring, and blood donation and recovery have become available. When considering the indications for surgical intervention, one must consider the ability of the surgery to achieve the goals of deformity correction, a solid arthrodesis, and a favorable alteration of the natural consequences of the deformity.

The indications for surgical intervention in idiopathic scoliosis are based upon characteristics of the curve and of the patient. The curve is assessed by magnitude, rotation, location, progression, and balance. The patient's age, either skeletal, physiologic (eg, history of menses), or chronologic, is of primary importance. The effect of each of these characteristics on the long-term consequences of untreated idiopathic scoliosis is a component of the natural history of this disease. While the functional outcome with regard to pulmonary compromise and incidence of back pain is the primary consideration, concerns regarding social and cosmetic outcomes must also be considered. These later concerns are often the most identifiable for the patient and family.

Surgical indications or surgical technique based solely on any single parameter, such as curve magnitude, are inappropriate. For instance, a juvenile idiopathic scoliosis may be followed or braced over a greater range, ie, to 50° or 55° for a thoracic curvature, in comparison to adolescent scoliosis. Such bracing is used to delay surgical intervention until a Risser 2 pattern is reached, in order to minimize the risk of the crankshaft phenomenon in younger children. On the contrary, prolonged bracing may have detrimental effects on chest wall deformity and dynamics as well as the patient's social development. The particular indications for fusion take into account multiple factors. In general terms, the skeletally immature patient who presents with curves beyond the limits of effective brace treatment (40°) or who demonstrates progression despite appropriate brace wear is a candidate for fusion. Mature patients with thoracic curves greater than 50°, thoracolumbar or lumbar curves greater than 30° with marked apical rotation or translatory shift, double major curves greater than 50°, or those with significant coronal imbalance may all be considered surgical candidates. Progression of such curves despite skeletal maturity has been documented in long-term follow-up studies.

Preoperative Assessment

The preoperative assessment is based on the patient's history, physical examination, and planar radiographs. The history must thoroughly cover all symptoms and organ systems. Any accompanying pain, functional difficulties, or neurologic symptoms are atypical and should alert the examiner to potential nonidiopathic causes. A history of congenital heart disease or pulmonary diseases may increase the risks associated with surgery. Previous treatment for the deformity, such as bracing or surgery, must be reviewed to assess its effect on the deformity.

The maturity of the patient may be assessed historically by physiologic changes of pubarche and menarche. These markers demonstrate considerable variability, and their usefulness is somewhat controversial. Authors have argued over the relative usefulness of Tanner staging, menarche, Risser sign, and wrist or elbow for bone age. Still, most natural history and treatment studies have been based on Risser sign and menarche. A family history of deformity and treatment may affect the physician's approach to these problems and the patient's perspective of these.

The physical examination in idiopathic scoliosis is essential to planning the surgical approach with regards to rib deformity, balance, and coronal and sagittal alignment. The presence of thoracic lordosis or a significant leg length discrepancy may result in alterations of the surgical approach. Abnormal neurologic signs point to nonidiopathic causes of the deformity and require further evaluation.

While planar radiographs remain the essential starting point, other radiographic studies have taken on increasing importance in the preoperative evaluation for the surgical

At the time of this writing, bone screws placed posteriorly into vertebral elements have not been cleared for use in this specific manner by the Food and Drug Administration (FDA). These are Class III devices. This category includes screws placed transfacetally, within pedicles, or in articular, lateral masses. Some bone screws for use within the sacrum have been approved as Class II devices. Some companies have received Class II clearance for use of screws in lumbar pedicles specifically to supplement fusions in the treatment of grade III and IV spondylolisthesis with the proviso that these devices are removed after the arthrodesis has healed. Anterior vertebral body screws (cervical, thoracic, and lumbar) are Class II devices and can be used as labeled in vertebral bodies. Many of the posterior screw-based devices have been shown in laboratory and clinical testing to be useful and may be used in an off-label manner if the physician feels this is appropriate and important for the treatment of the patient. As with all surgeries, informed consent should explain the procedure and why a particular technique has been chosen, as well as its risks and benefits. The question of whether informed consent regarding pedicle screws must include a discussion of the device's FDA clearance status is currently being litigated in several jurisdictions. In cases that have been included in the multidistrict litigation in the Eastern District of Pennsylvania, this additional requirement has not been imposed.

treatment of idiopathic scoliosis. Full length side-bending films have been shown to be most reproducible and beneficial when performed supine instead of upright. These side-bending films are used to assess overall and segmental flexibility, balance, and disk space mobility. All of these components are studied to determine which segments require instrumentation and fusion. Postoperative balance requires such assessments. Some authors have advocated preoperative traction radiographs, evaluated in a similar fashion.

The initial radiographic identification of curve type is often done based on the side-bending films, especially for King type II and type V curves. Failure to appropriately identify these curve types will often lead to postoperative imbalance, with potential for progression and cosmetically inferior results. Vertebral rotation is analyzed by the Nash-Moe classification or Perdriolle measurements. Vertebral rotation and rib deformity, which often represent the most obvious aspect of the scoliosis to the patient, are sometimes overlooked in surgical planning. In juvenile scoliosis, a rib vertebral angle difference of greater than 10° at the apex of the curve is associated with greater risk of progression, as is thoracic hypokyphosis.

Preoperative magnetic resonance imaging (MRI) is indicated for patients with atypical curve patterns, eg, left thoracic curvature, or for patients with neurologic findings and atypical presentations, such as unexplained pain. Studies have demonstrated that intraspinal abnormalities requiring neurosurgical intervention were identified in those patients who presented with neck pain, headache, or significant neurologic findings (ataxia, weakness, or limb deformity). Abnormalities have been most commonly identified in left thoracic juvenile curves. The discovery of Arnold-Chiari malformations, syringomyelia, tethered cord, or other abnormalities may necessitate neurosurgical intervention prior to orthopaedic intervention. The planned MRI must visualize the entire spinal axis from cerebellum to sacrum.

While preoperative pulmonary function tests are often obtained, they are generally indicated only for those patients who have significant radiographic thoracic hypokyphosis or pulmonary symptoms. Similarly, while some clinicians advocate coagulation profiles for all patients, these profiles can be restricted to patients with a history of bleeding disorders.

Preoperative blood donation by the patient or directed donations are often advocated. Preoperative autologous donation of 1 to 3 units has several advantages including safety, availability, and avoidance of other blood products. Directed donation is considered by many to present risk to the patient equal to or greater than that associated with generalized random donor bank blood. Yet designated donor blood is often preferred by patients and their families. The use of multi-dose erythropoietin has been shown to produce a rise in the preoperative hematocrit. However, its effect on the need for intraoperative transfusion has not been analyzed. To reduce the use of autologous blood products, intraoperative hypotensive anesthesia and acute hemodilution techniques have been utilized. Intraoperative and postoperative recovery and transfusion of shed red cells has been advocated. Intraoperative cell recovery is most effective when blood loss is anticipated to exceed 500 to 1,000 ml. Postoperative cell recovery and transfusion requires especially meticulous care and may best be confined to centers familiar with its use. A study of 101 spinal surgeries that used these techniques showed that administration of additional blood products was avoided in 90% of patients. Preoperative discussion and informed consent should include aspects of surgery that are related to blood products.

Curve Patterns

The selection of fusion levels has undergone closer scrutiny as different techniques and instrumentation have evolved. Fusion of fewer vertebral levels, restoration of sagittal balance, and correction of rotational deformity have been the impetus for most of these changes. Overall, spinal balance and potential for progression remain problematic, especially with shorter fusions. The concepts of stable and neutral end vertebrae remain important. The King classification continues to be useful for the description of various thoracic curve patterns (Fig. 1).

In the immature spine, several centers have reported the occurrence of the crankshaft phenomenon, which is progression of curvature and rotation after achievement of a solid posterior fusion with instrumentation. This phenomenon appears to be secondary to continued anterior vertebral growth. Such progression has not been prevented by segmental fixation. Consideration should be given to combined anterior and posterior arthrodesis in patients under age 10, or for those premenarcheal patients with Risser Grade 0. In addition, the presence of an open triradiate cartilage has been correlated with an even higher risk of progression. Although the crankshaft phenomenon is best appreciated by the changes seen in the clinical appearance over time, changes in the rib vertebral angle difference have been reported to be the most consistent radiographic markers.

Techniques/Instrumentation

Anterior spinal fusion, with or without instrumentation, is being used with increasing frequency in the treatment of idiopathic scoliosis. Anterior instrumentation for lumbar and thoracolumbar curves has many advantages, including greater correction, derotation, and the ability to limit the extent of fusion necessary. Sagittal plane deformity and the potential for visceral irritation or perforation have been concerns with traditional anterior constructs. Stronger constructs, such as anterior Texas Scottish Rite Hospital (TSRH) or Isola devices have resulted in better correction and maintenance of sagittal contours. As the importance of sagittal balance has become increasing well

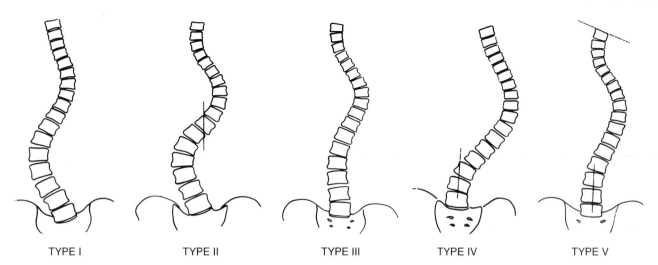

Fig. 1 Diagrammatic representation of King-Moe classification of idiopathic scoliosis. (Adapted with permission from King HA, Moe JH, Bradford DS, et al: The selection of fusion levels in thoracic idiopathic scoliosis. *J Bone Joint Surg* 1983;65A:1302–1313.)

TYPE I	TYPE II	TYPE III	TYPE IV	TYPE V

recognized, anterior release, with or without instrumentation, is being used in cases of thoracic hypokyphosis or curves with significant rigidity on side-bending. Although it has not been fully defined in the literature, this rigidity may be defined as a residual curve of $> 45°$ on side bending or correction of less than 50%. Such releases allow for better correction with either anterior or posterior instrumentation. The use of anterior fusion to prevent the crankshaft phenomenon in skeletally immature patients has recently been advocated in patients with significant skeletal immaturity, ie, those younger than 10 years of age or premenarcheal with Risser 0, particularly in the presence of open triradiate cartilages.

An emerging approach to the anterior spine has been developed by video-assisted thoracoscopic surgery at a number of centers. Thoracoscopic instruments use multiple intercostal portals. Resection of disk material; anterior release, including the anterior longitudinal ligament; osteotomy; and bone grafting have been performed. Extensive training is required to use these procedures, and the long-term benefit of this approach has yet to be established.

Studies of anterior instrumentation procedures have identified the potential for neurologic injury with ligation of the segmental arteries. In most instances, anterior release and fusion can be performed by dissection over the disk level, which avoids arterial ligation. In cases that require arterial ligation, such as in the placement of anterior instrumentation, the temporary occlusion of the segmental arteries while the patient undergoes intraoperative somatosensory-evoked potential (SSEP) monitoring may serve to avoid permanent neurologic injury.

Anterior instrumentation systems that evolved from the Dwyer technique used a flexible cable, which meant that they relied on the rigidity of bony compression for stability. This technique resulted in more kyphosis than is cur-

rently deemed acceptable. The Zielke technique uses a threaded rod, which provides somewhat greater rigidity, and corrects the deformity through a combination of derotation and compression across the intervening disk spaces. Correct placement of the Zielke screws and anteriorly placed bone graft blocks will minimize the tendency for kyphosis across the instrumented segments. The solid rod systems of TSRH and Isola allow contouring of the rod, so that, with rotation, better sagittal restoration can be achieved. Irritation and perforation of viscera and neurovascular structures have been reported with anterior spinal instrumentation. To avoid these problems, adequate soft-tissue coverage of the prominent hardware must be achieved. The use of muscular and pleural rotation flaps normally achieves this, but this requirement, which is of particular concern for anterior thoracic instrumentation, represents a potential significant disadvantage to this approach.

Posterior spinal instrumentation has evolved from Harrington rods in an attempt to address concerns over rotation, translation, and sagittal contours. Yet, Harrington distraction instrumentation, with or without compression instrumentation, has demonstrated consistent and satisfactory results, especially for thoracic fusions. Correction of greater than 40% of the coronal curve may be achieved consistently, with appropriate spinal balance and low rates of pseudarthrosis and neurologic injury. However, distraction can have a detrimental effect on sagittal alignment and does little to correct apical derotation. Specifically, the rib deformity changes minimally. In a recent review of Wisconsin instrumentation, which uses additional segmental spinous process wires and buttons, a 40% to 50% coronal correction was achieved with a loss of 10% to 25% of correction over 5 years. Sagittal curves were maintained and no incidences of pseudarthrosis were noted. Of these patients, 90% were satisfied. Digitized studies of pre- and postoperative radiographs have shown that vertebral axial rotation, vertebral translation, and vertebral tilt are minimally changed with Harrington or Wisconsin instrumentation.

Segmental instrumentation systems have evolved from the Luque and Harrington systems. Luque sublaminar wiring is used primarily to treat neuromuscular scoliosis. Cotrel-Dubousset (CD) and TSRH instrumentation rely primarily on rotational maneuvers to achieve correction and have become the standard in treating idiopathic scoliosis. Coronal corrections of 50% or more are reported, with correction beyond the flexibility noted on bending films. Rotational correction of 40% of the thoracic curves and 20% of the lumbar curves has been noted radiographically, but correction of the apical vertebrae has been less significant. Studies suggest that the perceived "rotation" is more realistically the product of translation in several planes. Unfortunately, the forces associated with the rotation maneuver may also contribute to significant postoperative decompensation and this must be understood during preoperative planning, particularly in King type II curves. More recent systems, such as the Isola, use sublaminar wires and hooks in a translational mode. These systems seek to correct the deformity through a series of sequential translational forces applied in each plane. The rigidity and strength of the rods used with each of these systems allows for correction of sagittal plane deformity in concert with coronal correction.

Preliminary reports of these segmental fixation systems indicate a significant learning curve and support the need for advanced training. Early reports for one of these systems has identified a 10% percent delayed deep infection rate in a series of 102 patients. This may be secondary to the increased bulk of the implants and consequent increased dead space. This has led one group of investigators to explore the possibility of a single-rod, multiple-hook fixation system. Most of these systems have adjunctive screws, which currently are not FDA approved for pedicle placement in scoliosis. Full disclosure of this fact and informed consent should be included in preoperative discussions when screws are planned for specific indications.

The achievement of adequate spinal fusion relies on appropriate and meticulous fusion technique. Facetectomy, as introduced by Moe, remains paramount. Although early studies with bone graft substitutes and osteogenic factors have been somewhat promising, autograft bone remains the current standard for spinal fusion. Autograft bone may be harvested from rib, iliac crest, and spinous processes, depending upon surgical approach and needs. The iliac crest may be approached through a separate incision, whether oblique or longitudinal, or along the dorsolumbar fascia. The longitudinal approach lessens the risk of cutaneous nerve injury.

The criterion for thoracoplasty in surgical correction of scoliosis remains controversial. Studies have demonstrated a persistent rib prominence in selected patients without rib resection compared to those who have had such resection, but this has not been correlated with patient satisfaction. Additionally, the resected rib serves as bone graft and can often alleviate the need for iliac crest graft. During anterior thoracic spinal surgery with thoracotomy, internal rib resection can achieve the same advantages with minimal additional morbidity.

In juvenile scoliosis that has progressed beyond 50° despite bracing, use of a subcutaneous rod, with cephalad and caudad hook placement and fusion of vertebrae adjacent to the hooks, has been successful. The rod is periodically distracted and occasionally replaced. Bracing is mandatory throughout this treatment. The method is temporizing until an appropriate age for definitive fusion is achieved. Subcutaneous rodding used in distraction increases hypokyphosis, while allowing increased kyphosis proximal to the rod. The procedure and follow-up carries with it an increased risk of neurologic injury, loss of fixation, loss of correction, and failure of instrumentation in addition to those risks inherent with other spinal surgeries.

Treatment by Curve Type

Type I curves (those with a predominant lumbar curve and secondary thoracic curve) are assessed for flexibility of both curves by side-bending films. In cases in which the right thoracic curve is sufficiently structural or rigid to affect skeletal balance, the use of posterior instrumentation and fusion of both curves is advocated. Several reports show satisfactory results of Harrington instrumentation, but its use is associated with a loss of sagittal contour, especially lumbar lordosis. Nevertheless, long-term results have been satisfactory, with relatively low rates of pain. The use of segmental systems has allowed for restoration of sagittal contour. Often the thoracic curve is less significant, allowing for primary lumbar anterior spinal instrumentation and fusion. Zielke instrumentation has given excellent coronal correction (near 70%) and balance when the fusion is carried to or beyond the neutral stable vertebrae. However, most series report increased sagittal plane deformity and higher rates of pseudoarthrosis in comparison to posterior instrumentation systems. Kyphosis of the instrumented segment is usually increased, but the remaining spine compensates in the sagittal plane. While traditional treatment requires anterior instrumentation and fusion of all levels within the measured curvature, recent limited fusions have shown early success. Selective instrumentation of three or four vertebrae centered at the apical vertebrae or apical interspace has allowed correction and balance with limited fusion. In preliminary reports, instrumentation systems with stiffer solid rods, such as the TSRH, allow better maintenance and correction of the sagittal plane deformity and have demonstrated excellent rates of fusion, with reports of 100% fusion at 8 months. These systems allow for rotational and translational correction as well. Postoperative bracing has been advocated, although some centers suggest that the larger rod systems may not require orthotic support.

Type II curves (those with a predominant thoracic curve and secondary lumbar curve) have presented the greatest difficulty with both analysis and treatment. The current trend is to distinguish type II curves (false double major) from a true double major curve. The flexibility index (the relative flexibility of the thoracic and lumbar curves) alone may not be sufficient to determine the efficacy of selective thoracic fusion. This distinction is made based on careful analysis of the lumbar curve for magnitude, rotation, and apical translation (from the plumbline), with the degree of each aspect compared with those of the thoracic curve. For these curves, selection of proper fusion levels is critical if one is to avoid decompensation. Selective thoracic fusion with segmental hook systems and rotational maneuvers has led to lumbar decompensation in 10% of cases that used King's fusion criterion. However, higher incidences of decompensation have been reported if these criteria were not followed. Such decompensation has been associated with persistent postoperative lumbar-sacral obliquity. Several authors cite correction of the thoracic curvature beyond flexibility demonstrated on side-bending films. This "overcorrection," achievable with current segmental instrumentation, leaves the uninstrumented lumbar curve unable to compensate appropriately and achieve coronal plane balance. Several authors postulate that this overcorrection is secondary to the 90° rod rotation maneuver used with Cotrel-Dubousset instrumentation. In type II curves undergoing selective thoracic fusion, many authorities now advocate fusion caudally to the stable vertebrae with distraction forces applied with segmental instrumentation, although this method remains controversial. Reversal of rod bend (into lordosis) and reversal of hook pattern (with the caudal two hooks placed in compression on the concave aspect and distraction on the convex aspect) have also been advocated to reduce decompensation and maintain lumbar lordosis. Posterior instrumentation of both components of true double major curves is necessary if one is to avoid decompensation. Although this procedure has been criticized for fusion of lumbar segments, several reports have cited satisfactory long-term results.

King type III curves (thoracic only) do not have a structural lumbar component and, therefore, are treated by limited thoracic fusion alone. The apex varies from T5 to T9, but usually is T7 or T8 with L1 or L2 within the stable zone. Thoracic hypokyphosis, a normal component of these curves, requires special attention for instrumentation and correction. Posterior spinal fusion with instrumentation remains the standard of treatment, with the fusion extending to the neutral stable vertebrae. Results of Harrington instrumentation remain satisfactory, despite the lack of significant sagittal correction. In the face of significant hypokyphosis, the "derotation" maneuver, with apical fixation using Cotrel-Dubousset instrumentation, has improved the sagittal alignment on postoperative CT studies. Translational correction with sublaminar wires or hooks is felt to have a similar result. Distally, this instrumentation should extend to the L1 or L2 level, because decompensation has been reported with instrumentation to T12. Because the fusion extends past the thoracolumbar junction, some authors recommend reversal of the rod bend and a caudal hook pattern when using segmental instrumentation systems. With rigid hypokyphosis, thoracotomy or thoracoscopy and anterior release of the apical disk spaces may result in improved sagittal correction. Paraspinal rib osteotomy has also been advocated. As noted above, anterior instrumentation of type III curves is being undertaken in some centers.

The King type IV curve (long thoracic curve extending to L4) is less common and is sometimes misdiagnosed. These curves have traditionally been treated with Harrington instrumentation and fusion from T4 to L4. Although this treatment involves a significant loss of lumbar lordosis, it has had relatively good results over time. The use of segmental systems, such as CD or TSRH, for type IV curves has gained popularity primarily because of the ability of these systems to maintain lumbar lordosis, especially in those cases in which preoperative loss of sagittal contours is noted. Reversal of the rod bend is essential to achieve lordosis. In cases demonstrating neutral rotation of L3 and reversal of L3-4 disk space wedging on side-bending films, the alternative of ending the fusion at L3 has been proposed.

The King type V curve (double thoracic curves) presents a dilemma for both recognition and treatment. The lower, right thoracic curve typically has greater magnitude, apical rotation, and length. The presence of the upper curve has been identified by different methods: tilt of T1 into the curve, elevation of the left 1st rib or shoulder, and rotation of the apical vertebrae of the upper curve. A structural upper thoracic curve should be suspected even when the left shoulder or 1st rib are level. Indications for inclusion of the upper thoracic curve in the instrumented segment have been controversial. The upper thoracic curve should be included in the fusion if the curve is either more rigid than the lower curve or fails to correct to < 20° on side-bending, or if the left shoulder is elevated on standing examinations. Rotation ($\geq$ Grade I by Nash-Moe) or translation ($\geq$ 1 cm) of the apical vertebrae of the upper thoracic curve is a relative indication for inclusion in the surgery. Positive T1 tilt remains a controversial indicator, which is best correlated to the other criterion. If the upper thoracic curve is not to be included in the instrumented fusion, great care must be taken not to overcorrect the lower thoracic curve, either with regard to coronal correction or the "derotation" maneuver, because the lower thoracic curve is often more flexible than the upper. The use of segmental fixation allows for greater correction of the lower thoracic curve, which may necessitate a lower threshold for inclusion of the upper curve. If instrumentation of the upper curve is elected, fusion to T2 cephalad has been the treatment of choice. Harrington rod instrumentation has been shown to give effective correction of

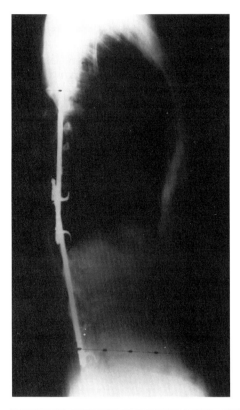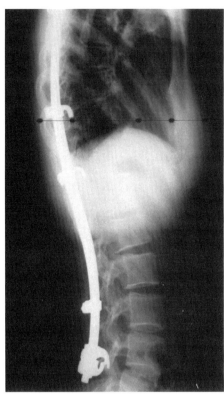

Fig. 2 **Left,** Harrington instrumentation to L4, demonstrating a flat back or loss of sagittal lordosis. **Right,** Segmental hook and rod instrumentation with maintenance of sagittal contour.

the coronal plane deformity, but sagittal plane analysis has not been reported. Hook patterns used in CD or segmental fixation (if hyperkyphotic) remain controversial, but compression across the convexity and distraction across the concavity of the upper thoracic curve is recommended.

Intraoperative Considerations

Neurologic and anesthetic considerations remain paramount intraoperatively. Somatosensory-evoked potentials (SSEP), used to monitor dorsal column pathways, may facilitate prevention or detection of most neurologic injuries intraoperatively. Temperature, blood pressure, and anesthetic agents affect the evoked potentials, but these effects may be lessened with use of epidural leads. Some centers have used motor-evoked potentials (MEP), often in combination with sensory-evoked potentials (SEP). MEP may be obtained either with magnetic coil or percutaneous monitoring. The MEP has less delay in alteration and records anterior pathways indicative of motor neuron injury. This combination (SEP/MEP) appears to be more sensitive to neurologic injury, but its specificity remains controversial. The Stagnara intraoperative wake-up test remains the gold standard, particularly if electrical monitoring changes are noted during instrumentation. Intraoperative blood loss may be minimized by proper positioning, careful surgical technique, and by deliberate hypotensive anesthesia.

Postoperative Considerations

In the immediate postoperative period, close observation neurologically and hemodynamically is necessary. If significant or progressive neurologic deficits are noted, strong consideration must be given to removal of instrumentation. While a standard regimen, ie steroids, hypervolemia, etc, for acute spinal cord injury may be followed, the efficacy in this setting has not been statistically proven.

Significant fluid retention is expected because of operative fluid volumes and inappropriate antidiuretic hormone syndrome in the postoperative period. Spontaneous diuresis is expected at 36 to 48 hours after surgery. Ileus and abdominal distention are normal components, but if they persist longer than 4 days, nutritional supplementation may be required, which may be the first indication of a superior mesenteric artery syndrome.

Postoperative limitations differ for each type of instrumentation and fusion. For all, activity is reduced to avoid significant lifting and bending for at least 9 months. Most anterior fusions have been supplemented with postoperative orthotics. For the current generation of posterior segmental instrumentation systems, bracing is used only in cases of questionable fixation, decompensation, or for progression of secondary curves. Long-term limitations on activity vary with the surgeon, the instrumentation, and the patient. Essentially full activity may be tolerated, but studies demonstrate that most patients are not engaged in full-time heavy manual labor. The use of Harrington instrumentation and fusion for adolescent idiopathic scoliosis has led to long-term satisfaction in 80% to 90% of patients surveyed. An increased risk of low back pain or arthritis is a concern, especially for those patients fused with Harrington instrumentation to the low lumbar (L4 or L5) region. Hopefully, the current emphasis on segmental fixation, maintenance of lumbar lordosis, and limiting the distal extent of fusion into the lumbar spine will minimize the long-term risks of low back pain and degenerative arthritis (Fig. 2).

Summary

The last decade has seen numerous attempts to better understand the deformity and natural history of idiopathic scoliosis. In response to these studies, there has been a proliferation of instrumentation that emphasizes the restoration of anatomic parameters, while allowing better fixation. The increased use of neurologic monitoring, along with new surgical and anesthetic techniques, has increased the safety of surgical intervention. These and other goals continue to evolve.

Annotated Bibliography

Preoperative Assessment

Oga M, Ikuta H, Sugioka Y: The use of autologous blood in the surgical treatment of spinal disorders. *Spine* 1992; 17:1381–1385.

A retrospective review of 101 spine surgeries with autologous donations, 48 of the patients were adolescents with scoliosis (38 idiopathic). In this group, an average of 2940 ml of cryopreserved blood was obtained preoperatively and 867 ml of cell saver. Ninety percent required no additional homologous blood, with a mean hematocrit of 40.1% 2 weeks postoperatively. No complications were noted.

Roye DP Jr, Rothstein P, Rickert JB, et al: The use of preoperative erythropoietin in scoliosis surgery. *Spine* 1992; 17(suppl 6):S204–S205.

A study of 10 patients treated preoperatively with erythropoietin in multiple doses. On average, the preoperative hematocrit rose from 37.9 to 46.7, with no increase in blood pressure. No statistical analysis of the need for transfusion was undertaken.

Tate DE Jr, Friedman RJ: Blood conservation in spinal surgery: Review of current techniques. *Spine* 1992;17: 1450–1456.

A review of the current technique of blood conservation. Pertinent studies of autologous blood donation/transfusion, intraoperative and postoperative autologous recovery and transfusion, and anesthetic techniques for reducing blood loss are reviewed. Despite these, emphasis must still be placed on operative techniques.

Curve Patterns

Sanders JO, Herring JA, Browne RH: Posterior arthrodesis and instrumentation in the immature (Risser-grade-0) spine in idiopathic scoliosis. *J Bone Joint Surg* 1995;77A:39–45.

A retrospective review of 43 patients with idiopathic scoliosis and Risser Grade 0 at the time of posterior spinal instrumentation and fusion. Crankshaft phenomenon is described. Eleven patients demonstrated this phenomenon. The change in rib-vertebral angle difference was the most consistent marker of progression. The patient younger than 10 years of age or premenarcheal and Risser 0 with open triradiate cartilages had significant risk for crankshaft phenomenon.

Techniques/Instrumentation

Bischoff R, Bennett JT, Stuecker R, et al: The use of Texas Scottish-Rite instrumentation in idiopathic scoliosis: A preliminary report. *Spine* 1993;18:2452–2456.

A retrospective review of 23 adolescent patients treated with TSRH instrumentation followed for 18 months (average). There were no failures of instrumentation, but four hooks pulled out. No statistical analysis of decompensation is given, but several cases are mentioned.

Harvey CJ Jr, Betz RR, Clements DH, et al: Are there indications for partial rib resection in patients with adolescent idiopathic scoliosis treated with Cotrel-Dubousset instrumentation? *Spine* 1993;18:1593–1598.

A retrospective study of rib cage deformity after spinal fusion with and without rib resection. By radiographic criteria, residual rib deformity was assessed as unsatisfactory in 12 of 83 patients who underwent CD instrumentation without rib resection. It is recommended that rib resection be performed in patients with > 15° prominence on forward bend radiographs, for curves > 60°, flexibility < 20% and correction of < 50% on intraoperative films. Correlation with patient satisfaction was not determined.

Herndon WA, Sullivan JA, Gruel CR, et al: A comparison of Wisconsin instrumentation and Cotrel-Dubousset instrumentation. *J Pediatr Orthop* 1993;13:615–621.

This retrospective study compared 36 patients treated with CD instrumentation with 26 patients with Wisconsin instrumentation. Although coronal curve correction was greater with CD instrumentation, neither instrumentation system gave statistically significant better results in regards to final rotation or sagittal alignment when used on type III and type II curves, either with selective or full fusion. In this study, CD instrumentation was related to greater blood loss, operating time, and instrumentation "problems" (none statistically significant), along with greater cost.

Jeng CL, Sponseller PD, Tolo VT: Outcome of Wisconsin instrumentation in idiopathic scoliosis: Minimum 5-year follow-up. *Spine* 1993;18:1584–1590.

A retrospective study with minimum 5-year follow-up of 35 patients who underwent correction of adolescent idiopathic scoliosis with Wisconsin instrumentation by the age of 46 (mean age 20). Only five had postoperative bracing. There was one hook dislodgement and two wire breaks, along with two significant infections. Thoracic curves were corrected by 40% to 50% initially, losing up to 10% correction over 5 years, while lumbar curves lost 23% of their initial 53% correction. The lordosis and kyphosis were maintained, but not improved significantly. All curves fused, with no pseudarthrosis evident. More than 90% of patients were satisfied.

Lowe TG, Peters JD: Anterior spinal fusion with Zielke instrumentation for idiopathic scoliosis: A frontal and sagittal curve analysis in 36 patients. *Spine* 1993;18:423–426.

A retrospective review of 36 patients undergoing anterior spinal fusion and instrumentation of lumbar or thoracolumbar curves. All vertebrae in the curve were instrumented (average of 4.5 segments). Average coronal correction was 69% of curve, with maintenance or improvement of frontal plane balance. Kyphosis in the instrumented segments increased by an average of 8°, but overall thoracic kyphosis was decreased by an average of 19°. Overall sagittal and coronal balance was maintained.

Moskowitz A, Trommanhauser S: Surgical and clinical results of scoliosis surgery using Zielke instrumentation. *Spine* 1993;18:2444–2451.

A retrospective review of 32 patients (13 adolescents) treated with anterior fusion and Zielke instrumentation for thoracolumbar and lumbar curves. Postoperative care included an average of 6 to 7 months in brace. Average coronal correction was 79%, maintained at 71% at 4-year follow-up. The thoracic curves corrected 49%. Sagittal alignment was not significantly improved. Overall patient satisfaction was good for both cosmesis and symptoms.

Regan JJ, Mack M, Picetti GD: A technical report on video assisted thoracoscopy in thoracic spinal surgery: Preliminary description. *Spine* 1995;20:831–837.

A preliminary study on the use of thoracoscopy in spinal surgery for 12 patients, including 3 scoliotic deformities. The methods and results were reviewed. The potential benefits of thoracoscopy were noted, although not directly compared to a matched control group. The technique is specialized and has a significant learning curve.

Richards BS, Herring JA, Johnston CE, et al: Treatment of adolescent idiopathic scoliosis using Texas Scottish Rite Hospital instrumentation. *Spine* 1994;19:1598–1605.

An initial retrospective report of 103 patients with idiopathic scoliosis treated with Texas Scottish Rite Hospital instrumentation. At minimum 2-year follow-up, all curve types corrected an average of 48% to 65%, with thoracic curves demonstrating the best correction. Thoracic hypokyphosis (< 20°) improved 43%, but sagittal alignment was otherwise unchanged. There were no neurologic complications, but 10% developed delayed deep infections.

Roye DP Jr, Farcy JP, Rickert JB, et al: Results of spinal instrumentation of adolescent idiopathic scoliosis by King type. *Spine* 1992;17(suppl 8):S270–S273.

In this retrospective study of 51 patients treated with a variety of approaches and instrumentation, the results were followed for decompensation. Decompensation was noted primarily in those patients treated with CD instrumentation, noting 30% decompensation in Type II curves. The authors recommended anterior instrumentation and fusion for "large, stiff, and highly rotated lumbar curves."

Shufflebarger HL, Smiley K, Roth HJ: Internal thoracoplasty: A new procedure. *Spine* 1994;19:840–842.

This prospective study of six patients undergoing same-day anterior release and posterior instrumentation and fusion of the spine for idiopathic scoliosis describes the technique of internal rib resection during thoracotomy and compares this to patients without rib resection. No additional morbidity was identified.

Stokes IA, Ronchetti PJ, Aronsson DD: Changes in shape of the adolescent idiopathic scoliosis curve after surgical correction. *Spine* 1994;19:1032–1038.

A study of the digitized pre- and postoperative radiographs of 36 patients, of whom 21 had undergone fusion with Harrington instrumentation and 16 with Wisconsin instrumentation. Both methods improved the Cobb measurement by nearly 50%, but no change in axial rotation of the apical vertebrae was noted. The curve "shape," as defined by position, translation, and tilt of the vertebrae, also changed little.

Turi M, Johnston CE II, Richards BS: Anterior correction of idiopathic scoliosis using Texas Scottish Rite Hospital instrumentation. *Spine* 1993;18:417–422.

In this study of the first 14 patients who underwent this procedure at TSRH on lumbar and thoracolumbar curves, four to six vertebrae were instrumented. Postoperative bracing was used in 13 of 14 patients, although the authors now felt no bracing was necessary. The average curve corrected 75% of the preoperative magnitude, representing 131% of the bending correction. Fusion was radiographically achieved at all disk spaces by 8 months. Spinal decompensation was corrected to near (1 mm) perfect balance, while rotation improved an average of 49%. Sagittal alignment was unchanged (within 5°) in seven patients, with increased kyphosis in six and lordosis in one. The advantage of an adjustable, but stiff, construct are discussed in obtaining and maintaining correction while achieving fusion.

Willers U, Hedlund R, Aaro S, et al: Long-term results of Harrington instrumentation in idiopathic scoliosis. *Spine* 1993;18:713–717.

In this retrospective study, with a 10-year follow-up, of 33 patients with Harrington instrumentation, plane radiographs and computed tomography demonstrated lasting correction of the coronal deformity, but no improvement of rotational or sagittal deformities. There was little change in the rib hump or translation.

Treatment by Curve Type

Lee CK, Denis F, Winter RB, et al: Analysis of the upper thoracic curve in surgically treated idiopathic scoliosis: A new concept of the double thoracic curve pattern. *Spine* 1993;18:1599–1608.

This retrospective review of 246 patients with upper thoracic curves of > 20°, divided the patients into groups who had a positive T1 tilt and fusion of both thoracic curves (138 patients), and those who had only lower thoracic fusion with positive T1 tilt (43 patients) or negative or neutral T1 tilt (65 patients). Positive T1 tilt did not correlate preoperatively with left shoulder elevation nor with curve flexibility on side bending. Approximately 25% of the unfused upper thoracic curves corrected spontaneously, with correction corresponding to the bending flexibility, not to T1 tilt. None of these curves progressed more than 5°. The authors suggest fusion of the upper thoracic curve in the face of preoperative left shoulder elevation, with care taken not to over-correct the lower thoracic curve if balanced or right shoulder elevation is noted. An upper thoracic curve that is more rigid than the lower one should be included in the fusion.

Lenke LG, Bridwell KH, Baldus C, et al: Preventing decompensation in King type II curves treated with Cotrel-Dubousset instrumentation: Strict guidelines for selective thoracic fusion. *Spine* 1992;17(suppl 8):S274–S281.

In this retrospective study of 50 patients with type II and type III curves, after selective thoracic fusion, 10% of type II curves were decompensated in the immediate postoperative period, despite a positive flexibility index. These type II curves, which demonstrated greater lumbar curve magnitude (relative to the thoracic component) and apical rotation and apical translation (from the plumbline), should be considered true double major curves.

Lenke LG, Bridwell KH, Baldus C, et al: Cotrel-Dubousset instrumentation for adolescent idiopathic scoliosis. *J Bone Joint Surg* 1992;74A:1056–1067.

In this retrospective study of 95 patients with adolescent idiopathic scoliosis, some type II or type III curves demonstrated postoperative decompensation. The criterion for selecting caudal end vertebra and modifying techniques to avoid decompensation are given. Overall, the CD instrumentation gave good correction in all planes, but little rotational correction (11%). Pulmonary function also improved.

Lenke LG, Bridwell KH, O'Brien MF, et al: Recognition and treatment of the proximal thoracic curve in adolescent idiopathic scoliosis treated with Cotrel-Dubousset instrumentation. *Spine* 1994;19:1589–1597.

In this retrospective review, which compared results of 27 type III curves and 27 type V curves to determine the appropriate criteria for treatment of upper thoracic curves, the authors felt that multiple criteria such as curve magnitude (> 30°), side bending correction (≥ 20°), apical rotation (≥ Grade I), or translation of ≥ 1 cm indicated the need to include the upper thoracic curve.

McCall RE, Bronson W: Criteria for selective fusion in idiopathic scoliosis using Cotrel-Dubousset instrumentation. *J Pediatr Orthop* 1992;12:475–479.

In this retrospective review of 52 patients treated with CD instrumentation, 23 patients had type II curves, with the thoracic curves fused selectively either one level cephalad to the stable vertebra or to that vertebra, all either to or beyond the neutral vertebra. Four of the 23 had progressive decompensation, with a mean flexibility index of 20% (increased stiffness of lumbar versus thoracic curve) and lumbar curve of > 45° as opposed to a mean index of 40% for the nonprogressive group.

Puno RM, Grossfeld SL, Johnson JR, et al: Cotrel-Dubousset instrumentation in idiopathic scoliosis. *Spine* 1992;17(suppl 8):S258–S262.

In this retrospective study of 82 patients (mostly adolescent) treated with CD instrumentation, 35% of type II curves demonstrated > 10-mm decompensation when fused short of or to the stable vertebrae, and 15% when fused beyond the stable vertebrae. While results suggest that decompensation may be improved by fusing caudal to the stable vertebrae or avoiding over-correction, there was no statistical significance between choice of distal fusion level and amount of decompensation.

Richards BS: Lumbar curve response in type II idiopathic scoliosis after posterior instrumentation of the thoracic curve. *Spine* 1992;17(suppl 8):S282–S286.

In this retrospective study of 24 patients with type II curves, all patients had lumbar curves of > 40° (average 49°) with average flexibility of 73%. Despite the flexibility, selective thoracic fusion and correction was accompanied by a persistent lumbar deformity larger than the postoperative thoracic curve and persistent lower lumbar obliquity relative to the pelvis. These findings were independent of the preoperative lumbar rotation and curve magnitude and of the selected fusion level above, at, or below the stable vertebra. Preoperative lumbar flexibility was not helpful in predicting balance.

Thompson JP, Transfeldt EE, Bradford DS, et al: Decompensation after Cotrel-Dubousset instrumentation of idiopathic scoliosis. *Spine* 1990;15:927–931.

In this prospective study of 30 patients undergoing treatment of scoliosis with Cotrel-Dubousset instrumentation, preoperative and postoperative radiographs and CT scans were evaluated for response to instrumentation, especially regarding torsional changes and decompensation. Decompensation occurred with correction of the major curve beyond the preoperative flexibility and with instrumentation of the distal mobile segments. Type II curves were especially susceptible to decompensation, presumably from excessive derotation.

14

Congenital Spine Deformities

Introduction

Congenital deformities of the spine result from a wide range of anomalies in the development of vertebrae. Some deformities have little or no effect on the health and well-being of the patient, although others result in dramatic deformity of the spine, cor pulmonale, neurologic defects, and premature death. The orthopaedic surgeon will see some patients with remarkable deformities, but the majority of patients will have only mild deformities. The orthopaedist will need to assess the patient, calculate the risk of progression, and apply treatment when warranted.

By definition, congenital vertebral deformities are the result of anomalous embryo vertebral development and may be classified by the area of the spine affected, the pattern of deformity, or the type of anomalous vertebral development involved. Patterns of development include scoliosis, kyphosis, and lordosis, or combinations of patterns, such as kyphoscoliosis and lordoscoliosis. Basic types of anomalous vertebral development include failure of formation of vertebrae and failure of segmentation of adjacent vertebrae. These two basic errors can vary significantly and probably occur more frequently as combinations than alone. Formation defects that occur anteriorly result in kyphosis and defects that occur laterally result in scoliosis. Complete segmentation errors result in a solid block of two or more vertebrae. Partial segmentation errors occur laterally, posteriorly, or anteriorly.

Evaluation

The presence of a congenital vertebral anomaly should prompt a careful and complete physical examination of the child. The embryologic development of the spinal column coincides with the development of numerous other organs and systems, and it is not unusual for patients with congenital vertebral anomalies to also have congenital anomalies elsewhere. As many as 60% of individuals with vertebral malformations have associated malformations that may be present as anomalies outside the spinal column, elsewhere in the bony structure of the spine, or within the spinal canal and the neural tissue. The type of vertebral anomaly that occurs does not predict the type or location of any associated anomalies.

Structural abnormalities of the urinary tract occur in 18% to 37% of individuals with congenital vertebral anomalies and renal agenesis, duplication, ectopia, and fusion are the most common abnormalities, followed by ureteral anomalies and reflux. Renal agenesis and ectopia are also frequently associated with genital anomalies. All urinary tract anomalies occur more often in patients with congenital scoliosis than in the general population. The great majority of renal tract anomalies are asymptomatic in childhood, but some of these asymptomatic anomalies may have serious consequences. Hydronephrosis that is caused by reflux or ureteral obstruction can silently destroy renal function.

Until recently, intravenous pyelography (IVP) has been the most common imaging technique used to search for abnormalities in the renal tract. Recent studies suggest that ultrasonography has 95% of the accuracy of an IVP and may also be used as an acceptable screening tool.

In 1972, the acronym VATER was created to group together vertebral anomalies, anal anomalies, tracheoesophageal fistula, and radial limb dysplasias. Since that time, the term VATER association has been used to describe the nonrandom association of multiple malformations of the vertebrae, lower gastrointestinal tract, trachea and esophagus, renal tract, lungs, heart, radius, ear, and lip and palate. There is no clear embryologic explanation for this phenomenon, and no clear pattern of inheritance. This association confirms the importance of a thorough physical examination of children who have congenital vertebral anomalies, although the examiner need not expect to discover multiple anomalies. The list of possible musculoskeletal anomalies is extensive. It has been demonstrated in reviews that 2% to 5% of individuals with diverse upper limb anomalies will also have congenital vertebral anomalies.

A disconcerting finding among children with congenital scoliosis and kyphosis is the high incidence of congenital cervical vertebral anomalies. Cervical vertebral anomalies were recently reported in 298 of 1,215 patients who had congenital scoliosis and kyphosis. These anomalies may occur at single or multiple sites, have no clear correlation with particular forms of congenital scoliosis, and are usually asymptomatic in early childhood. Imprecisely referred to as Klippel-Feil syndrome, cervical congenital vertebral anomalies represent sites of potential instability and may necessitate restrictions in athletic activities (Fig. 1).

The last group of associated anomalies includes lesions of the spinal canal and its contents. Intraspinal anomalies are found in 18% to 38% of individuals with congenital spine deformities. Diastematomyelia, the most common and troublesome intraspinal anomaly, is present in 5% to 16% of cases (Fig. 2). Other intraspinal anomalies are tethered cord, low conus, diplomyelia, syrinx, and lipoma. The estimated prevalence of these anomalies is increasing with wider use of magnetic resonance imaging (MRI).

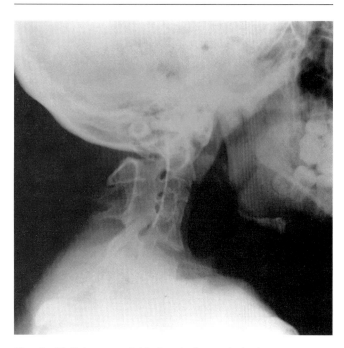

Fig. 1   Multiple congenital fusions in the cervical spine.

Diastematomyelia may be defined as a complete or partial osseous or fibrocartilaginous spinal canal septum that invaginates or splits the neural tissue. When results of several studies are combined, 9% of diastematomyelias occur between T1 and T6, 27% between T7 and T12, and 64% in the lumbar spine. The female to male ratio for diastematomyelia is 8 to 1, compared to 2.5 to 1 for congenital scoliosis. Although the overall prevalence of diastematomyelia in congenital vertebral anomalies is 5% to 16%, one author reported that 46% of those patients who had a hemivertebra and same-level unsegmented bar also had a diastematomyelia.

Clinical findings associated with diastematomyelia have been consistent. Cutaneous lesions (especially hair patches) are found in 55% to 75% of patients; anisomelia (usually calf or thigh circumference asymmetry) is found in 52% to 58% of patients; foot deformity (most commonly cavus) is found in 32% to 52% of patients, and is almost always unilateral; neurologic deficits, such as reflex changes, weakness, and sensory deficits are found in 58% to 88% of patients; and significant scoliosis has been reported in 60% to 100% of patients. Important radiographic findings consistent with diastematomyelia include spina bifida occulta, which occurs in 76% to 94% of cases and widened interpedicular distance at the level of diastematomyelia, which occurs in 94% to 100% of cases.

It is not necessary to obtain a diagnostic study (MRI or myelogram) of the spinal canal in every child with congenital vertebral anomaly. Diagnostic studies should be obtained when significant back or leg pain, neurologic deficit, foot deformity, radiologically evident diastematomyelia or interpedicular widening, or combined unsegmented bar and hemivertebra are present. Studies should also be obtained for all spine fusion candidates.

Commonly cited reasons to excise a diastematomyelia include progressive neurologic deficit and impending spine fusion surgery with instrumentation. Most authors do not recommend excision of a diastematomyelia in the absence of a neurologic deficit or with a stable neurologic deficit, although one investigator recommends excision in all children in whom it is predicted that growth will create a spine deformity that will require spine fusion.

Natural History

Deformity of the spine may be the result of local vertebral architecture, unbalanced growth potential, or compensatory curves. Accurate predictions of growth potential based on imaging studies such as plain radiographs, tomograms, and MRI can be difficult to formulate, but natural history studies have identified some disturbing patterns of deformity. Results of two studies, one with 251 patients, and one with 234 patients, all with congenital scoliosis, showed that approximately 75% of the patients required treatment before they reached maturity. The rate of deformity formation and its final severity depended on the type and site of the deformity. Incarcerated or unsegmented single hemivertebrae show the lowest rate of progression. Fully segmented hemivertebrae with a contralateral bar, particularly at the thoracolumbar junction, always result in severe deformity. Scoliosis at the cervicothoracic junction causes shoulder height asymmetry and head tilt, and scoliosis at the lumbosacral junction can result in severe trunk decompensation. In general, progression is most rapid from time of birth to 3 years of age, and during early adolescence. The most difficult deformities to predict are those that involve failures of both formation and segmentation of numerous vertebrae, such as the spondylothoracic dysplasia syndrome. In any congenital spine deformity, high quality radiographs and meticulous measurements are essential to detect and quantify deformity progression.

Treatment

Braces have a limited role in the management of congenital scoliosis. An open-frame brace that carefully applies pressure to the soft thorax may help control early deformities in infants. In older children, braces may be useful to help control long flexible curves, curves resulting from multiple anomalies, or compensatory curves. Braces may slow the progression of deformity, but they cannot be expected to halt growth-related deformity. Most brace failures result from procrastination of use in the face of relentless deformity progression.

There are many surgical options to treat congenital scoliosis. Surgical options include posterior spine fusion, an-

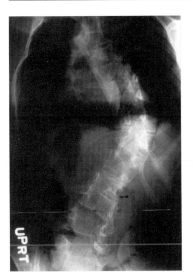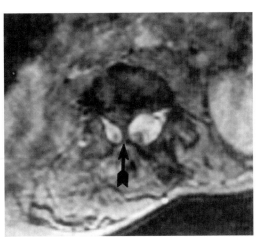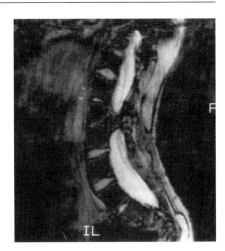

Fig. 2 Congenital scoliosis in a teenage girl. Diastematomyelia is noted at the L2–3 region **(left)**. MRIs demonstrate a split in the neural elements in the transverse plane **(center)** and sagittal plane **(right)**.

terior spine fusion, combined anterior and posterior spine fusion, partial fusion in the form of convex growth arrest or hemiepiphysiodesis, vertebral excision, and instrumentation as a part of fusion or as a temporary means of curve control while delaying fusion. The surgeon chooses the best surgical procedure according to the vertebral pathology, the behavior of the deformity, and evaluation of the child with the deformity.

Posterior spine fusion is the oldest surgical technique, as well as the simplest and safest, and is the benchmark against which to compare all other methods. The posterior spine fusion technique should include facetectomy and copious bone graft so that the result is a thick, wide fusion mass that will resist later growth deformity. When the technique is combined with use of a cast, some curve correction can be expected without risk of neurologic deficit. Instrumentation will produce a higher percentage of correction and less dependence on postsurgical casts and braces, but it also includes a higher risk of neurologic deficit that includes paralysis, particularly in patients with significant kyphosis, such as type I congenital kyphosis. Instrumentation should never be used without presurgical imaging of the spinal canal, and must be done with spinal cord monitoring or an intraoperative "wake-up" test. Indications for posterior spine fusion for congenital scoliosis include small or moderate size curves and curves with slow progression. The procedure should be performed on children in adolescence with limited growth potential. Lordotic scoliosis is a relative contraindication to posterior fusion. Indications for posterior fusion for congenital kyphosis include patients who have anterior bar formation and wedged vertebrae (type II deformities) and less than 50° of angulation. The fusion should include the entire kyphotic area plus one level above and one below, when fea-

sible. This may result in some spontaneous correction of the kyphosis and lead to a very satisfactory cosmetic appearance.

Anterior spine fusion as a single surgical solution outside the cervical spine is only applicable for progressive congenital lordosis caused by posterior segmentation defects. Anterior spine fusion is commonly used in combination with posterior spine fusion. Anterior spine fusion is more surgically complex, but it may improve deformity correction, reduce the incidence of pseudarthrosis, and prevent the bending of the posterior fusion from future growth (crankshaft phenomenon). Combined anterior and posterior spine fusion for congenital scoliosis is indicated for children with substantial growth potential; deformities with marked growth imbalance, such as both hemivertebrae and a bar; large rigid curves; and excessive kyphosis. Indications for a combined anterior and posterior spine fusion for congenital kyphosis include failure of anterior vertebral formation (type I deformities) or other deformities that occur with severe kyphosis.

In carefully selected patients, instrumentation without fusion may be a prelude to the definitive spine fusion. In patients with congenital scoliosis without spinal canal lesions, instrumentation may be used to control long curves with mixed anomalies or compensatory curves; however, there are significant risks associated with this method and repeated surgeries to modify rod length may be needed. Possible complications associated with the use of the instrumentation method include hook dislodgment, rod fracture, junctional kyphosis at the upper end of the instrumentation, and soft-tissue fibrosis from repetitive incisions and dissection. Repeated surgery for rod length modification or replacement is necessary every 6 to 9 months. Use of a brace is mandatory.

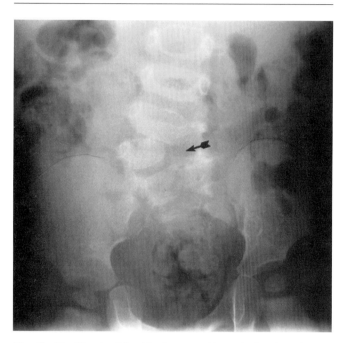

Fig. 3 Significant pelvic obliquity caused by an L5 hemivertebra is seen in a 2 1/2-year-old child.

Convex hemiarthrodesis and hemiepiphysiodesis is a procedure designed to prevent deformity progression and allow deformity improvement by surgically creating an anterior and posterior bar on the convexity of the scoliosis. This procedure is best performed on curves of limited length (five or fewer vertebrae), limited magnitude (less than 70°) with little or no kyphosis, and real concave growth potential. The entire curve segment must be included when performing this procedure and it may be appropriate to also include one level above and one level below the curve. The best demonstration of curve correction after surgery occurs in children younger than 5 years of age. The procedure generally consists of partial diskec-

tomy and bone grafting, with convex posterior facetectomy and fusion included. Some authors report success achieving the anterior growth arrest by a transpedicular vertebral body decancellation.

One of the most controversial surgical procedures for congenital scoliosis is hemivertebra excision. The hemivertebra excision may be considered the equivalent of an apical wedge excision and may be used when that type of curve correction is needed. The best indication for the procedure is a lumbosacral hemivertebra that causes an oblique angulation of the lumbar spine and significant trunk decompensation (Fig. 3). The entire hemivertebra must be removed and the entire curve fused in order for the procedure to be successful. Failure to remove all of the hemivertebra increases the risk of nerve root impingement, and failure to fuse the whole curve may result in progressive deformity. Extensive vertebrectomy is performed as an attempt to create correction through instability, although stable internal fixation is essential. This procedure carries with it the highest risk of neurologic deficit.

Although traction is rarely used in congenital scoliosis, it may be appropriate at times. A thorough evaluation of the spinal canal is essential before traction is used. Traction may be a means to gain slow, gradual deformity correction in a patient who is awake and whose neurologic function can be closely monitored. Indications for the use of traction include severe complex deformities, some compensatory curves with marked decompensation (between anterior and posterior procedures), and also following osteotomies of unilateral bars before final fusion.

The care of children with congenital vertebral anomalies begins with a careful patient evaluation that includes physical examination and spine deformity assessment. Treatment solutions are selected based on what is best for the particular deformity and results of the patient evaluation. The physician must be open-minded and able to offer the patient a number of treatment options. Finally, children with congenital spine deformities must be followed to maturity. Often, patients with congenital spinal deformity may need two or more episodes of treatment to achieve the best possible results for correction of the deformity.

Annotated Bibliography

Evaluation

Beals RK, Robbins JR, Rolfe B: Anomalies associated with vertebral malformations. *Spine* 1993;18:1329–1332.

This article is an extensive examination of 218 patients with a wide range of vertebral malformations, of which 61% were found to have anomalies affecting seven systems. No correlation could be found between extraspinal anomalies and the type and location of vertebral malformations.

Beals RK, Rolfe B: VATER association: A unifying concept of multiple anomalies. *J Bone Joint Surg* 1989;71A:948–950.

This extensive review of medical literature pertains to the collection of system anomalies associated with congenital vertebral anomalies that is frequently referred to as VATER association.

Bradford DS, Heithoff KB, Cohen M: Intraspinal abnormalities and congenital spine deformities: A radiographic and MRI study. *J Pediatr Orthop* 1991; 11:36–41.

Results of a study of nonconsecutive patients with congenital vertebral anomalies showed that 16 of 42 patients (38%) were found to have abnormalities of cord structure or location. The authors list possible indications for MRI examination of the spine in patients with congenital vertebral anomalies.

Day GA, Upadhyay SS, Ho EK, et al: Pulmonary functions in congenital scoliosis. *Spine* 1994;19:1027–1031.

Extensive pulmonary function tests on 28 consecutive patients with a mean curve magnitude of 43° were evaluated. The patients demonstrated reduced vital capacity, particularly in cases of multiple vertebral anomalies, indicating a restrictive pattern of lung function. The authors advocated early surgical intervention before significant deformity progression.

Drvaric DM, Ruderman RJ, Conrad RW, et al: Congenital scoliosis and urinary tract abnormalities: Are intravenous pyelograms necessary? *J Pediatr Orthop* 1987;7:441–443.

In this study, 100 congenital scoliosis patients were examined by intravenous pyelograms (IVP), and 25 additional patients were examined by IVP and ultrasonography (US). The authors detected a 37% incidence of structural urinary tract anomalies and concluded that US is a sufficiently accurate method of renal tract examination that can replace IVP as the primary screening tool for renal tract anomalies.

McMaster MJ: Occult intraspinal anomalies and congenital scoliosis. *J Bone Joint Surg* 1984;66A:588–601.

This article is an extremely thorough review of 251 patients from Scotland that was previously reported in a study of the natural history of congenital scoliosis. Findings reported by other investigators are confirmed and studied in detail. In addition to the commonly accepted indications for resection of diastematomyelia, the author recommends resection in all children in whom congenital scoliosis is detected before 6 years of age, regardless of neural status, and in children in whom it is predicted that future deformity of the spine will require surgical intervention.

Miller A, Guille JT, Bowen JR: Evaluation and treatment of diastematomyelia. *J Bone Joint Surg* 1993;75A:1308–1317.

In this careful review of 43 consecutive patients with diastematomyelia discovered over a 35 year period at the AI duPont Institute, the authors characterize the clinical presentation of individuals with diastematomyelia and review the literature. The authors recommend resection of the diastematomyelia if any progressive neurologic deterioration is documented.

Winter RB, Moe JH, Lonstein JE: The incidence of Klippel-Feil syndrome in patients with congenital scoliosis and kyphosis. *Spine* 1984;9:363–366.

This paper reports that in an exhaustive study of 1,215 patients with congenital vertebral anomalies, 25% of the patients have cervical vertebral anomalies. The cervical anomalies were diverse, and had no clear relationship with the particular form of vertebral anomalies found more distally in the spine.

Natural History

McMaster MJ, Ohtsuka K: The natural history of congenital scoliosis: A study of two hundred and fifty-one patients. *J Bone Joint Surg* 1982;64A:1128–1147.

This study is important reading material for any serious student of congenital vertebral anomalies. The authors carefully evaluate the patients and group them by types of vertebral anomalies. The natural history of each type of anomaly is presented, and the authors provide an invaluable table that demonstrates the risks of progression for each type of deformity, related to the location of the deformity in the spine.

Treatment

Bradford DS, Boachie-Adjei O: One-stage anterior and posterior hemivertebral resection and arthrodesis for congenital scoliosis. *J Bone Joint Surg* 1990;72A:536–540.

The authors report the outcomes of hemivertebra resection, combined with arthrodesis, in seven children with hemivertebra in the lumbar spine. Early results showed stable deformities without pseudarthrosis or neurologic deficit.

Winter RB, Lonstein JE, Denis F, et al: Convex growth arrest for progressive congenital scoliosis due to hemivertebrae. *J Pediatr Orthop* 1988;8:633–638.

In this study of the effects of "hemiepiphysiodesis-hemiarthrodesis" in the treatment of congenital vertebral anomalies in children, a slow reduction in curve magnitude as a result of this technique was demonstrated. The authors outline their prerequisites for this type of surgery.

Winter RB, Moe JH: The results of spinal arthrodesis for congenital spinal deformity in patients younger than five years old. *J Bone Joint Surg* 1982;64A:419–432.

Patients who undergo spinal arthrodesis at a very young age are the focus of this study. The authors examine the efficacy of spinal arthrodesis for serious early congenital vertebral deformities, and the effect on body proportions.

Winter RB, Moe JH, Eilers VE: Congenital scoliosis: A study of 234 patients treated and untreated. I: Natural history and II: Treatment. *J Bone Joint Surg* 1968:50A:1–47.

This is the first truly comprehensive study of individuals with congenital vertebral anomalies. Although some aspects of surgical care have changed with time, notably spinal instrumentation, the natural history of congenital scoliosis and the principles of care put forth in this article remain valid.

Winter RB, Moe JH, Lonstein JE: Posterior spinal arthrodesis for congenital scoliosis: An analysis of the cases of two hundred and ninety patients, five to nineteen years old. *J Bone Joint Surg* 1984;66A:1188–1197.

In this companion study to the article from the same center that reported treatment of children with congenital vertebral deformities younger than 5 years of age, an extremely large number of individuals between 5 and 19 years of age at the time of their surgery are examined retrospectively. None of these patients had an anterior spinal arthrodesis. Bending of the fusion mass occurred in only 14% of patients, and pseudarthrosis was detected in only 7% of patients.

15

Scheuermann's Disorder

Introduction

There are few physical features of a child that concern parents as much as increased rounding of the back, or thoracic kyphosis. Most parents consider it unsightly and believe it is the result of poor posture. They seek to have thoracic kyphosis corrected during childhood because they fear it will become a stigma for their child during adulthood.

A single Cobb angular measurement value cannot describe a "normal" thoracic kyphosis. Instead, normal is defined by a range of measurements obtained from the standardized standing lateral radiographs of a large number of individuals. Studies suggest that approximately 95% of normal individuals have between 20° and 45° of thoracic kyphosis in their early adult years. Thoracic kyphosis slowly increases as part of the natural aging process, particularly in postmenopausal women.

A "postural" thoracic hyperkyphosis is a flexible curvature with normal vertebral structures and intervertebral disks. There is no evidence that such curvatures predispose individuals to pain or disability. One type of thoracic hyperkyphosis, however, commonly referred to as Scheuermann's disease, includes abnormalities of vertebral and disk structures and may be associated with problems in adulthood. The definition of Scheuermann's disease, its consequences, and treatment are controversial.

In 1920, Holger Scheuermann, a Danish radiologist and orthopaedist, described the radiographic characteristics of the deformity that now bears his name. His findings included increased thoracic kyphosis in adolescence, wedging of vertebral bodies, and irregularity of vertebral end plates. He speculated that these findings were the result of aseptic necrosis. In 1964, Sorenson proposed the criteria by which the term Scheuermann's kyphosis could be applied: three adjacent vertebrae with wedging of at least 5°.

More recently, several more abnormal radiographic findings in the spines of children have been described. These include wedging, irregular end plates, protrusion of disk material into the vertebral body (Schmorl's nodes), narrowing of disk height, and the development of spinal stiffness (Fig. 1). Although these findings are generally associated with hyperkyphosis, they are also seen in spines with sagittal curves that are well within accepted normal ranges.

Theories about the causes of these abnormal radiographic findings include familial predisposition, hormonal abnormalities, collagen defects, juvenile osteoporosis, excessive manual labor, athletic injuries, and vitamin deficiencies. Ultrastructural studies of children in whom these abnormal findings appear have shown that the vertebral end plates and physes are thinned or absent. Chondrocytes are disorganized and variable in size and shape. Proteoglycan content in the spinal area is altered and there is a reduction in thick collagen fibrils. Ossification is abnormal, with distorted vertebral growth.

Recent publications about Scheuermann's kyphosis have become inconsistent regarding patient material and terminology. The term Scheuermann's kyphosis has been used to describe individuals who meet Sorenson's criteria, in addition to those with a single vertebra wedged at least

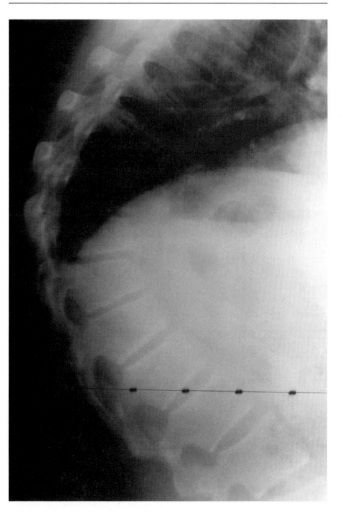

Fig. 1 Scheuermann's disorder in a male teenager. Note the vertebral wedging and narrowed thoracic disk spaces.

125

5°, diffuse minor vertebral wedging, or even stiff hyper-kyphosis with end-plate irregularities and no wedging. Uncertainty about the etiology of Scheuermann's kyphosis has allowed the use of terms such as disease, disorder, or condition. It has become very difficult to apply the information in the medical literature to the problems of a particular individual.

Use of a single term, Scheuermann's disorder, that would represent a spectrum of clinical presentations may be the best solution to the problem of inconsistency. At one end of the spectrum would be those individuals with spinal deformity caused by focal wedging of vertebral bodies. At the other end of the spectrum would be those individuals who have normal sagittal contours, but who also experience disk narrowing, end plate irregularities, and Schmorl's nodes. Such a spectrum may be artificial and bring together unrelated conditions, but, because definitive explanations for these findings are lacking, it would provide a reasonable framework to organize patients and their problems.

Natural History

Most adolescents with Scheuermann's disorder are evaluated because of excessive rounding of the back. When pain does exist, it is usually associated with rapid growth, activities that emphasize forward flexion or lifting, or athletic activities. Symptoms may be present for weeks or months, and are often described as dull, aching, annoying, or non-radiating pain. The pain is usually at the apex of deformity or in the lumbar region. Neural defects are not found in this age group.

Significant kyphosis or pain in adolescence is often cited as evidence that adult disability is impending and treatment should be started. Recent natural history studies challenge the belief that adult disability is common in Scheuermann's disorder. Pain in two groups of individuals in Iowa, one group with Scheuermann's disorder and the other a control group, was compared. All of the participants were between 25 and 82 years of age. Patients with Scheuermann's disorder had pain that was more intense and in a different location than in individuals in the control group. The most intense pain was experienced by individuals with more severe kyphosis, especially if the apex of the deformity was above level T8. Overall, the effect of this pain was not remarkably different from that experienced by the control group. Individuals in the group with Scheuermann's disorder demonstrated less trunk flexibility and usually held less physically demanding jobs. Otherwise, their education, total amount of time absent from work, recreational activities, pain medication use, and self-esteem were similar to those of the control group. Restrictive lung disease was found only in those individuals with kyphosis greater than 100°, with a deformity apex above level T8.

Other studies have focused on individuals with normal sagittal curves but who have disk narrowing, end-plate ir-regularities, and Schmorl's nodes, particularly in the lower thoracic and upper lumbar regions. Diagnostic imaging centers, where many individuals with back pain are evaluated with magnetic resonance scans and computed tomography, have reported a possible relationship between Scheuermann's disorders, radiographic findings, and early adult degenerative disk disease. Many of the individuals who undergo diagnostic imaging have already undergone surgical procedures, and show degenerative changes in disks above the fusions in the mid and lower lumbar spine.

Nonsurgical Treatment

Stretching and strengthening exercises and brace treatment are the only nonsurgical methods available to treat Scheuermann's disorder. Stretching and strengthening exercises for the trunk may improve pain symptoms but will not improve the deformity.

Brace treatment can improve the kyphosis. Studies of brace treatment of Scheuermann's disorder suggest that bracing, with or without preceding extension cast correction, initially reduces the magnitude of the kyphosis and that progression occurs during brace use and continues after cessation of bracing. Studies also suggest that a large number of adolescents fail to complete an adequate course of brace treatment.

This overview may be excessively gloomy. Several factors may be used to predict success or failure of brace treatment in children. Factors that suggest brace success include a moderate deformity (< 70°), a lower apex (level T9 or below), flexibility, diffuse kyphosis instead of severe focal deformity, meaningful growth potential (≥ 2 years), and the child's genuine interest in treatment of the deformity. The most effective brace is the Milwaukee brace. A skilled orthotist is needed to adjust the brace in the first 6 weeks of wear, to adapt the brace to the gradual improvement in the deformity.

Surgical Treatment

Currently, the acceptable indications for spine fusion treatment of Scheuermann's disorder include a deformity of greater than 70°, progressive deformity, pain, and the patient's genuine concern about appearance. Spine fusion may consist of a combined anterior and posterior procedure or a posterior procedure only. Several studies demonstrate that good outcomes may be achieved with either technique. The role of multilevel disk excision and bone grafting with release of the anterior longitudinal ligament remains controversial. The best indications for a multilevel disk excision and bone grafting appear to be large, stiff deformities, especially those with very focal kyphosis.

In the past, the traditional spinal instrumentation used for Scheuermann's disorder was dual Harrington compression rods. This type of instrumentation was not particularly strong and as a result, curve progression, rod breakage, and pseudarthrosis were often reported. Today, stronger dual rod, multiple hook, and segmental fixation systems are used with reports of better and more durable correction and lower pseudarthrosis rates.

Short segment kyphosis immediately above or below the fusion region is a troublesome complication of spine fusion in Scheuermann's disorder. Failure to include all vertebrae in the kyphotic segment during a spine fusion is a common cause of progressive kyphosis above or below the fusion segment. Excessive deformity correction, to a magnitude less than 50% of the original measurement, appears to be associated with increased risk of proximal kyphosis. Failure to include the first lordotic disk space and nonwedged vertebrae below the kyphotic segment appears to be associated with an increased risk of short segment kyphosis below the fusion.

Annotated Bibliography

Heithoff KB, Grundry CR, Burton CV, et al: Juvenile discogenic disease. *Spine* 1994;19:335–340.

Patients in this study were referred to a diagnostic imaging center for either computed tomographic radiographs or magnetic resonance scans of the thoracolumbar and lumbar spine. The authors point out the correlation between a relatively early onset of lumbar degenerative intervertebral disk disease and the presence of findings usually associated with Scheuermann's disease. They speculate that such patients are at risk for degenerative change, and may not respond to fusion surgery in the same manner as patients lacking the Scheuermann-like changes.

Ippolito E, Bellocci M, Montanaro A, et al: Juvenile kyphosis: An ultrastructural study. *J Pediatr Orthop* 1985;5:315–322.

Vertebral end plates and intervening intervertebral disk material from seven individuals with severe juvenile kyphosis were examined by histologic and histochemical methods. Abnormalities in gross structure, chondrocytes, proteoglycans, and collagen fibrils were found when compared to an age-related normal individual.

Lowe TG, Kasten MD: An analysis of sagittal curves and balance after Cotrel-Dubousset instrumentation for kyphosis secondary to Scheuermann's disease: A review of 32 patients. *Spine* 1994;19:1680–1685.

This is a study of 32 individuals with kyphosis greater than 75° who were treated by combined anterior and posterior spine fusion and multiple hook, dual rod, and segmental instrumentation. Junctional kyphosis proximal to the fused segment was associated with correction that exceeded 50% of the original curve magnitude and failure to include all of the vertebrae in the upper half of the kyphotic segment. Junctional kyphosis distal to the fused segment was associated with failure to include the vertebrae immediately below the first lordotic intervertebral disk space.

Murray PM, Weinstein SL, Spratt KF: The natural history and long-term follow-up of Scheuermann's kyphosis. *J Bone Joint Surg* 1993;75A:236–248.

The authors studied 67 individuals with a diagnosis of Scheuermann's kyphosis. The mean age of the participants was 52 years. Methods included a questionnaire, examination, radiographs, and pulmonary function tests. Statistically significant differences for some factors were found between the participants and a control group, especially for very large curves with an apex above level T8. The authors do not believe that the differences are a major interference in their patients' lives and they questioned the value of spine fusion surgery.

Reinhardt P, Bassett GS: Short segmental kyphosis following fusion for Scheuermann's disease. *J Spinal Disord* 1990;3:162–168.

This is a review of 14 individuals with Scheuermann's kyphosis who were treated by spine fusion. The fusions were intended to include all vertebrae in the measured kyphotic segment. Despite inclusion of the wedged distal end vertebrae, progressive junctional kyphosis developed in three of 12 patients. The authors state that the distal end of the fusion must include an unwedged or "square" vertebra to eliminate this problem.

Sachs B, Bradford D, Winter R, et al: Scheuermann kyphosis: Follow-up of Milwaukee-brace treatment. *J Bone Joint Surg* 1987;69A:50–57.

This is an important study of the effects of Milwaukee brace treatment of Scheuermann's kyphosis, with minimum of 5 years follow-up after completion of bracing. Half of the original patient group was lost to follow-up during brace treatment. The study demonstrates a consistent response to the Milwaukee brace that included significant reduction of kyphosis initially, some progression during brace use, and further progression after cessation of bracing. Numerous factors affecting results were analyzed. The factors that were predictive of poor brace outcome were large magnitude of deformity (>70°), poor brace wear or inadequate use of the brace, and initiation of brace treatment too late in adolescence.

Sturm PF, Dobson JC, Armstrong GW: The surgical management of Scheuermann's disease. *Spine* 1993; 18:685–691.

Scheuermann's kyphosis in 39 individuals was treated by posterior spine fusion with Harrington compression instrumentation and outcomes were analyzed. The average presurgical kyphosis of 71° was reduced to 32° immediately, and was found to be 37° at follow-up. The authors discussed problems of hook or rod failure and concluded that anterior longitudinal ligament release and interbody fusion are rarely needed.

16

Spondylolysis and Spondylolisthesis

Introduction

Spondylolysis and spondylolisthesis, although relatively frequent in the general population (4% to 6%), are often asymptomatic and may go undiagnosed. Many times, however, these conditions cause problems such as pain, progressive deformity, or neurologic problems, which require specific treatment. In the 1980s, successful and reliable methods of treatment were reported for the mild or moderate conditions. For severe degrees of spondylolisthesis, especially in children, spine surgeons have not clearly defined the specific roles of various treatment modalities. Many authors have addressed these issues in the early 1990s, and as our knowledge and experience grow, more exact indications for specific treatment measures will be identified.

Definitions and Classification

The words spondylolysis and spondylolisthesis are derived from the Greek words *spondylo* (spine), *lysis* (breakdown) and *Olisthanerin* (to slip). Although bilateral spondylolysis is more common, unilateral spondylolysis also occurs, especially in association with trauma. In children, the most common site for spondylolisthesis is L5 on S1, but slippage of L4 on L5 does occur. Spondylolisthesis in the cervical and thoracic spine has also been reported.

In cases of severe spondylolisthesis of L5 on S1, the L5 vertebral body angulates (angular slippage and sagittal rotation) and loss of trunk height occurs. When the posterior portion of the body of L5 falls off the anterior lip of the sacrum, associated with severe sagittal rotation and vertical sinking, the terms total spondylolisthesis and spondyloptosis are used.

Spondylolisthesis is classified into five subtypes: dysplastic, isthmic, degenerative, traumatic, and pathologic. In the pediatric age group, the majority of deformities are either dysplastic or isthmic. The dysplastic type is associated with congenital abnormalities of the upper sacrum or of the posterior arch of L5. In the isthmic type, the defect occurs in the pars interarticularis. This defect may be lytic (fatigue fractures), elongated (pars remains intact), or the result of an acute fracture. This current review in children is limited to the dysplastic and isthmic types of spondylolysis and spondylolisthesis.

Prevalence and Etiology

Spondylolysis and spondylolisthesis are commonly, but incorrectly, referred to as congenital abnormalities. Rarely have pars defects been reported in infants or in those younger than 5 years of age. More commonly, it is noted after 7 to 8 years of age. The prevalence of spondylolysis and spondylolisthesis gradually increases in the general population until age 20 and then is stationary. The reported prevalence is between 4% and 6%.

Genetic, traumatic, and developmental etiologies have all been reported as causing spondylolysis. Prevalences ranging from 27% to 69% have been reported in first degree relatives, with it being more common in the dysplastic type (33%) than in the isthmic type (15%). A high prevalence (54%) of spondylolysis exists in certain Eskimo tribes. Racial differences have also been noted between African-Americans (1% in females) and Caucasians (6% in males). Finally, there is an increased prevalence of sacral spina bifida and congenital lack of development of the proximal part of the sacrum and superior sacral facets in spondylolysis. This is seen in 94% of the dysplastic and 32% of the isthmic types. Even with these abnormalities in the anatomy, a defect of the pars interarticularis in very young children is rare.

Repetitive trauma as a cause of spondylolysis has been widely supported. The upright position of man strongly suggests that repetitive forces acting on the lower lumbar spine may produce the pars defect. Spondylolysis and spondylolisthesis are conditions known only in humans and are not found in other species, including semierect primates. Increased lumbar lordosis in the posture of young children during the early phases of gait development may place increased stresses on the pars and neural arch areas ultimately leading to the pars fracture. A prevalence of 50% of spondylolysis has been reported in Scheuermann's disorder, presumably because of the excessive lumbar lordosis that is present secondary to the thoracic or thoracolumbar kyphosis. More specifically, a traumatic etiology is supported by an 11% prevalence of spondylolysis in adolescent athletes, including female gymnasts, weight lifters, and football players (Fig. 1).

Spondylolisthesis also occurs in children affected by neuromuscular conditions. A recent study evaluated the prevalence of spondylolisthesis in patients with myelodysplasia. In a group of 305 myelomeningocele patients with congenital absence of the posterior neural arch, the prevalence was 6%, which is identical to that of the normal population. However, the frequency of spondylolisthesis increased as the child's level of function increased. Those with minimal function (L1-L2 level) had a 2% prevalence while those with L5-S1 function had a 16% prevalence. Increased lumbar lordosis and body weight were also associated with an increased prevalence. None of the children

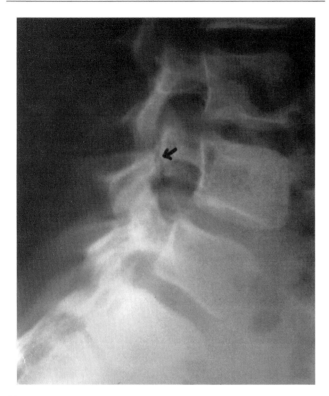

Fig. 1 Lateral radiograph showing an acute pars fracture in a 10-year-old injured while high-jumping.

with thoracic level function had spondylolisthesis. Rather, only those patients who exhibited some degree of ambulation were affected. Ambulatory children with spastic diplegia also have an increased prevalence of L5-S1 spondylolisthesis (14%).

Natural History

Although dysplastic spondylolisthesis may be seen before age 4 or 5, isthmic spondylolisthesis is uncommon before then. Isthmic spondylolysis commonly occurs between 5 and 8 years of age and, as previously mentioned, results from multiple fatigue fractures in the pars interarticularis of L4 or L5. These fatigue fractures either heal (leading to an elongated pars) or progress to nonunion. If only one pars is affected, sclerosis of the opposite pars may develop as a result of stress concentration. If involvement of the pars is bilateral, spondylolisthesis may occur. With spondylolisthesis, premature disk degeneration may occur and disk herniation, although rare, has been reported in the adolescent. For reasons unknown, girls are more prone to severe displacement. During the adolescent growth spurt, the likelihood for rapid worsening of the slippage increases (Fig. 2). However, if the slip is mild (less than 50%), the chances of progression are low. In one study of 47 children

with low-grade spondylolisthesis (50% or less), only 4% (two patients) progressed over a 7-year span. The intervertebral disk above the spondylolisthesis may be affected. Using diskography and magnetic resonance imaging (MRI), abnormalities have been demonstrated both at the level of the slip and at the disk above. The clinical significance of this in the adolescent remains unknown.

New information from large series of patients with long follow-up suggests that progression of severe spondylolisthesis (greater than 50%) is common and cannot be predicted. At the very least, follow-up every 6 months during the adolescent growth spurt is warranted in patients with spondylolisthesis of greater than 50%. Progression of the slip or refractory pain are the primary indications for fusion. Fusion to prevent progression of mild (25%) or moderate (50%) spondylolisthesis is not indicated.

Clinical Findings

Symptoms are relatively uncommon in children, but when they do develop, they usually occur at the onset of the adolescent growth spurt. In addition to back discomfort, children also present because of postural deformity or abnormal gait from tight hamstrings. Pain, if present, is frequently related to activities. Radicular symptoms are uncommon but, on a rare occasion, a disk herniation may occur, making physical examination necessary. Back pain may be a result of localized inflammation from the defect, may be associated with instability of the affected segment, or may be secondary to degeneration of the disk at the slip level. Radicular symptoms are more common with higher degrees of slip (grades III through V).

The physical findings correlate with the degree of slippage. In the child with minimal slippage (grades I and II) and few symptoms, spinal appearance and gait may be normal. As slippage increases, a visible and palpable step-off at the affected level may be evident and may be painful to palpation. There may be restricted motion of the lumbar spine with limitation of straight leg raising secondary to hamstring tightness. With high degrees of slip and associated lumbar kyphosis, hyperlordosis of the lumbar spine develops above the slip and the upper torso is shifted backward to compensate for the anterior translation of the slipped vertebra. As the degree of lumbosacral kyphosis increases, the pelvis and sacrum rotate posteriorly, creating a loss of buttock contour (Fig. 3). Torso shortening may occur as lumbar lordosis increases or spondyloptosis develops. A significant gait disturbance may develop and has been described as a pelvic waddle. The neurologic examination may reveal motor, sensory, or reflex abnormalities. Up to one third of those with spondylolisthesis of more than 50% may display these findings.

Three types of scoliosis can be seen in patients with spondylolisthesis—sciatic, olisthetic, and idiopathic. The first two are related to the spondylolisthesis directly. Sciatic scoliosis, a nonstructural lumbar curve caused by muscle spasm, resolves with recumbency or with relief of

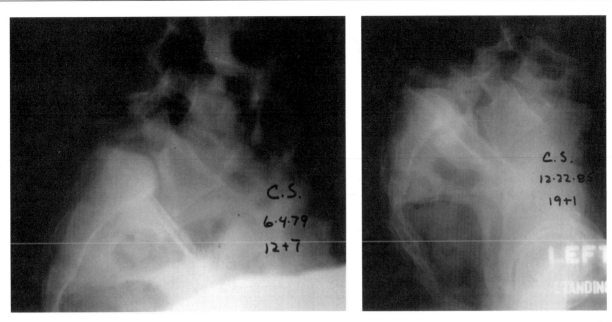

Fig. 2 **Left,** Grade III L5-S1 spondylolisthesis at age 12 years, 7 months. **Right,** In 6 years, the L5 slippage has increased to grade IV, and vertical sinking has occurred.

pain (Fig. 4). Olisthetic scoliosis is a torsional lumbar curve that begins at the spondylolytic area. Most sciatic and olisthetic curves resolve after surgical stabilization of the spondylolisthesis. Idiopathic scoliosis is a structural curve in the thoracic or thoracolumbar spine, and these curves do not correct with stabilization of the spondylolisthesis in patients with spondylolisthesis. A standing posteroanterior radiograph of the entire spine is obtained to evaluate this possible association.

Radiologic Evaluation

Plain radiographic evaluation includes standing anteroposterior, lateral, and oblique views of the lumbosacral spine. Flexion and extension lateral radiographs may be helpful in assessing lumbosacral instability. For patients in whom no clear delineation of the anatomic pathology can be seen, oblique tomograms or computed tomography (CT) may be useful. Enhanced CT scanning or MRI should only be considered if findings suggest nerve root compression from an associated rare herniated disk.

Unilateral pars defects occur in 20% of patients with spondylolysis. Oblique tomograms or CT may be needed to visualize these lesions adequately. The associated reactive sclerosis of the opposite pars interarticularis or lamina may be further delineated with CT. Radionuclide bone scans may demonstrate increased activity in either of these pars interarticularis conditions.

MRI evaluation of symptomatic children and adoles-

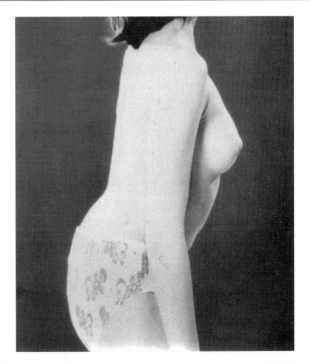

Fig. 3 Lateral clinical photograph showing severe grade IV L5-S1 spondylolisthesis.

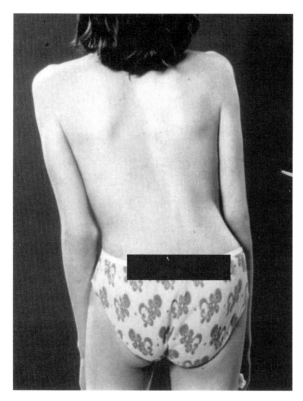

Fig. 4   Posterior view of the same patient as in Fig. 3. Note list from sciatic scoliosis.

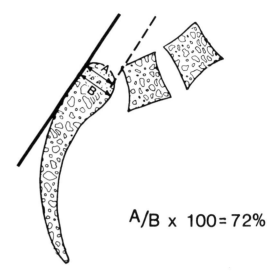

A/B x 100=72%

Fig. 5   Percent slip (Taillard classification). (Reproduced with permission from Bradford DS: Spondylolysis and spondylolisthesis in children and adolescents: Current concepts in management, in *The Pediatric Spine.* New York, NY, Thieme, 1985, p 406.)

cents with spondylolisthesis may show disk degeneration at or above the slip level in a large percentage of patients. This information may be helpful in planning treatment. Furthermore, SPECT (single-photon emission CT) imaging can be useful in the early diagnosis of spondylolisthesis. In the predisruptive phase, edema and hemorrhage from microfracture of the pars may be detected.

There are many methods for measuring the deformity associated with spondylolisthesis on standing lateral radiographs. For translational or tangential displacement, the Meyerding grading system is most commonly used and is based on the percentage of slippage: grade I, 0 to 25%; grade II, 25% to 50%; grade III, 50% to 75%; and grade IV, greater than 75%. Taillard also measures the percent slippage by comparing the anterior displacement of the posterior edge of L5 on the sacrum as a percentage of the L5 vertebral body width (Fig. 5). Slip angle, or the angle of lumbosacral kyphosis, is calculated by measuring the angle between a line perpendicular to the posterior aspect of S1 and a second line parallel to the endplate of L5 (Fig. 6). Occasionally, the inferior endplate of L5 is too deformed to measure accurately. In this instance, the superior endplate of L5 can be used. Sacral inclination is the angle that the sacral reference line makes with a line perpendicular to the floor. Normally this should be greater than 30° (Fig. 7).

Treatment

Spondylolysis

Asymptomatic spondylolysis requires observation only. Symptomatic spondylolysis in the adolescent is uncommon, and, when present, it is necessary to rule out other causes of pain, such as disk space infection, herniated disk, tumor, or osteoid osteoma. Initial treatment of the symptomatic spondylolysis should be conservative, and includes rest and activity modifications, nonsteroidal anti-inflammatory drugs, exercises, traction, bracing, and casting. All children or adolescents with symptomatic bilateral spondylolysis should be followed for the possible development of spondylolisthesis, although this would be uncommon. If an acute pars fracture from a hyperextension injury is documented, thoracolumbosacral orthosis (TLSO) or cast immobilization is recommended because healing of the acute pars interarticularis may occur.

A small percentage of symptomatic children with bilateral defects who do not respond to conservative treatment may require surgical stabilization. An L5 to S1 posterolateral fusion provides relief of symptoms. An alternative to the L5-S1 posterolateral fusion is direct repair of the spondylolitic defect. Some authors recommend that MRI evaluation be done preoperatively to determine whether L5-S1 disk degeneration is present. If degenerative disk disease is present at the defect level, a conventional posterolateral segmental fusion is recommended, not direct repair of the pars defect. Several techniques of direct pars defect repair have been advocated, including screw fixation, hook-screw fixation, pedicle screw wiring, and the modified Scott wiring technique. If a pedicle screw is used for the proximal

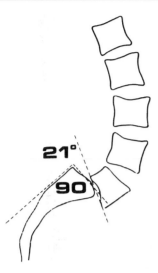

Fig. 6 Slip angle. (Reproduced with permission from Bradford DS: Spondylolysis and spondylolisthesis in children and adolescents: Current concepts in management, in *The Pediatric Spine*. New York, NY, Thieme, 1985, p 406.)

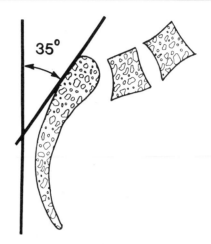

Fig. 7 Sacral inclination. (Reproduced with permission from Bradford DS: Spondylolysis and spondylolisthesis in children and adolescents: Current concepts in management, in *The Pediatric Spine*. New York, NY, Thieme, 1985, p 406.)

anchor for the wiring, it eliminates the need to pass wires around the transverse process, thereby avoiding nerve root injury.

Asymptomatic Spondylolisthesis

In asymptomatic patients with grade I or II slips, observation alone is recommended. Only 4% of grade I or II slips are expected to progress. If progression does occur, in-situ posterolateral fusion is recommended. For more severe spondylolisthesis (>50%), the likelihood of progressive worsening is greater. Consideration should be given for surgical stabilization.

Symptomatic Spondylolisthesis

In those with mild spondylolisthesis, a conservative treatment program as outlined above will often provide pain relief. However, nonsurgical management is much less successful in controlling symptoms in those with grade III or IV slips. Other risk factors associated with unsuccessful conservative management include young age, female gender, persistent symptomatology, dysplastic type slip, increasing slip angle, kyphosis greater than 40°, or flexion/extension instability. For the symptomatic patient with associated risk factors, fusion should be considered. In grade I or II slips, an in-situ posterolateral fusion is recommended. If the slip is greater than 50% (grade III or IV), extension of the posterolateral fusion to L4 is needed. In these high-grade slips, a pantaloon cast for 3 to 4 months postoperatively is recommended to optimize the fusion rates, prevent progressive deformity and improve the lumbosacral kyphosis. Excellent long-term results (without

neurologic deficits) have been reported using this technique.

Continued slip progression may occur after surgery even if the patient is kept supine, especially if the slip angle is more than 55° with more than 50% slippage. Progression has been shown to occur in spite of an apparently solid fusion. In this circumstance, reduction with or without supplemental anterior fusion may be beneficial. Several authors report that the presence of L5-S1 kyphosis is prognostic for the potential success of a posterolateral fusion alone.

If the kyphosis is reducible, then posterolateral fusion with pantaloon casting is indicated. For patients with spondylolisthesis of Meyerding grade IV or greater, with a slip angle of more than 45° and a rigid kyphosis, then combined anterior release and fusion with posterior reduction techniques and fusion have been reported to achieve stability in the older adolescent. Maintenance of reduction may be accomplished with a combination of casting and instrumentation.

In the 1990s, the concept of reduction and instrumentation has been reported with increasing frequency as newer fixation devices have become available. Advantages of instrumentation include deformity correction, partial or complete reduction, and maintenance of the reduction. Pedicle segmental instrumentation (L4-S1) has distinct advantages in correcting both the lumbosacral kyphosis as well as the translation of L5. However, the main goal is reduction of the kyphosis and a solid arthrodesis rather than correction of translational displacement. Older adolescents, who are approaching skeletal maturity and who have very severe spondylolisthesis (grade IV spondylolisthesis and rigid kyphosis greater than 45°), may benefit from these newer techniques of reduction, instrumentation, and fusion. However, these salvage procedures are fraught with a myriad of complications and should be performed only by the experienced spine surgeon. The most common complications are secondary to pedicle screw placement with both motor and sensory neurologic deficits. Neurologic deficits may also occur with aggressive reduction either by hyperextension casting or with instrumentation that stretches contracted lumbar nerve roots. In addition, disk herniation may occur with aggressive reduction. In order to avoid complications associated with nerve root contraction from prolonged L5-S1 kyphosis, some authors have advocated L5 vertebrectomy before reduction. Nevertheless, neurologic complications are still high for these salvage procedures. Although most of the deficits are transient, permanent deficits are reported in series by experienced spine surgeons.

Long-Term Follow-up

Controversy continues concerning the best treatment for severe spondylolisthesis when the slip is greater than 50%. Most authorities agree that surgical treatment is indicated when the patient is symptomatic and, because of the risk of progression in the immature child or adolescent, many would consider surgical treatment in the asymptomatic patient. While arthrodesis without reduction of the slip angle or translation has been successful in grade I or II slips, progression after arthrodesis in grade III or IV slips may be a problem. Reduction either by casting or surgical reduction with instrumentation has been advocated, but major complications have been associated with reduction. The issue then hinges on whether the results of reduction justify the increased risks.

Since 1990, a number of authors have attempted to elucidate the issue of risk versus benefit in their long-term review of large series of patients treated by various techniques. In a report on 105 patients treated with in situ fusion, 39 had grade III or IV slips (of more than 50%) that were treated with combined anterior and posterior in situ fusion. After 8 years follow-up, postoperative progression was uncommon. Their data suggested that grade III or IV slips can be successfully treated surgically without reduction or instrumentation. In another series reporting the results of posterolateral fusion without reduction for patients with slips greater than 50%, lumbosacral kyphosis was increased in 45% at follow-up. Other authors have compared the results of in situ fusion alone with reduction, fusion, and cast immobilization. In these reports, the authors found that reduction and fusion resulted in decreased progression of the deformity postoperatively (without neurologic deficit) in comparison to the in situ fusion group alone. Nevertheless, further progression did occur in several patients in the reduction and fusion group. Despite this, nearly all of the patients were without low back complaints or activity restrictions in long-term follow-up. Because of concern regarding progressive clinical and radiographic deformity that can occur following posterolateral fusion and cast immobilization alone, sev-

eral authors state that for severe symptomatic slips with significant kyphotic deformities that reduction, fusion, and instrumentation may be indicated.

Reducing the spondylolisthesis and associated lumbosacral kyphosis with gradual traction followed by anterior and posterior fusion without instrumentation has been reported. A good result was achieved in 86% of the patients. Although complete reduction of the spondylolisthesis was not achieved with traction, the lumbosacral kyphosis was significantly improved. The complication rate was high and included radiculopathy and footdrop. Others have reported successful results in the adolescent with severe spondylolisthesis following reduction, instrumentation, and fusion. Associated minor neurologic deficits, most of which are transient, are present in each report. Grade V slips (spondyloptosis) and certain grade IV slips with higher slip angles (greater than 45°) would most likely benefit with instrumentation for maintenance of reduction along with anterior and posterior fusion.

When deciding whether to reduce a grade IV slip or fuse in situ it is helpful to review long-term gait abnormalities with in situ fusions. A recent study reported that four of seven patients fused in situ during adolescence for grade IV spondylolisthesis had slight residual forward trunk lean with increased hip flexion on gait analysis. Residual knee crouch could not be demonstrated. With regard to cosmesis, three patients noted their backs appeared the same as their peers, but four felt their backs looked worse. The authors concluded that the patients had acceptable cosmetic results in terms of trunk alignment, although some shortening was noted.

In conclusion, the evaluation and treatment of spondylolisthesis is challenging as well as rewarding. Careful planning, both in the selection of patients for surgical intervention and the surgical techniques used, is mandatory. Unfortunately, surgical complication rates, including permanent neurologic deficits, increase dramatically when reduction is undertaken in the more severe slips. Because of these factors, it is advised that these particular patients be treated by spine surgeons experienced in these techniques.

At the time of this writing, bone screws placed posteriorly into vertebral elements have not been cleared for use in this specific manner by the Food and Drug Administration (FDA). These are Class III devices. This category includes screws placed transfacetally, within pedicles, or in articular, lateral masses. Some bone screws for use within the sacrum have been approved as Class II devices. Some companies have received Class II clearance for use of screws in lumbar pedicles specifically to supplement fusions in the treatment of grade III and IV spondylolisthesis with the proviso that these devices are removed after the arthrodesis has healed. Anterior vertebral body screws (cervical, thoracic, and lumbar) are Class II devices and can be used as labeled in vertebral bodies. Many of the posterior screw-based devices have been shown in laboratory and clinical testing to be useful and may be used in an off-label manner if the physician feels this is appropriate and important for the treatment of the patient. As with all surgeries, informed consent should explain the procedure and why a particular technique has been chosen, as well as its risks and benefits. The question of whether informed consent regarding pedicle screws must include a discussion of the device's FDA clearance status is currently being litigated in several jurisdictions. In cases that have been included in the multidistrict litigation in the Eastern District of Pennsylvania, this additional requirement has not been imposed.

Annotated Bibliography

Prevalence and Etiology

Harada T, Ebara S, Anwar MM, et al: The lumbar spine in spastic diplegia: A radiographic study. *J Bone Joint Surg* 1993;75B:534–537.

This is a random sample (84 patients) of a spastic diplegia population. Forty-three patients were 19 years of age or under and all were ambulatory. Six of 43 patients between the ages of 10 and 19 had spondylolysis between L5 and S1, a prevalence of 14%. A definite correlation was found between increased lumbar lordosis and spondylolysis suggesting repetitive micro-trauma from posterior element compressive forces.

Ogilvie JW, Sherman J: Spondylolysis in Scheuermann's disease. *Spine* 1987;12:251–253.

Spondylolytic defects were noted radiographically in 9 of 18 patients with Scheuermann's disease.

Stanitski CL, Stanitski DF, LaMont RL: Spondylolisthesis in myelomeningocele. *J Pediatr Orthop* 1994;14:586–591.

Myelomeningocele was reviewed in 305 patients, and a 6% incidence of asymptomatic spondylolisthesis was reported. Of those with spondylolisthesis, the vertebral translation averaged 37%. Patient age averaged 12.2 years. Lumbar lordosis, thoracic kyphosis, neurosegmental level of involvement, and the ratio of body weight to height were all examined to determine whether there was a correlation with the incidence and degree of spondylolisthesis. Positive correlations were noted for increased lumbar lordosis and the incidence of spondylolisthesis, as well as for increased body weight and increased severity of spondylolisthesis. More importantly, a positive correlation was noted between the patient's level of function and the incidence of spondylolisthesis. A progressive rise in the prevalence of spondylolisthesis was seen with increasing function (2% at the L1-L2 level, 16% at the L5-S1 level). Only 11% of those with slips showed progression. None of the patients with thoracic level myelomeningocele showed spondylolisthesis.

Natural History

Frennered AK, Danielson BI, Nachemson AL: Natural history of symptomatic isthmic low-grade spondylolisthesis in children and adolescents: A seven-year follow-up study. *J Pediatr Orthop* 1991;11:209–213.

This is a retrospective analysis of 47 patients up to 16 years of age with spondylolysis or spondylolisthesis. Slip angle, lumbar index, lumbosacral disk height, sacral inclination, and lumbar lordosis were measured. At the time of diagnosis, 31 of the 47 had back pain or sciatica. The rest were asymptomatic. There were no neurologic deficits. Forty-six of the 47 patients had a Meyerding grade II slip or less and one had a grade III slip. Follow-up averaged 7 years. At follow-up, only 4% (two patients) had a progression of slip. A favorable prognosis is expected for mild slips.

Schlenzka D, Poussa M, Seitaslo S, et al: Intervertebral disc changes in adolescents with isthmic spondylolisthesis. *J Spinal Disord* 1991;4;344–352.

Twenty-seven patients undergoing surgery for L5-S1 isthmic spondylolisthesis were evaluated by plain radiographs (27 patients), diskography, (23 patients) and MRI (16 patients). The purpose was to select those patients for whom direct repair of the pars defect would be more suitable than segmental fusion. The mean slip of L5 was 33% ±22%. On plain radiographs, 59% of the patients had narrowing of the L5-S1 disk. Diskograms were done at L3, L4, and L5. Four of the nine (44%) diskograms at L3, 18 of the 22 (82%) diskograms at L4, and all 11 (100%) of the diskograms at L5 were abnormal. On MRI evaluation of 16 patients, one L3 disk, nine L4 disks, and all 16 L5 disks were abnormal. The authors concluded that this information may be helpful in future surgical decision-making. The authors recognize this to be a theoretical, rather than practical, consideration.

Radiologic Evaluation

Lusins JO, Elting JJ, Cicoria AD, et al: SPECT evaluation of lumbar spondylolysis and spondylolisthesis. *Spine* 1994; 19:608–612.

Fifty patients with back pain and spondylolysis were evaluated using SPECT. The test was positive in acute cases of spondylolysis. SPECT was also positive when spondylolisthesis was present, but the increased uptake was noted in the vertebral body-disk location, suggesting microfracture of the vertebral endplate. As the process stabilized, the SPECT scan became negative.

Yamane T, Yoshida T, Mimatsu K: Early diagnosis of lumbar spondylolysis by MRI. *J Bone Joint Surg* 1993; 75B:764–768.

When 79 patients (younger than 19 years of age) with low back pain were screened with plain radiography, CT, and MRI, 44 were found to have spondylolysis. The authors noted that a hypointense area in the pars interarticularis was present on the T1-weighted MRI images before the spondylolysis became evident on plain radiographs or CT. This may be due to edema or hemorrhage. The authors concluded that MRI may be useful as an early diagnostic tool.

Treatment and Long-Term Follow-Up

Bell DF, Ehrlich MG, Zaleske DJ: Brace treatment for symptomatic spondylolisthesis. *Clin Orthop* 1988;236: 192–198.

Twenty-eight symptomatic patients with grade I or II spondylolisthesis were treated with antilordotic braces for a mean duration of 25 months. Brace treatment relieved pain in all patients and no progression was evident at the time of brace discontinuation. However, it remains unproven that bracing had any influence on the lack of slip progression.

Boos N, Marchesi D, Zuber K, et al: Treatment of severe spondylolisthesis by reduction and pedicular fixation: A 4–6-year follow-up study. *Spine* 1993;18:1655–1661.

Ten patients (8 adolescent or young adults) with severe spondylolisthesis averaging 78% and a slip angle averaging 43° underwent reduction, pedicle screw fixation, and posterolateral fusion. Four of the 10 had spondyloptosis and also had interbody fusion. Five of six who had a single-stage posterolateral fusion and instrumentation lost reduction and had nonunion and implant failure. All four patients who had both anterior and posterior fusion had a solid fusion without loss of reduction. Two patients had temporary foot drop postoperatively. Ultimately, all patients had resolution of pain. These data suggest that anterior fusion should be combined with posterior fusion and instrumentation if reduction of severe spondylolisthesis is to be undertaken.

Bradford DS, Boachie-Adjei O: Treatment of severe spondylolisthesis by anterior and posterior reduction and stabilization: A long-term follow-up study. *J Bone Joint Surg* 1990;72A:1060-1066.

Nineteen patients with severe spondylolisthesis (greater than 75%) underwent posterolateral fusion and a Gill procedure, followed by gradual reduction by haloskeletal traction and then a second stage anterior fusion, followed by cast immobilization. Fourteen of the 19 patients were 18 years of age or younger. Of the 19 patients, six had a grade IV slip and 13 had grade V slip (spondyloptosis). The slip angle was reduced from 71° preoperatively to 28° at follow-up, but the percent of slippage did not change. Pseudarthrosis developed in four patients, cauda equina syndrome in one, and L5 neuropathy in two. Sagittal alignment was improved in 17 patients and pain was relieved in all but one. The authors recommend this technique only in severe slips.

Burkus JK, Lonstein JE, Winter RB, et al: Long-term evaluation of adolescents treated operatively for spondylolisthesis: A comparison of in situ arthrodesis only with in situ arthrodesis and reduction followed by immobilization in a cast. *J Bone Joint Surg* 1992;74A: 693–704.

These authors compared 18 adolescents with in situ posterolateral arthrodesis without reduction to a similar group of 24 adolescents with Scaglietti's cast reduction technique. Cast reduction was performed 5 to 14 days postoperatively. All slip grades (I through IV) were treated in each group. No neurologic problems occurred. Follow-up ranged from 2 years to 27 years. Regardless of the grade of the spondylolisthesis, adolescents treated with reduction and casting had less evidence of deformity progression compared with the group fused without reduction. Complication rates were comparable in both groups. At most recent clinical follow-up examination, 38 of the 42 patients had no complaints of back pain or any restriction of activities. These authors recommend in situ posterolateral fusion and reduction followed by cast immobilization for all grades of slip in skeletally immature patients.

Frennered AK, Danielson BI, Nachemson AL, et al: Midterm follow-up of young patients fused in situ for spondylolisthesis. *Spine* 1991;16:409–416.

These authors followed 105 patients younger than 25 years of age with spondylolisthesis for a mean of 8 years, 2 months. Sixty-six patients had an in situ posterolateral fusion alone (slip less than 50%) and 39 patients had combined posterolateral and anterior fusion (slip greater than 50%). Age at surgery averaged 15.5 years. The patients with posterior fusion alone were immobilized in a Boston brace; and those with combined fusion were immobilized in a pantaloon cast for 3 months, followed by a Boston brace for 3 more months. Sixty-four percent had removal of a loose lamina, which had no effect on the postoperative results of sciatica. There was a 6% pseudarthrosis rate. Postoperative progression was rare and complications were few. These authors report good results in all grades of slips with fusion and effective immobilization without the need for instrumentation or reduction.

Hardcastle PH: Repair of spondylolysis in young fast bowlers. *J Bone Joint Surg* 1993;75B:398-402.

Ten patients (mean age 21 years) had persistent back pain after conservative treatment for pars defects resulting from fast bowling in the game of cricket. All had a direct repair of the pars defect with screw fixation across the defect. This technique was first described by Burk in 1970 with 88% to 93% success rate. All ten returned to this sport painfree. The longest follow-up was 3 years, 11 months. Longer term follow-up is needed to determine if fusion had indeed occurred.

Hefti F, Seelig W, Morscher E: Repair of lumbar spondylolysis with a hook-screw. *Int Orthop* 1992; 16:81–85.

Thirty-three patients were treated by direct surgical repair of the spondylitic pars defect by a new hook-screw device and followed for at least 2 years. Of the 16 patients younger than 20 years of age, 14 had satisfactory results with relief of pain and 15 achieved fusion of the defect. The authors recommend MRI evaluation to rule out degenerative disk disease and, if it is present, they recommend a conventional segmental fusion (for the adult). The best results were in patients under age 20 years.

Johnson GV, Thompson AG: The Scott wiring technique for direct repair of lumbar spondylolysis. *J Bone Joint Surg* 1992;74B:426–430.

Twenty-two patients (who had failed conservative treatment for symptomatic spondylolysis) had a direct repair of the pars defect by a modified Scott wiring technique. The mean age at surgery was 15.5 years. All of the 19 patients under age 25 had excellent results despite incomplete or failed fusion in three. Because of the close proximity of the nerve root to the lower border of the transverse process, the authors recommend passing a wire through a hole drilled on the lower edge of the transverse process and passing it cephalad and then around the spinous process before tightening. The authors suggest MRI evaluation preoperatively to rule out disk degeneration in older patients.

O'Brien JP, Mehdian H, Jaffray D: Reduction of severe lumbosacral spondylolisthesis: A report of 22 cases with a ten-year follow-up period. *Clin Orthop* 1994;300:64–69.

Twenty-two patients with severe spondylolisthesis (50%) were treated by posterior decompression, posterolateral fusion, halo-femoral hyperextension traction, anterior fusion with or without AO screw fixation and hyperextension pantaloon cast. Of the 22, 18 were adolescents at the time of surgery. Good results were reported for 19 patients who had a normal lifestyle and excellent cosmetic result. Two patients had permanent neurologic deficits.

Pizzutillo PD, Hummer CD III: Nonoperative treatment for painful adolescent spondylolysis or spondylolisthesis. *J Pediatr Orthop* 1989;9:538–540.

Eighty-two adolescent patients with symptomatic spondylolysis or spondylolisthesis were treated conservatively for 1 to 55 months. Conservative treatment included rest, traction, exercises, bracing, and casting. Follow-up ranged from 1 to 14 years. Of patients with grade I or II slips, 67% had pain relief, but only 8% of patients with grade III or IV slip had pain relief. Twenty-five of the 82 patients ultimately required surgical treatment for pain. Although nonsurgical treatment of the mild symptomatic spondylolisthesis can reliably relieve pain, surgical stabilization is more appropriate for painful grade III or IV slips.

Salib RM, Pettine KA: Modified repair of a defect in spondylolysis or minimal spondylolisthesis by pedicle screw, segmental wire fixation, and bone grafting. *Spine* 1993;18:440–443.

These authors describe a technique using a pedicle screw as the proximal anchor for wiring of the iliac graft over the pars defect. This technique avoided passing the wire around the transverse process. The patient was immobilized in a TLSO and fusion occurred.

Schwend RM, Waters PM, Hey LA, et al: Treatment of severe spondylolisthesis in children by reduction and L4-S4 posterior segmental hyperextension fixation. *J Pediatr Orthop* 1992;12:703–711.

Twenty children (average age 14 years) with severe spondylolisthesis averaging 76% had reduction and posterior stabilization with rectangular Luque rod technique with posterolateral fusion. The slip severity reduced to 55%. All patients had solid fusion at 6 months with no progression of deformity at 43-month follow-up. All had cosmetic improvement. Neurologic complications included seven transient L5 or S1 neuropathies and one permanent residual L5 weakness.

Seitsalo S: Operative and conservative treatment of moderate spondylolisthesis in young patients. *J Bone Joint Surg* 1990;72B:908–913.

This study compares the results of surgical and nonsurgical treatment in 149 young patients with moderate (30% or less) spondylolisthesis. Seventy-seven were treated by fusion (posterior or posterolateral) and 72 conservatively. Follow-up averaged 13.3 years. At final review, there was no significant difference in the progression of the slip between the two groups though the clinical results were slightly better in those treated surgically. The authors conclude that moderate spondylolisthesis in adolescents usually has a benign course. It seems that spontaneous segmental stabilization occurs as a result of degeneration of the disk at the level of slip.

Seitsalo S, Osterman K, Hyvarinen H, et al: Severe spondylolisthesis in children and adolescents: A long-term review of fusion in situ. *J Bone Joint Surg* 1990;72B:259–265.

Eighty-seven children and adolescents with spondylolisthesis of greater than 50% (mean 76% slip) had in situ posterolateral fusion (30 patients), posterior fusion (54 patients), or anterior fusion (three patients). The mean age at surgery was 14.8 years; follow-up averaged 14 years. Only a 2% increase in slip progression occurred after surgery. However, 45% of patients had increased kyphosis (increased sagittal rotation angle) after

surgery. At follow-up, 77 of 82 patients were subjectively improved. The authors were concerned that posterior fusions alone cannot prevent progression of severe spondylolisthesis and that surgical reduction of the L5 kyphosis may be indicated in severe cases.

Seitsalo S, Osterman K, Hyvarinen H, et al: Progression of spondylolisthesis in children and adolescents: A long-term follow-up of 272 patients. *Spine* 1991;16:417–421.

Two hundred seventy-two symptomatic children and adolescents with spondylolisthesis were first diagnosed at an average age of 14.3 years. Eighty-two patients (33%) were treated nonsurgically. One hundred ninety patients (66%) were treated with spinal fusion for stabilization (posterior in situ in 112, posterolateral in 65, and anterior fusion in three). Of those treated surgically, no reduction was attempted and 34 had concomitant laminectomies. Follow-up averaged 14.8 years (range 5 to 32 years). This large series with extensive follow-up showed that the tendency for slip progression (whether they were treated surgically or nonsurgically) increased markedly when the slip was greater than 20% at the time of diagnosis. More than 10% slip progression occurred in 62 patients (no statistical difference between surgical and nonsurgical). For those treated surgically, this progression usually occurred within the first year postoperatively. The only radiologic variable with predictive value for progression was the percentage amount of the primary slip.

Shelokov A, Haideri N, Roach J: Residual gait abnormalities in surgically treated spondylolisthesis. *Spine* 1993;18:2201–2205.

Seven patients were studied with gait analysis 10.5 years after successful in situ fusion in adolescence for grade IV spondylolisthesis. Four patients had slight persistent forward trunk lean with increased hip flexion. Residual knee crouch could not be demonstrated. With regard to cosmesis, three patients noted their backs appeared the same as their peers, and four thought their backs looked worse. The authors concluded that the seven patients had good cosmetic results in terms of trunk alignment although some shortening was noted.

17

Pediatric Cervical Spine

Introduction

A variety of conditions in children lead to significant abnormalities of the cervical spine with associated functional, neurologic, and cosmetic consequences. Although broad classifications of the etiologies of these conditions (such as congenital, developmental, inflammatory, or traumatic causes) have been used, considerable overlap often occurs. For example, rotatory subluxation may be the result of either traumatic or inflammatory processes. Atlantoaxial instability secondary to odontoid hypoplasia in a patient with a skeletal dysplasia is usually considered developmental, although certainly the underlying chondroosseous abnormality has been present since birth. Apart from these difficulties with classification, it is important to recognize the unique differences between the pediatric and adult cervical spine.

An understanding of the anatomic development of the cervical spine is essential to accurately differentiate normal variants from abnormal conditions and avoid unnecessary investigations and treatment. This knowledge should include the location and appearance of the primary and secondary ossification centers as well as the timing of closure of the numerous synchondroses for the atlas, axis, and lower cervical vertebrae. The normal and physiologic radiographic variants of childhood also should be recognized. These include absent cervical lordosis, apparent anterior wedging in young children secondary to immature ossification, pseudosubluxation of C2 on C3, and a normal atlanto-dens interval of 4 to 5 mm in children. Apart from immature ossification and increased ligamentous laxity in childhood, the more horizontal orientation of the upper cervical facets (30 to 35) in comparison to adults (75 to 80) allows for greater degrees of translation in both flexion and extension.

Klippel-Feil Syndrome

Klippel-Feil syndrome is a congenital failure of segmentation of two or more cervical vertebrae. The classic form includes a short neck, low posterior hairline, and limited cervical motion. This triad is seen in less than half of the individuals who have cervical synostosis. Klippel-Feil syndrome is associated with a number of other orthopaedic and nonorthopaedic conditions, including Sprengel's deformity, scoliosis, congenital heart disease, urogenital abnormalities, and conductive or neural hearing deficits. In the child with cervical synostosis, appropriate diagnostic studies should be performed for concomitant abnormalities.

Congenital cervical synostosis may lead to increased motion and stress concentration on adjacent open vertebral motion segments. In a study of patients with Klippel-Feil syndrome, in which the kinematics of cervical spine motion were evaluated in comparison to normal controls, the investigators found significantly increased motion per open segment in the upper cervical spine. Increased motion per segment may lead to disk degeneration, neck pain, segmental instability, and either acute or chronic cord compression. Cord compression and instability, when not directly related to acute trauma, generally do not develop until adulthood in the patient with congenital cervical synostosis.

Three patterns of congenital cervical synostosis that have the potential for neurologic compromise have been identified. The first pattern is the occipitalization of C1 combined with a C2-C3 fusion. The second pattern is subaxial multilevel synostosis combined with an abnormal occipitocervical junction. The third pattern is an open motion segment between two long sections of fused cervical vertebrae. Neurologic symptoms and signs may include radiculopathy, myelopathy, or quadriplegia. Patients with instability related to excessive motion at an open segment should strongly be considered for posterior fusion.

Apart from the obvious segmentation defects, several recent reports have documented the increased incidence of subluxation, spondylolysis, disk herniation, and either brain stem or intraspinal abnormalities in patients with Klippel-Feil syndrome evaluated by computed tomography (CT) myelography or magnetic resonance imaging (MRI). Of 24 patients in one series, co-existing spinal cord or brain abnormalities, including cervical cord dysplasia, diastematomyelia, and Arnold-Chiari I malformations, were identified in seven. Cervical spondylolysis or disk herniations were identified in 42%. In another series of 20 pediatric-aged patients evaluated by MRI, 25% had subluxation greater than 5 mm; 25% had stenosis of 9 mm or less, and 12% had cord abnormalities (diplomyelia and hydromyelia with Arnold-Chiari I malformation). Therefore, the etiology of neurologic deficits in patients with Klippel-Feil syndrome is potentially multifactorial and not necessarily related to abnormal motion segments or disk degeneration. The possibility of stenosis or intraspinal abnormalities must be considered.

Familial Cervical Dysplasia

Of 12 family members from three generations, nine were found to have abnormalities of the atlas, and six had ab-

139

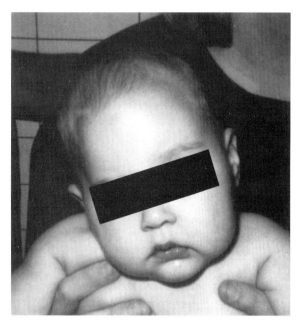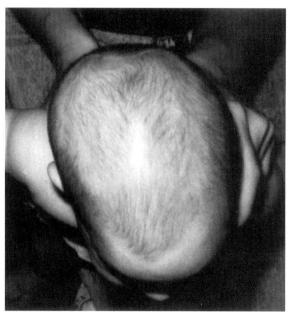

Fig. 1   **Left** and **Right,** A 4-month-old infant with torticollis and plagiocephaly.

normalities of the axis. Four patients had associated hypermobility of the atlanto-occipital articulation. Two patients were symptomatic. The mode of transmission for these kindred was autosomal dominant with complete penetrance and variable expressivity.

Congenital Muscular Torticollis

The term "torticollis" is used to delineate those deformities of the head and neck consisting of a combination head tilt and abnormal rotation. If one considers all pediatric groups at initial presentation, the differential diagnosis of torticollis is large, including typical congenital muscular torticollis and torticollis secondary to such causes as osseous malformations, inflammation, and ocular, neurogenic, and neoplastic disorders.

Congenital muscular torticollis is most typically discovered in the first 2 months of life, is painless, and is associated with a contracture of the sternocleidomastoid muscle. A fibrous mass (pseudotumor) is frequently palpable in the substance of the sternocleidomastoid on the side of the torticollis. This pseudotumor disappears with time. Classically, the cause of torticollis has been postulated to be an injury during birth with intramuscular hemorrhage in the sternocleidomastoid muscle. The hemorrhage or hematoma then organizes, resulting in a fibrous contracture of the sternocleidomastoid muscle.

Recently, another theory regarding the etiology of muscular torticollis has been proposed. One group of investigators used MRI to study ten patients with congenital

muscular torticollis between the ages of 4 weeks and 5 years. Nine of the ten patients were age 4 to 12 weeks at the time of imaging. The entire involved muscle was found to exhibit an abnormal signal. In the single older patient (5 years old), the signal produced was consistent with atrophy and fibrosis of the entire muscle. These signals were similar to those seen in compartment syndromes of the forearm and leg. Injection studies and pressure measurements were obtained at the time of bipolar release of the sternocleidomastoid muscle in three patients. This muscle and sheath did indeed represent a discreet compartment. Therefore, these authors have postulated that congenital muscular torticollis is the result of an intrauterine compartment syndrome.

If the sternocleidomastoid contracture persists, deformation of the face and skull occurs within the first year of life (Fig. 1). This plagiocephaly is most likely the result of prone positioning from sleeping with flattening of the face and head. Twenty percent of children with congenital muscular torticollis have coexistent hip dysplasia. All children with congenital muscular torticollis thus should be carefully screened for hip abnormalities.

With proper treatment, the prognosis is excellent in children with congenital muscular torticollis, with the majority resolving by 12 months of age. During the first year of life, stretching of the sternocleidomastoid combines rotation of the chin toward the same shoulder with tilting the head toward the contralateral side. For resistant cases, usually in children older than 1 year of age, the use of a custom-molded brace holding the face and head in a corrected position may be efficacious. Occasionally, this has been combined with the use of a helmet specially designed by plastic surgeons in an attempt to remodel significant plagiocephaly. Those children who have persistent head tilt or significant plagiocephaly by 2 years of age tend to have persistent deformities into adult life. Thus, the 5% to 10% of children who have not had satisfactory resolution of their torticollis and plagiocephaly should have surgical treatment of the tight sternocleidomastoid muscle before the age of 3.

The surgical treatment is either a unipolar release of the sternocleidomastoid just above the clavicle or a bipolar release with release of the sternocleidomastoid muscle at the mastoid process proximally and clavicle distally. The surgical skin incision should be transverse and 1 cm above the clavicle to avoid an unsightly scar. A recent review of 55 patients was reported, for whom bipolar release of the sternocleidomastoid muscle was used to treat recalcitrant torticollis deformity. A recurrence rate of 2% was reported and 50% had satisfactory improvement in the plagiocephaly. Forty-eight of the 55 patients had no functional or cosmetic impairment following the bipolar release at follow-up. When performing this surgery, care should be taken not to injure the greater auricular nerve lying below the mastoid process, the spinal accessory nerve in the midsubstance of the muscle, the anterior and external jugular veins, the carotid sheath, or the carotid vessels.

Previous authors have emphasized the addition of Z-plasty lengthening of the sternal attachment of the sternocleidomastoid muscle coupled with the bipolar release. It has been suggested that the Z-plasty lengthening maintains the "V" contour of the neck and results in an improved cosmetic appearance of the neck over a simple bipolar release.

Sternocleidomastoid contracture has been reported in association with vertebral abnormalities. Radiographs may initially be interpreted as normal in the immature spine. In one recently reported series of four patients with both sternocleidomastoid contracture and vertebral abnormalities, the torticollis recurred following what was considered to be a successful surgical release of the contracted muscle.

Benign Paroxysmal Torticollis of Infancy

Benign paroxysmal torticollis is characterized by periodic episodes of wry neck, usually alternating from side to side. It is a self-limited process of unknown etiology that presents in infancy and usually resolves by 2 or 3 years of age. It is sometimes associated with ataxia, vomiting, irritability, or drowsiness. There is no known treatment for this condition.

Rotatory Subluxation

Rotatory atlantoaxial subluxation, an uncommon cause of torticollis, occurs in children following infections in the

neck or pharynx (Grisel's syndrome), pharyngeal surgery, or minor trauma. An increased laxity of the alar and transverse ligaments as well as capsular constraints following inflammatory processes or traumatic events is the presumed etiology of this condition. The normal rotation of the atlantoaxial joint becomes fixed in a rotated and subluxated position. Children present with torticollis and limited range of motion of the neck, with or without pain.

Plain radiographs are difficult to interpret because of the head tilt and rotation. Radiographic documentation is best obtained by dynamic CT with the head maximally rotated to each side. This study will demonstrate a loss of normal rotation of the first and second cervical vertebrae, which move as a unit rather than independently.

Treatment remains controversial. Based on a retrospective review of 23 children treated for rotatory atlantoaxial subluxation, treatment recommendations have been made by several authors and are dependent on the duration of torticollis prior to treatment. Patients who have had a rotatory subluxation for less than 1 week can usually be treated successfully with immobilization of the neck in a soft collar and rest for a week. Those whose symptoms persist for longer than 1 week but less than 1 month or who fail to respond to the soft collar and bed rest regimen require hospitalization and traction. Traction may be applied either by a head halter or by application of a halo device for refractory cases. If reduction is achieved, some form of cervical immobilization should be used for 4 to 6 weeks to prevent recurrent subluxation. Reduction is rarely achieved if the rotatory subluxation has been present for more than a month. If resolution of the torticollis does not occur, posterior C1-C2 arthrodesis could be considered.

Cervical Disk Calcification

Cervical disk calcification is an uncommon disease in childhood. It is characterized by calcification of the nucleus pulposus of one or more intervertebral disks, affecting the cervical spine more commonly than the thoracic spine (Fig. 2). The incidence of this disorder is unknown because many patients may be asymptomatic. Symptoms, when they do occur, include pain, muscle spasm, decreased range of motion, and fevers. Elevation of the erythrocyte sedimentation rate and peripheral white blood cell count have been noted in some. Disk protrusion has been identified in more than one third of patients, although neurologic symptoms and signs are usually absent.

The disease is self-limited with eventual resorption of the calcification. Treatment consists of a soft cervical collar and anti-inflammatory agents with a resolution of symptoms in two thirds of children within 3 weeks, and 95% within 6 months. Occasionally, a calcified disk will herniate with a resultant compressive myelopathy. In these circumstances, anterior cervical decompression and fusion is indicated.

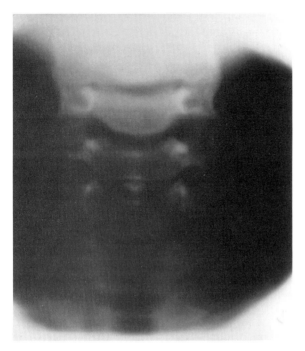

Fig. 2 A 13-year-old girl with a calcified cervical disk. (Courtesy of Ronald L. DeWald, MD, Chicago, IL)

Osteochondrodysplasias

Many dwarfing conditions are associated with significant abnormalities of the cervical spine. Patients with these heritable osteochondrodysplasias frequently initially have complaints or conditions unrelated to the neck. Nevertheless, during the course of a comprehensive evaluation, they are found to have a potentially severe abnormality of the cervical spine. For the skeletal dysplasias, it is helpful to classify these problems regionally into three types: foramen magnum, atlantoaxial, or lower cervical. For example, patients with achondroplasia have a high incidence of foramen magnum stenosis. Atlantoaxial instability is frequently observed in the spondyloepiphyseal dysplasias, pseudoachondroplasia, chondrodysplasia punctata, Kneist dysplasia, metatrophic dysplasia, chondrometaphyseal dysplasia, and Morquio-Brailsford's disease. Finally, severe cervical kyphosis is found in diastrophic dysplasia and Larsen's syndrome.

Children with achondroplasia may develop cervicomedullary compression during the first 2 to 3 years of life secondary to stenosis of the foramen magnum. Achondroplasia is a disorder of endochondral ossification and therefore the foramen magnum may be stenotic at birth because growth of the foramen magnum is also through endochondral ossification. The resulting stenosis of the foramen magnum and upper cervical spine may result in quadriplegia, hypertonia, hypotonia, delayed developmental mile-

stones, sleep apnea, or respiratory compromise. Apart from a careful clinical examination, it is recommended that infants with achondroplasia should have an MRI evaluation of the brain stem during the first 6 months of life if the patient is not meeting growth and developmental milestones normally for achondroplasia. Somatosensory-evoked potentials and sleep apnea studies are also indicated for many patients. For achondroplastic infants with evidence of cervicomedullary compression, foramen magnum decompression and duraplasty by a neurosurgeon is indicated. Arthrodesis is not required. In one reported series of 15 patients undergoing this combined procedure, improvement in the presenting neurologic or respiratory complaints was noted in all patients.

Atlantoaxial instability frequently occurs in many of the dwarfing conditions, including spondyloepiphyseal dysplasia, pseudoachondroplasia, chondrodysplasia punctata, metatrophic dysplasia, Kneist dysplasia, metaphyseal chondrodysplasia, with the highest incidence occurring in Morquio-Brailsford's disease. A feature common to most is an abnormality of development of the dens and varying degrees of ligamentous laxity. Odontoid hypoplasia, aplasia, and os odontoideum have all been described. The instability may be flexion, extension, or both, as determined by lateral flexion-extension radiograph. Although standard measurements of the atlanto-dens interval and space available for the cord on lateral radiographs are helpful, the most diagnostic of the available imaging studies is an MRI obtained in both flexion and extension.

Patients with atlantoaxial instability may be asymptomatic or may present with signs and symptoms of a myelopathy. Though extremely rare, vertebral artery insufficiency has also been reported in patients with severe instability. In most disorders, the neurologic abnormalities are thought to be secondary to the instability itself. However, in Morquio's disease, the severity of the spinal cord compression is determined by the thickness of the anterior extradural soft tissues. In a recent study of 13 patients with Morquio's disease evaluated by CT myelography, the degree of spinal cord involvement correlated with these soft-tissue abnormalities and not with the magnitude of the atlantoaxial instability. All 13 patients had odontoid hypoplasia.

Treatment of atlantoaxial instability is posterior fusion of the atlas and axis (Fig. 3). If extension instability is present with odontoid hypoplasia, care must be taken at the time of surgery not to overreduce the ring of C1 on C2 with any of the posterior wiring techniques. Internal fixation is not necessary in children and excellent results have been achieved with the use of halo immobilization. Frequently, the posterior synchondrosis of C1 will be quite wide in these patients with a skeletal dysplasia. This synchondrosis may necessitate extension of the fusion to the occiput in order to achieve a satisfactory arthrodesis.

Severe cervical kyphosis, secondary to anterior wedging of the third and fourth vertebral bodies and ligamentous laxity, has been reported in diastrophic dysplasia. In a re-

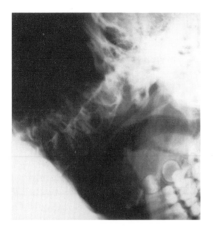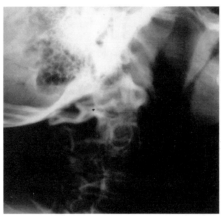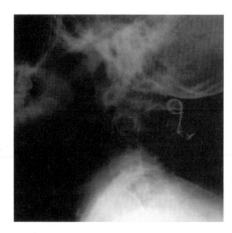

Fig. 3 A 12-year-old child with spondyloepiphyseal dysplasia congenita and C1-C2 flexion instability. **Left,** In flexion. **Center,** In extension. **Right,** Reduced and fused in extension.

view of 101 patients from Finland, over one third had cervical kyphosis of varying degrees. Severe deformities have been reported even in very young children. These patients are at high risk for spinal cord compression with resultant quadriplegia. Many diastrophic dwarfs will have wedging of the midcervical vertebra without instability on lateral flexion radiographs. These patients may be observed if neurologically normal. If instability is noted, flexion-extension MRI is useful to document the presence or absence of cord compression. Surgical stabilization is indicated for patients with symptoms or signs of a myelopathy or for those with kyphosis, instability, and evidence of cord compression by MRI, even if asymptomatic at presentation.

Trisomy 21 (Down Syndrome)

Upper cervical instability is a recognized problem in children with trisomy 21. Twenty percent of individuals with trisomy 21 have a varying degree of C1-C2 instability. This instability is thought to be secondary to laxity of the transverse ligament of the atlanto-dens interval; however, in a recent study of 78 children with Down syndrome, skeletal abnormalities of the upper cervical spine were identified in 48 patients, and 39 had radiographic evidence of atlantoaxial instability. A longitudinal study of 141 patients from this same center found only minor changes (1.0 mm to 1.5 mm) in the atlanto-dens interval with time in 130 (92%) patients. Eleven patients (8%) developed increasing instability with documented changes of 2.0 mm to 4.0 mm. Children with more than 7.0 mm of C1-C2 instability are considered to be at high risk for developing symptomatic atlantoaxial instability.

Apart from the increased incidence of atlantoaxial instability in Down syndrome, there is an increasing awareness of the potential for atlanto-occipital instability as well. In a recent study of 64 children with Down syndrome, 43 demonstrated greater than 4 mm of posterior subluxation of the atlanto-occipital articulation. Twenty-one percent of these patients had concomitant atlantoaxial instability measuring greater than 5 mm.

For many years, children with Down syndrome have been integrated into the Special Olympics programs. Each state has its own regulations for the participation of these children in the Special Olympics. Traditional guidelines have required screening of these children prior to allowing the child with Down syndrome to participate in these sports events. Typically, lateral flexion-extension radiographs of the cervical spine have been obtained. The need for routine, serial radiographs has recently been called into question by pediatricians based upon the long history of the safety of these events. From the orthopaedic surgeon's vantage point, children with mild degrees of instability (more than 7 mm) should be followed closely for progressive instability with periodic radiographic examinations. Certainly, children with signs of neurocompression should not be allowed to participate in athletic events and strong consideration should be given for surgical stabilization.

The child with symptomatic C1-C2 instability should be treated with a posterior C1-C2 arthrodesis. Although still controversial, the opinion of most authorities is that any instability of C1-C2 greater than 10 mm should be stabilized with a posterior C1-C2 arthrodesis. A fixed subluxation of C1 on C2 should not be reduced but fused in situ.

Posterior C1-C2 fusion in a child with Down syndrome is associated with a high rate of complications, including infection, resorption of the bone graft, and intraoperative neurologic injury to the spinal cord. In a recent review of ten patients with Down syndrome who required posterior arthrodesis of the upper cervical spine, complications related to the procedure were identified in all ten patients.

A posterior arthrodesis at C1-C2 in a child with Down syndrome should be approached with great caution, and the parents should be fully informed before the procedure of potential complications.

Deformity Following Decompression

Instability and deformity of the cervical spine are recognized complications of decompression of the cervical spine in the growing child, particularly if decompression distal to the axis is required. Excessive lordosis, kyphosis, or laxity have all been reported in the orthopaedic literature. Of 20 myelodysplastic patients studied, 19 developed instability of the cervical spine following suboccipital craniectomy and cervical decompression of an Arnold-Chiari type II malformation. Excessive translation (4 mm) occurred between the second and third cervical vertebrae. Angulation averaging 17 occurred between the third and fourth cervical vertebrae.

Deformity of the cervical spine following decompression was documented in 46 of 89 patients (53%) reviewed in another series. Thirty-three developed a cervical kyphosis (mean, 30) and 13 had hyperlordosis (mean, 62) of the cervical spine, the latter correlating with a younger age (4 years) at the time of decompression.

Clearly, there is a need for careful monitoring of these children following cervical decompression. Prophylactic bracing and osteoplastic laminotomy with reconstruction of the posterior arch have been proposed in an attempt to prevent instability or deformity. To date, the results of these techniques have not been reported. Once instability and/or deformity occur, surgical stabilization is generally required, usually anterior arthrodesis.

Trauma

There are several characteristics of the cervical spine in children that distinguish it from the adult cervical spine. Soft tissues in children are much more elastic than those of adults, which, when traumatic events occur, allows for greater displacement of the spine in childhood than is possible in the adult. This results in a much higher incidence of spinal cord injuries without radiographic abnormalities in the child. The orientation of the upper cervical facets (C2-C4) changes from a horizontal inclination of 30 to 35 in the child to a more vertical 75 to 80 inclination in adolescents. Greater excursion or translation is permitted with a more horizontal orientation. An additional characteristic of children younger than 8 years of age is that the fulcrum for flexion centers at C2-C3 as a result of the child's larger head size relative to the neck. After the age of 8, the fulcrum for flexion is similar to the adult pattern and centers around C5-C6. These factors result in a much higher percentage of upper cervical spine injuries in the child as compared to the adult. One center recently reported the results of a retrospective review of 143 children and adolescents seen following an injury to the cervical spine.

Children younger than 11 years of age, most commonly injured in falls, had a higher incidence of upper cervical injuries and mortality secondary to cord injuries in comparison to 11- to 15-year-olds. This latter group had a higher incidence of lower cervical injuries and were most commonly injured during sports or recreational events.

Another center reported the results of nonsurgical treatment of cervical spine injuries in 24 children. Reduction was achieved by Crutchfield or Gardner-Wells tongs followed by external immobilization with a 95% success rate, although 14% developed a kyphotic deformity measuring between 5 and 24. Forty-three percent of their patients with neurologic injury recovered function.

Finally, the preadolescent child who sustains a cervical spinal cord injury has a high likelihood of developing a scoliosis or abnormal kyphosis that will require surgical treatment. After adolescence the likelihood of developing a symptomatic spinal deformity as a result of a cervical spinal cord injury is extremely small.

Surgical Techniques and Results

The results of posterior fusion of the cervical spine in children and adolescents have generally been excellent apart from the high complication rate reported for patients with Down syndrome. Common elements in reported series include the use of a high-speed burr for decortication, the liberal use of autogenous iliac crest bone graft, and postoperative immobilization, most commonly halo vest or cast. Internal fixation is generally minimal. Care must be taken at surgery to expose only those segments intended for arthrodesis, because extension of the fusion mass has been reported for greater than 30% of patients reviewed.

Halo-dependent traction has long been used for gradual correction of severe spinal deformities. The use of a halo-Ilizarov distraction cast technique for correction of severe cervical spine deformities was found to be efficacious in six patients (three of whom were children) studied.

Summary

The cervical spine in children has certain characteristics that differ from those of the adult spine, including greater degrees of soft-tissue elasticity and anatomic differences with regard to facet joint orientation and fulcrum. A variety of problems secondary to disturbances of growth, development, inflammation, and trauma are associated with instability or deformity of the child's cervical spine. Neurosurgical procedures for decompression of the cord or resection of spinal cord tumors in the growing child are associated with long-term structural sequelae. Early recognition of cervical abnormalities or conditions associated with potential problems involving the cervical spine is critical in order to avoid or minimize the long-term consequences of deformity or instability in the pediatric population.

Annotated Bibliography

Klippel-Feil Syndrome

Hall JE, Simmons ED, Danylchuk K, et al: Instability of the cervical spine and neurological involvement in Klippel-Feil syndrome: A case report. *J Bone Joint Surg* 1990;72A:460–462.

This is a case review of an adolescent with Klippel-Feil syndrome who presented with intermittent neurologic symptoms. Neurologic findings in patients with cord compression secondary to congenital cervical synostosis are presented, and recommendations for diagnosis are discussed.

Pizzutillo PD, Woods M, Nicholson L, et al: Risk factors in Klippel-Feil syndrome. *Spine* 1994;19:2110–2116.

Kinematic evaluation of cervical spine radiographs was performed for 111 patients with Klippel-Feil syndrome. Increased motion per open interspace was noted for the upper cervical spine.

Ritterbusch JF, McGinty LD, Spar J, et al: Magnetic resonance imaging for stenosis and subluxation in Klippel-Feil syndrome. *Spine* 1991;16(suppl 10):S539–S541.

Twenty patients with Klippel-Feil syndrome were evaluated by MRI and lateral flexion-extension radiographs. Subluxation measuring greater than 5 mm was found in 25% and stenosis measuring less than 9 mm was found in 25%. Three patients (12%) had cord abnormalities.

Ulmer JL, Elster AD, Ginsberg LE, et al: Klippel-Feil syndrome: CT and MR of acquired and congenital abnormalities of cervical spine and cord. *J Comput Assist Tomogr* 1993;17:215–224.

MRI and CT studies were reviewed in 24 patients with Klippel-Feil syndrome. Cervical spondylosis or disk herniations were seen in ten. Congenital defects of the cord or brain, including dysraphism, diastematomyelia, and Chiari I malformations, were observed in seven patients.

Familial Cervical Dysplasia

Saltzman CL, Hensinger RN, Blane CE, et al: Familial cervical dysplasia. *J Bone Joint Surg* 1991;73A:163–171.

In this study, nine of 12 family members from three generations had an inherited form of cervical vertebral dysplasia. Affected people had abnormalities of the first cervical vertebra. Some also had defects of the axis and caudad to it. The mode of transmission of the disorder is autosomal dominant, with complete penetrance and variable expressivity.

Congenital Muscular Torticollis

Brougham DI, Cole WG, Dickens DR, et al: Torticollis due to a combination of sternomastoid contracture and congenital vertebral anomalies. *J Bone Joint Surg* 1989;71B:404–407.

Four patients with sternomastoid contractures combined with torticollis secondary to congenital vertebral anomalies are discussed. The clinician should be aware of these conditions and should also realize that the radiographs of the very immature spine may not disclose the bony abnormalities.

Davids JR, Wenger DR, Mubarak SJ: Congenital muscular torticollis: Sequela of intrauterine or perinatal compartment syndrome. *J Pediatr Orthop* 1993;13:141–147.

Ten patients with congenital muscular torticollis were studied by MRI and were found to have changes involving the entire sternocleidomastoid muscle consistent with prior compartment syndrome. Pressure measurements obtained at surgery in three patients confirmed the potential of this muscle and accompanying sheath as a true compartment.

Wirth CJ, Hagena FW, Wuelker N, et al: Biterminal tenotomy for the treatment of congenital muscular torticollis: Long-term results. *J Bone Joint Surg* 1992;74A:427–434.

These authors recommended that a biterminal release be performed at the age of 3 to 5 years in all patients who do not respond to nonsurgical treatment for congenital muscular torticollis.

Benign Paroxysmal Torticollis of Infancy

Bratt HD, Menelaus MB: Benign paroxysmal torticollis of infancy. *J Bone Joint Surg* 1992;74B:449–451.

Benign paroxysmal torticollis is a self-limiting condition occurring during infancy. It resolves by the age of 2 to 3 years. Periodic episodes of torticollis may randomly alternate from side to side and may be associated with other symptoms. The etiology is unknown and no treatment is effective.

Rotatory Subluxation

Phillips WA, Hensinger RN: The management of rotatory atlanto-axial subluxation in children. *J Bone Joint Surg* 1989;71A:664–668.

These authors present a management protocol for atlanto-axial subluxation in children based on the duration of the torticollis prior to treatment. Subluxation of less than 1 week duration can be treated with immobilization of the neck in a soft collar and rest for a week. Those with symptoms longer than 1 week or who failed to respond to the soft collar and bed rest require hospitalization and traction for up to 3 weeks. If resolution of the torticollis does not occur and the patient remains symptomatic, posterior C1-C2 arthrodesis should be considered.

Cervical Disk Calcification

Girodias JB, Azouz EM, Marton D: Intervertebral disk space calcification: A report of 51 children with a review of the literature. *Pediatr Radiol* 1991;21:541–546.

Data on 51 children with intervertebral disk calcifications are presented. Regression of the calcifications was seen in 33 (66%), persistence or progression in 21 (39%), and disk herniation in 21 (39%).

Mohanty S, Sutter B, Mokry M, et al: Herniation of calcified cervical intervertebral disk in children. *Surg Neurol* 1992;38:407–410.

Two patients with cervical disk calcification had rapid neurologic deterioration requiring urgent anterior diskectomy and fusion with subsequent recovery.

Wong CC, Pereira B, and Pho RW: Cervical disc calcification in children: A long-term review. *Spine* 1992;17:139–144.

Four patients were presented, three of whom had follow-up greater than 10 years. In general, regression of the calcifications were noted but persistent mild flattening of adjacent vertebral bodies and loss of lordosis were noted in two patients.

Osteochondrodysplasias

Aryanpur J, Hurko O, Francomano C, et al: Craniocervical decompression for cervicomedullary compression in pediatric patients with achondroplasia. *J Neurosurg* 1990;73:375–382.

Congenital osseous abnormalities associated with achondroplasia includes stenosis of the foramen magnum and upper cervical spinal canal. In the pediatric achondroplastic patients, such stenosis may lead to cervicomedullary compression with serious sequelae, including paresis, hypertonia, delayed motor milestones, and respiratory compromise. The authors present the results of 15 children with achondroplasia treated by cervicomedullary compression by craniocervical decompression and duraplasty. In their series, this treatment proved to be an effective and safe treatment for young achondroplastic patients with cervicomedullary compression.

Hecht JT, Horton WA, Reid CS, et al: Growth of the foramen magnum in achondroplasia. *Am J Med Genet* 1989;32:528–535.

The growth of the foramen magnum in achondroplasia is characterized by markedly diminished growth, resulting not only from abnormal enchondral bone growth, but also because of abnormal placement and premature fusion of the synchondroses.

Krecak J, Starshak RJ: Cervical kyphosis in diastrophic dwarfism: CT and MR findings. *Pediatr Radiol* 1987;17:321–322.

The authors discuss the results of a 3-year-old child with diastrophic dwarfism and truncal and upper extremity weakness. A severe cervical gibbus was found. Cord compression was documented on MRI.

Nelson FW, Hecht JT, Horton WA, et al: Neurologic basis of respiratory complications in achondroplasia. *Ann Neurol* 1988;24:89–93.

An evaluation of 32 individuals with achondroplasia revealed that 28% had a history of apnea and 22% had respiratory abnormalities on polysomnography. The study suggested that brain stem compression was common in achondroplasia and could account in part for the abnormal respiratory function in this disorder, including obstructive apnea, central apnea, and hypoxemia.

Poussa M, Merikanto J, Ryoppy S, et al: The spine in diastrophic dysplasia. *Spine* 1991;16:881–887.

In a review of 101 patients with diastrophic dysplasia, one third of the patients had cervical kyphosis. In the most severe case, the kyphosis led to quadriplegia during anesthesia.

Reid CS, Pyeritz RE, Kopits SE, et al: Cervicomedullary compression in young patients with achondroplasia: Value of comprehensive neurologic and respiratory evaluation. *J Pediatr* 1987;110:522–530.

A prospective study of 26 patients with achondroplasia revealed respiratory abnormalities in 85% of these children.

The majority of respiratory problems were caused by a primary problem of the pulmonary system, such as a small thoracic cage or obstructed airway. In three patients, respiratory problems were explainable only by cervicomedullary cord compression. In each patient, respiratory problems were alleviated by decompressive surgery.

Stevens JM, Kendall BE, Crockard HA, et al: The odontoid process in Morquio-Brailsford's disease: The effects of occipitocervical fusion. *J Bone Joint Surg* 1991;73B:851–858.

High-definition, computed cervical myelograms have been made in flexion and extension in 13 patients. Odontoid dysplasia was present in every case. Atlanto-axial instability was mild. Severe spinal cord compression, when present, was caused by anterior extradural soft-tissue thickening. This compression was not relieved by flexing or extending the neck and was manifested early in life. Posterior occipitocervical fusion resulted in disappearance of the soft-tissue thickening and normalization of subsequent development of the dens.

Trisomy 21 (Down Syndrome)

American Academy of Pediatrics Committee on Sports Medicine and Fitness: Atlantoaxial instability in Down syndrome: Subject review. *Pediatrics* 1995;96:151–154.

Davidson RG: Atlantoaxial instability in individuals with Down syndrome: A fresh look at the evidence. *Pediatrics* 1988;81:857–865.

In this case review of children with Down syndrome, there was little support for the hypothesis that instability is a predisposing factor to dislocation. The study suggests that there is a need for carefully designed longitudinal studies of cervical spine instability in children with Down syndrome.

Gabriel KR, Mason DE, Carango P: Occipito-atlantal translation in Down's syndrome. *Spine* 1990;15:997–1002.

This study presents a retrospective analysis of 102 flexion and extension lateral cervical spine radiographs of 73 patients with Down syndrome. Normal occiput-C1 translation should be no more than 1 mm. Only 29% of patients showed anterior posterior translation of 1 mm or less. The authors data suggest that the prevalence and magnitude of occipitoatlantal instability in Down syndrome is greater than previously appreciated.

Pueschel SM, Scola FH, Tupper TB, et al: Skeletal anomalies of the upper cervical spine in children with Down syndrome. *J Pediatr Orthop* 1990;10:607–611.

This study showed that a significantly greater number of children with Down syndrome have cervical spine anomalies than an age- and gender-matched group of children without Down syndrome. Moreover, children with Down syndrome who had atlanto-axial instability had an increased frequency of cervical spine anomalies as compared with an age- and gender-matched group of children with this chromosomal disorder who did not have atlanto-axial instability.

Pueschel SM, Scola FH, Pezzullo JC: A longitudinal study of atlanto-dens relationships in asymptomatic individuals with Down syndrome. *Pediatrics* 1992;89:1194–1198.

One hundred and forty-one patients with Down syndrome were followed longitudinally with regard to atlanto-axial instability. One hundred and thirty patients (92%) developed minor changes measuring 1.0 mm to 1.5 mm, while 11 patients (8%) developed changes in the atlanto-dens measurement of 2.0 mm to 4.0 mm over time.

Segal LS, Drummond DS, Zanotti RM, et al: Complications of posterior arthrodesis of the cervical spine in patients who have Down syndrome. *J Bone Joint Surg* 1991;73A:1547–1554.

Ten patients who had Down syndrome and had a posterior arthrodesis of the upper cervical spine are presented. Complications related to the operation occurred in all patients. They included infection, wound dehiscence, incomplete reduction of the atlanto-axial joint, instability of the adjacent motion segment, neurologic sequelae, resorption of the autogenous bone graft, and death in the postoperative period. The authors recommend nonsurgical management for patients who have Down syndrome and atlanto-axial instability without neurologic signs or symptoms. If the severity of symptoms necessitates a posterior arthrodesis, a high rate of complications must be anticipated.

Tredwell SJ, Newman DE, Lockitch G: Instability of the upper cervical spine in Down syndrome. *J Pediatr Orthop* 1990;10:602–606.

The generalized ligamentous laxity of the upper cervical region in Down syndrome allows multidirectional instability. This study demonstrates that the instability at the atlanto-occipital level is common and must be considered in addition to the well-documented instability at the atlanto-axial level. Rotatory instability may also exist and should be examined. Treatment in these patients should depend on the amount of room available for the spinal cord rather than on the absolute value of displacement.

Deformity Following Decompression

Aronson DD, Kahn RH, Canady A, et al: Instability of the cervical spine after decompression in patients who have Arnold-Chiari malformation. *J Bone Joint Surg* 1991;73A:898–906.

Stability of the cervical spine was studied in two groups of children who had myelomeningocele. One group consisted of 20 children with an Arnold-Chiari type II malformation in whom a suboccipital craniectomy and cervical laminectomy was done to decompress the brain stem. Of the 20 patients, 19 had instability on postoperative follow-up on lateral flexion-extension radiographs. The instability was noted between C2-C3. The second group consisted of 20 children who had myelomeningocele, but had not had surgery for decompression. This group of patients developed no instability of the cervical spine.

Bell DF, Walker JL, O'Connor G, et al: Spinal deformity after multiple-level cervical laminectomy in children. *Spine* 1994;19:406–411.

Eighty-nine patients with a mean radiographic follow-up of 5.1 years were reviewed. Significant postlaminectomy deformity developed in 47 patients (53%), of whom 33 developed a mean kyphosis of 30 and 13 developed a mean hyperlordosis of 62. The development of hyperlordosis (swan-neck deformity) was strongly correlated with a peak age of surgery of 4 years. The high overall frequency of postoperative deformity after multiple level cervical laminectomy supports the necessity for careful monitoring of these patients, even if the facet joints are preserved.

Trauma

Bhatnagar M, Sponseller PD, Carroll C IV, et al: Pediatric atlantoaxial instability presenting as cerebral and cerebellar infarcts. *J Pediatr Orthop* 1991;11:103–107.

Neurologic findings in pediatric atlanto-axial instability have most commonly included signs of cord compression with hypertonia or hypotonia in tetraplegia. However, the patient's presenting symptoms were most consistent with infarcts in the cerebellum and occipitoparietal lobes, which correlated angiographically with vertebral artery narrowing at the level of the axis and subsequent low flow to the posterior cerebellum. After stabilization and fusion of the cervical spine, the patient regained normal neurologic function and remained free of symptoms at 2 years of follow-up.

Birney TJ, Hanley EN Jr: Traumatic cervical spine injuries in childhood and adolescence. *Spine* 1989;14:1277–1282.

Sixty-one children and adolescents with cervical spine injuries treated within a 10-year period of time were available for review. Ages ranged from newborn to 17 years. Analysis of injury types revealed four groups of roughly equal incidence. Atlanto-axial rotatory subluxation, upper cervical spine fracture or dislocation, lower cervical injury, and spinal cord injury without radiographic abnormality. Forty-four percent of the patients incurred an neurologic injury. Apart from those patients with complete neurologic deficits, the prognosis of these injuries is good.

de Beer JD, Hoffman EB, Kieck CF: Traumatic atlantoaxial subluxation in children. *J Pediatr Orthop* 1990;10:397–400.

Four patients with traumatic C1-C2 subluxation were reported, three of whom were treated nonsurgically and one treated surgically. All had satisfactory outcomes. Two had neurologic deficits, which resolved.

Evans DL, Bethem D: Cervical spine injuries in children. *J Pediatr Orthop* 1989;9:563–568.

Twenty consecutive cases of cervical spine injury in children were reviewed. Associated injuries occurred in 38% and neurologic injuries occurred in 29%. Forty-three percent of children with neurologic injuries recovered. Nonsurgical treatment was successful in 95%; however, 14% later developed kyphotic deformities. Anterior approach for cervical stabilization is inadequate, and indeed led to neurologic deficits in three of 16 patients. Cervical laminectomy has clearly been shown not to be helpful. Posterior spine fusion with interspinous wiring and autogenous bone graft proved to be reliable in this study.

McGrory BJ, Klassen RA, Chao EY, et al: Acute fractures and dislocations of the cervical spine in children and adolescents. *J Bone Joint Surg* 1993;75A:988–995.

One hundred and forty-three pediatric patients with cervical spine injuries were reviewed. Children younger than 11 years of age were more commonly injured in falls, were more likely to have upper cervical spine injuries, and had a higher incidence of mortality from spinal cord injury.

Surgical Techniques & Results

Graziano GP, Herzenberg JE, Hensinger RN: The Halo-Ilizarov distraction cast for correction of cervical deformity: Report of six cases. *J Bone Joint Surg* 1993; 75A:996–1003.

Six patients, three in the pediatric age group, had gradual correction of severe cervical spine deformities utilizing a halo connected to a body cast with Ilizarov components.

Letts M, Slutsky D: Occipitocervical arthrodesis in children. *J Bone Joint Surg* 1990;72A:1166–1170.

The authors present a technique for occipitocervical arthrodesis that uses spinous process wiring and postoperative halo fixation. It was found to be safe and effective in the seven patients treated.

McGrory BJ, Klassen RA: Arthrodesis of the cervical spine for fractures and dislocations in children and adolescents: A long-term follow-up study. *J Bone Joint Surg* 1994;76A:1606–1616.

Forty-two patients who had an arthrodesis for instability of the cervical spine resulting from trauma were followed clinically for a minimum of 7 years. The ages of the patients at the time of injury range from 1 year and 11 months to 15 years and 11 months. The spinal arthrodesis for fractures and dislocations of the cervical spine in children and adolescents can be accomplished safely, with an acceptable clinical outcome, a low rate of complications, and minimal morbidity after long-term follow-up. Pain, neurologic status, and function do not change markedly, but morbidity may decrease with longer follow-up.

Smith MD, Phillips WA, Hensinger RN: Fusion of the upper cervical spine in children and adolescents: An analysis of 17 patients. *Spine* 1991;16:695–701.

A retrospective review of 17 immature patients who underwent posterior spinal fusion of C1-C2 or C1-C3 was performed. Etiologies included os odontoideum, fixed rotatory subluxation, atlanto-axial subluxation, two dens fracture nonunion, and nonunion of the Hangman's fracture. The authors concluded that, in general, posterior spinal fusion of the upper cervical spine was a reliable, safe, and predictable procedure, but extra caution should be employed when considering arthrodesis in patients with ongoing spinal cord compression, fixed dislocation and inherited ligamentous laxity.

III
Lower Extremity

W. Timothy Ward, MD
Deborah Stanitski, MD
Section Editors

18

Slipped Capital Femoral Epiphysis

Description

Slipped capital femoral epiphysis (SCFE) is a disorder in which the epiphysis becomes posteriorly displaced on the femoral neck. This disorder, which occurs in adolescence, may lead to osteoarthritis in adults or may be complicated by chondrolysis or osteonecrosis in the adolescent. Important principles of treatment unique to this problem need to be understood in order to minimize complications.

Epidemiology

The prevalence of SCFE varies greatly by geographic locale. A prevalence of 0.2/100,000 is reported in eastern Japan, whereas American rates are reported to vary from 2.13/100,000 in the Southwest to 10.08/100,000 in Connecticut for the at-risk population of boys 10 to 17 years of age, and girls 8 to 15 years of age. The reason for this apparent regional difference is not known. SCFE is approximately twice as common in boys as in girls. The median age of onset is 14 years for boys and 12 years for girls. The black population appears to be more commonly affected than the white or Oriental populations, but in contradistinction to older literature, recent evidence suggests that the results of treatment are comparable and that the incidence of complications is no higher in blacks than in whites. No definitive environmental differences are obvious. Most children with SCFE are obese, with at least half of affected individuals weighing more than 95% of children in their age group. Excluding the rare case of acute physeal fracture following extreme trauma, the child generally does not recall a specific traumatic event. The prevalence of bilaterality was recently reported as 37% for symptomatic slips. However, if asymptomatic slips (noted on incidental follow-up radiographs) are included, the prevalence may be even higher. Nearly all of those who develop a contralateral slip after initial diagnosis do so within 18 months.

Clinical Findings

The onset of symptoms may be abrupt or may occur insidiously over many months. An abrupt onset of hip or groin pain typically is associated with a sudden large amount of epiphyseal displacement. A longer duration of symptoms, particularly medial thigh or knee pain, can be associated with either small or large amounts of epiphyseal displacement. Traditional clinical classification systems divided SCFE into acute (symptoms for less than 3 weeks), chronic (symptoms longer than 3 weeks), or acute on chronic (recent exacerbation of long-standing symptoms) categories. A recently introduced, more meaningful classification for SCFE differentiates between a stable and an unstable slip. A stable slip is one in which gentle movement at the hip does not result in independent fluoroscopic movement of the capital epiphysis with respect to the femoral neck. Clinically, the child is able to walk and bear weight, although crutches may be necessary. Radiographic signs of chronicity (callus formation at the periphery of the physis) typically will be present in a stable slip. In an unstable slip, there is independent fluoroscopic movement of the capital epiphysis with respect to the femoral neck when the hip is gently moved into internal rotation. Clinically, the child has such severe pain that walking is not possible, even with crutches. Radiographic signs of chronicity will not be present if the pathologic process is of short duration, but may be present in cases in which a recent exacerbation of a longer-standing process has occurred. This newer classification system is particularly useful in determining the patient's prognosis regarding osteonecrosis, which is the most devastating complication.

Pain is localized to the anterior hip, groin, or medial thigh and knee. If the slipping is abrupt and results in severe displacement, the child will be in marked pain and unable to walk. If the pain is not severe, it is common for the family to wait several weeks or months before seeking medical attention. The physical examination typically demonstrates an obese child who walks with a mild antalgic gait with the leg in external rotation. Sudden attempts at internal rotation of the hip will cause increased pain. Commonly, the severity of the slip correlates to the amount of obligatory external rotation during passive flexion of the hip.

Imaging Studies

Anteroposterior (AP) and lateral radiographs are the most important imaging studies for diagnosis and treatment. On the AP projection, the earliest radiographic evidence (preslip) is characterized by slight widening and fuzzy irregularity of the physis. When the slip is mild, the central epiphyseal height may be slightly decreased compared to that of the contralateral side. Normally, a line drawn tangent to the superior femoral neck (on the AP view) should intersect the lateral aspect of the femoral head. In most cases of even minor slipping this line (Klein's line) will pass more lateral on the capital epiphysis. The metaphyseal blanch sign on AP radiographs has been described as a crescent shaped area of increased density overlying the metaphysis adjacent to the epiphyseal plate. This line represents the posteriorly slipped epiphyseal edge. The lateral radiographic projection provides the most useful informa-

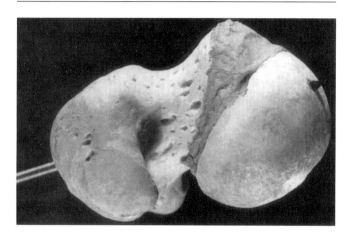

Fig. 1 Model of a moderately severe slipped capital femoral epiphysis, viewed from a cephalad orientation, demonstrating pure posterior displacement. (Reproduced with permission from Nguyen D, Morrissy RT: Slipped capital femoral epiphysis: Rationale for the technique of percutaneous in situ fixation. *J Pediatr Orthop* 1990; 10:341–346.)

tion and is mandatory when SCFE is suspected because it will show the posterior position of the capital epiphysis.

The true position of a slipped epiphysis has been shown to be posterior to the femoral neck, and not inferior as initially believed (Fig. 1). The apparent inferior or varus position of the capital epiphysis is explained by the radiographic phenomenon of parallax, which is created by the superimposed position of the femoral neck on the posteriorly positioned capital epiphysis. Slipping of brief duration will not show any radiographic evidence of callus formation or other signs of remodeling. Slipping of longer duration, commonly referred to as a chronic slip, will show callus formation at the inferomedial head–neck junction; callus formation is seen best on the lateral radiograph. The superior proximal edge of the head–neck junction will also show callus formation and a "rounding off" with chronic slips.

Slip severity can be classified radiographically by several methods. These are based on the amount of epiphyseal displacement (absolute or percentage) or on the angular measurements of the SCFE with respect to either the femoral neck or shaft (Fig. 2). These classifications divide the slipping into mild, moderate, or severe categories, depending on the amount of capital slipping. A slip is typically described as being *mild* if the epiphysis is displaced less than one third of the neck width or if the head–shaft angle is less than 30°; *moderate* if the epiphysis is displaced from one third to one half the neck width or if the head–shaft angle is between 30° and 50°; and *severe* if the epiphysis is displaced greater than one half the neck width or if the head–shaft angle is more than 50°. The head–shaft angle classification system currently is used most commonly. SCFE may also be evaluated using computed tomography (CT), which may provide more quantitative accuracy.

However, the routine use of CT for diagnosis or treatment is not necessary or recommended. CT, with three-dimensional reconstruction, may be helpful for planning complex osteotomies in certain salvage situations. Bone scans may show increased uptake at the physis but are of no more value than a good history, physical examination, and plain radiograph.

Pathophysiology

The capital epiphysis is positioned posteriorly with respect to the femoral neck. There is histologic evidence of hip joint synovitis, including round cell infiltration. Light microscopic examination of the physis indicates that the slipping occurs through the hypertrophic zone of the growth plate. The hypertrophic zone is abnormally widened and composed of large disarrayed clusters of chondrocytes. Electron microscopy reveals extensive disarray of the normally ordered thick and thin collagen fibrils in the hypertrophic zone. The loss of the normal longitudinal and transverse collagen septae is associated with significant structural weakness. Increased proteoglycan and glycoprotein staining in the hypertrophic region has been reported. Histology of the chondrocytes in the resting zone of the growth plate appears normal.

Etiology

The etiology of SCFE remains unknown. Several theories explain some cases of SCFE but certainly not all. In reality, many of the proposed etiologic factors may, in combination, lead to this condition. Most cases of SCFE are not associated with significant trauma. In fact, the pathophysiology of growth plate fractures differs from that of a slip. The disorganized histology and abnormal matrix formation of the growth plate in SCFE may imply a collagen formation defect that results in inherent weakness in this area. However, there is no evidence to prove whether these abnormalities are primarily causative or are produced secondarily because of the slip.

Although endocrine abnormalities, the most common of which is hypothyroidism, are known to be associated with SCFE, the vast majority of children with SCFE do not have an identifiable endocrine abnormality. SCFE has been reported in individuals with hypogonadism, parathyroid adenoma, hypopituitarism, pituitary tumor, growth hormone abnormality, and renal osteodystrophy. It has also been postulated that a subtle imbalance in the ratios between growth hormone and testosterone may result in physeal weakening, leading to SCFE. Patients with bilateral SCFE should be tested for thyroid insufficiency.

Immunologic abnormalities are also found in patients with SCFE, but again, whether these findings are causative or are a consequence of the slip is unclear. Both elevated serum and synovial immunoglobulin levels and elevated synovial complement C3 levels have been reported. Abnormal levels of these products have also been reported to be potential markers for children who are at increased risk of developing chondrolysis following SCFE.

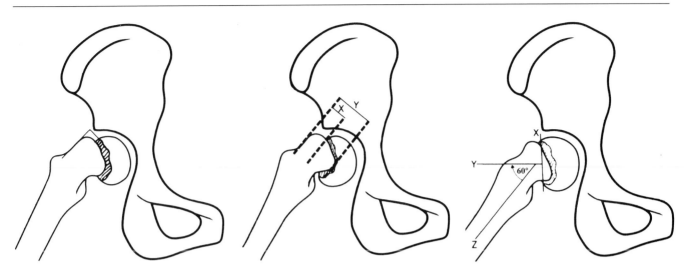

Fig. 2 Schematic representations of slip severity measured on the frog-lateral radiograph. **Left,** Absolute epiphyseal displacement. **Middle,** Percent epiphyseal displacement. **Right,** Lateral head-shaft angle. (Reproduced with permission from Cohen MS, Gelberman RH, Griffin PP, et al: Slipped capital femoral epiphysis: Assessment of epiphyseal displacement and angulation. *J Pediatr Orthop* 1986;6:259–264.)

Mechanical factors may play a significant role in the etiology of SCFE. The large size of many of the affected children supports the theory that abnormally high shear forces applied to a normal physis may overcome its inherent stability and lead to a slip. Excessive proximal femoral retroversion, common in SCFE, may contribute to the abnormal shear forces on the physis. However, as in the case of other proposed etiologies, it is unclear how significant this biomechanical explanation is in the causation of SCFE.

Treatment

The primary treatment goals in SCFE are to stabilize the slipping process and to achieve premature closure of the physis. A secondary treatment goal is the reorientation of the femoral head into a more normal weightbearing position. Reorientation of femoral head position, achievable by osteotomy, is generally reserved for severe cases and considered to be a salvage goal by most surgeons. The treatment methods reported are numerous and include immobilization, single screw fixation, multiple screw/pin fixation, physeal neck osteotomy, base of the neck osteotomy, and osteotomy at the inter or subtrochanteric level.

Stabilization Methods

Cast Immobilization This treatment method is rarely used in current practice. After casting, children require special home care as well as homebound schooling, and problems with skin care and hygiene may occur in more obese children. Because cast immobilization is not com-monly used, the results of this treatment have not been reported as frequently as those of other types of treatment. Current literature documents that the incidence of osteonecrosis and chondrolysis probably is no greater following cast immobilization than is commonly reported for internal fixation, although progression of the slip following cast removal can occur infrequently. The logistic problems of casting, concern about the implications of an open physis after cast removal, and, in particular, the improved techniques of screw fixation have made cast immobilization a rarity.

Screw Fixation At present, in situ single screw fixation using fluoroscopic control during insertion is the most common treatment for patients with SCFE. The risk of unrecognized joint penetration with multiple pins or screws has been widely appreciated since 1980. It is now understood that to avoid this complication, the safest position for metallic pin or screw placement is in the exact center of the femoral head, as seen on both AP and lateral radiographic views. After more than 10 years' experience with use of a single screw for treatment of stable SCFE, the results uniformly have been reported to be very good, regardless of the degree of slip severity. The rates of osteonecrosis and chondrolysis, typically significant following multiple pin insertion, have diminished considerably, and screw penetration into the joint is very uncommon with use of a single screw. A 6- to 7-mm cannulated screw, either fully or partially threaded, is positioned in the center of the epiphysis. Because the capital epiphysis rests purely posteriorly in SCFE, not in varus as in an adult femoral neck fracture, screw insertion must begin on the anterior aspect of the femoral neck if the screw is to pass

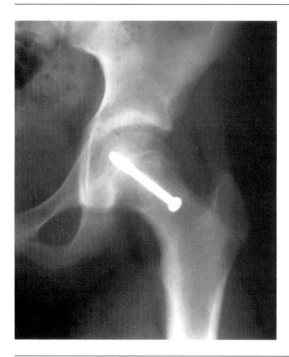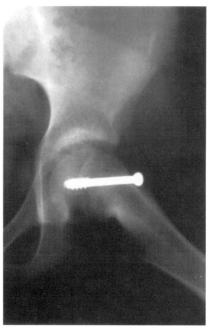

Fig. 3 **Left** and **right,** Anteroposterior and frog lateral radiographs showing anterior starting point and good central placement of a single screw.

centrally into the epiphysis on both AP and lateral radiographic views (Fig. 3). The more severe the slip, the more anteriorly the screw must be inserted, as can easily be seen when viewing the lateral fluoroscopic projection. The screw tip should end at least 5 mm from the subchondral surface. The cannulated screw can be inserted percutaneously over a properly positioned guide pin. Clinical experience has shown that fixation with a single 6- to 7-mm screw is sufficient to prevent further slipping of a stable slip and does induce premature closure of the proximal femoral physis. Radiographic physeal closure may take as long as 12 to 14 months following single screw fixation. However, clinical experience has shown that patients can resume their normal activities much sooner than this without sustaining further slipping. Many surgeons encourage the child to use crutches for 6 weeks postoperatively, although this protocol may not be necessary based on the number of children who do not comply and do not experience any apparent ill effects. There currently is not enough experience with single screw fixation for treatment of an unstable slip to uniformly recommend its use in this setting.

Multiple pin fixation was the most common treatment for SCFE prior to 1980. With the more recent understanding of the problems associated with multiple pin fixation (unrecognized pin penetration into the joint, chondrolysis, osteonecrosis, femoral neck fracture, or traumatic joint degeneration), its use has diminished substantially. However, an acutely painful, unstable SCFE may still represent an indication for the use of two screws because such use increases the strength of the internal fixation by one third.

Abandonment of multiple pin fixation for stable SCFE has had a dramatically favorable impact on the short-term complications associated with its treatment (Fig. 4).

Open Bone Graft Epiphysiodesis Open bone graft epiphysiodesis (OBGE) was initially described in the North American literature in 1931. Routine use of this technique has been infrequent in the United States despite reports of excellent results with low complication rates of osteonecrosis and chondrolysis. The primary objection to OBGE when compared to single screw fixation is that it is a much larger surgical intervention that requires more surgical expertise. When compared to treatment with multiple pins, OBGE offered the distinct advantage of predictable physeal closure (within 12 weeks) without the attendant complications. Indications for OBGE have decreased with the advent of single-screw fixation.

Realignment Osteotomies

Subcapital Wedge Osteotomy The subcapital wedge osteotomy has been used for moderate or severely displaced stable SCFE in which the physis remains open. This procedure is contraindicated when the proximal femoral physis is closed. Prior to physeal closure, the capital femoral circulation is provided by the posterior retinacular vessels, which travel in the periosteum of the femoral neck to enter the capital epiphysis at the level of the physis. By the time of physeal closure, the retinacular blood supply is less important and most of the capital femoral blood flow is through the metaphyseal circulation. With proper surgi-

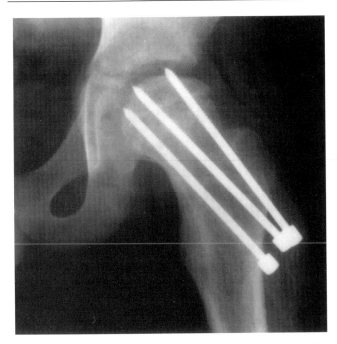

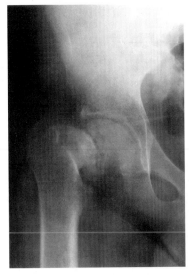
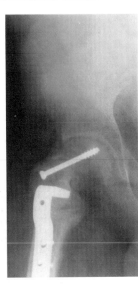

Fig. 5 **Left,** Preoperative severe, stable slip. **Right,** Postoperative intertrochanteric flexion, valgus osteotomy fixed with a blade plate. Supplemental screw fixation across the physis is also seen.

Fig. 4 Multiple pin fixation in which pin spread is too wide and all pins penetrate the joint surface.

cal technique, wedge osteotomy in the region of an open physis should not interfere with capital femoral blood supply, whereas osteotomy through a closed physis will significantly impair capital femoral circulation. Wedge osteotomy at the subcapital level is attractive because it can restore normal head–neck alignment. Restoration of normal alignment should diminish the probability of developing early onset osteoarthritis. A severe deformity can be corrected better at the subcapital region than at either the intertrochanteric or subtrochanteric level. When successfully performed for patients with moderate or severe SCFE, subcapital wedge osteotomy probably provides more optimal long-term results than all other interventions. However, associated with this procedure, there is a substantial reported risk of osteonecrosis, which approaches 35% in some series. This procedure cannot currently be recommended for the general orthopaedic surgeon treating SCFE; it should be considered only by surgeons who are fully aware of pediatric hip blood supply and skilled in pediatric hip surgical techniques.

Base of Neck Osteotomy In this osteotomy, a wedge of bone at the junction of the base of neck and intertrochanteric region is removed for treatment of moderate or severe SCFE. This procedure can be used to correct a head–neck deformity up to 50°. Base of neck osteotomy is believed to be safer than subcapital wedge osteotomy because the bone cut is distal to the medial femoral circumflex blood supply to the capital epiphysis. Osteonecrosis and chon-

drolysis have been reported only rarely after this procedure. The disadvantages of this procedure are that it produces a compensatory deformity and must shorten the femoral neck to a certain degree. This procedure has not been reported as commonly as either subcapital or subtrochanteric osteotomy for treatment of moderate or severe SCFE.

Intertrochanteric or Subtrochanteric Osteotomy This osteotomy is designed to provide biplane correction for both varus and posterior displacement of the capital epiphysis. Because it has recently been acknowledged that most slips are purely posterior displacements, the need for an osteotomy that provides varus correction is debatable. However, intertrochanteric or subtrochanteric osteotomy can provide good reorientation of the capital epiphysis without the risk of osteonecrosis (Fig. 5). Internal fixation of these osteotomies should be secure enough that supplemental cast immobilization is not required. The need to include supplemental screw fixation across an open physis at the time of osteotomy is unresolved. Intertrochanteric or subtrochanteric osteotomies are performed with the expectation that reestablishment of a more normal head–shaft angle will delay or possibly prevent the onset of osteoarthritis later in adult life. These osteotomies may also provide pain relief and favorably change the arc of motion of the hip. Their primary disadvantage is that the compensatory deformity produced at the osteotomy sites makes subsequent total hip replacement more difficult.

Long-Term Follow-up of SCFE Treated by In Situ Methods The natural history of SCFE treated by in situ meth-

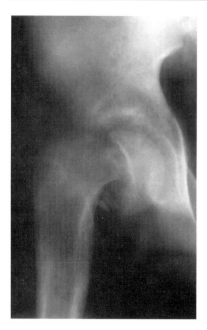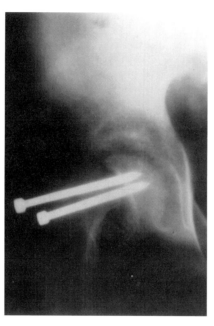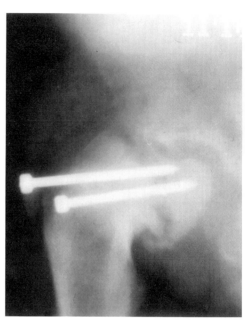

Fig. 6 Example of severe osteonecrosis following in situ fixation of a severe, unstable slip. **Left,** Preoperative radiograph showing severe slip. **Middle,** In situ fixation with two pins. **Right,** Significant osteonecrosis noted postoperatively.

ods appears to be related to the severity of the slip, length of follow-up, and associated complications, particularly osteonecrosis and chondrolysis. After treatment, the majority of patients, regardless of slip severity, function satisfactorily without serious clinical complaints or radiographic evidence of significant osteoarthritis. None of the long-term follow-up studies have specifically addressed how well these individuals are functioning with more demanding recreational activities. However, evidence of osteoarthritis tends to increase as longitudinal follow-up of severe slips is increased. The presence of osteonecrosis and chondrolysis, related or unrelated to treatment, worsens the long-term functional and radiographic results. If these complications are avoided, the majority of patients with SCFE can be expected to function satisfactorily at least until middle age.

Hip range of motion improves following all treatments for SCFE. The external rotation gait, so pronounced at the time of diagnosis, can be expected to improve over time even if a displaced slip had been stabilized in situ. On plain radiographs, the femoral neck remodels and appears to improve the head–neck alignment. However, more detailed CT analysis of the head–neck anatomy following in situ stabilization suggests that the head–neck orientation changes less than it appears to on plain radiographs. Notwithstanding the uncertainty of true head–neck remodeling, the majority of slip patients with in situ stabilization will demonstrate improved hip motion, gait, and functioning as long as osteonecrosis and chondrolysis are avoided. Reports that a significant percentage of patients with primary osteoarthritis of the hip (undergoing total hip replacement) actually demonstrate radiographic evidence of a prior unrecognized SCFE are not universally accepted as valid.

When reduction of a moderate or severely displaced SCFE has been successfully performed, and osteonecrosis and chondrolysis have been avoided, the natural history of that particular hip should be improved. Successful performance of any type of realignment osteotomy should also improve the natural history of that slip. Unfortunately, forceful reduction maneuvers and realignment osteotomies frequently have been associated with complications. This association makes it difficult to determine whether the potential benefit of these interventions outweigh the risks when evaluating available reports of long-term studies. Longer follow-up of reduced slips and realignment osteotomies using modern-day techniques is needed to determine whether these interventions provide a better long-term outcome than does in situ fixation alone.

Complications

The most serious complication associated with SCFE is osteonecrosis, which can occur without treatment, but more commonly is associated with treatment, such as aggressive reduction maneuvers applied to stable slips, subcapital osteotomy, gentle longitudinal reduction in severely unstable slips, and even after fixation in situ of severe, unstable slips (Fig. 6). In situ fixation of stable slips rarely results in osteonecrosis; however, a recent study reports an osteonecrosis rate approaching 47% following fixation of unstable slips without a formal reduction maneuver. Gentle longitudinal reduction of an unstable slip during placement on a fracture table often unavoidably changes the femoral head orientation. In this situation, damage to the capital blood supply may have already occurred at the time of sudden slippage, and any change in position of the slip is probably not contributory to further impairment of blood supply. Aggressive, manipulative reduction of stable slips can disrupt the tenuous blood supply to the capital epiphysis and should not be done. Clustering of pins or screws in the antero or posterolateral femoral head can cause segmental osteonecrosis.

Chondrolysis has a reported incidence between 3% and 7% in most series. It is a poorly understood condition that currently is believed to have an immunologic basis. Chondrolysis may be associated with unrecognized permanent pin/screw placement into the joint space; however, transient guide wire joint penetration is not associated with the problem. Recent reports show that the condition affects blacks and whites equivalently. Aggressive active

and passive motion treatment is recommended in the hope that cartilage nutrition and function will be improved following the diagnosis of chondrolysis. However, no specific treatment intervention has proven to definitively alter its course. Many cases of chondrolysis do appear to improve with time, although progression to ankylosis can occur.

Decreased articulotrochanteric distance (ATD) is commonly observed in severe slips treated with in situ screw fixation and following screw fixation for mild SCFE in which the physis intentionally is prematurely closed. Decreased ATD may result in abductor insufficiency although most children do not have complaints related to a small decrease in ATD. Leg length discrepancy may also occur, but is not typically a clinical problem. Pathologic fracture can occur through drill holes, created for screw or pin insertion, on the lateral cortex of the femur. This complication can be kept to a minimum by using only one screw and by avoiding any unnecessary drill holes in the femoral cortex. Initial insertion of a small guide wire to identify the correct screw insertion point should minimize pathologic fracture through empty drill holes.

Annotated Bibliography

Description: Epidemiology

Aronson DD, Loder RT: Slipped capital femoral epiphysis in black children. *J Pediatr Orthop* 1992;12:74–79.

In this retrospective review of 74 black children with 97 slips treated by either multiple or single screw fixation, state-of-the-art treatment with a single screw gave 91% satisfactory results. Only 3% of the entire group experienced chondrolysis. Results for black children were equivalent to reported results for white children.

Jerre R, Billing L, Hansson G, et al: The contralateral hip in patients primarily treated for unilateral slipped upper femoral epiphysis: Long-term follow-up of sixty-one hips. *J Bone Joint Surg* 1994;76B:563–567.

Sixty-one patients with SCFE were reviewed at skeletal maturity for the presence of bilateral slipping. Fourteen (23%) had simultaneous bilateral slips, while an additional 11 patients (18%) demonstrated sequential slipping (41% total bilaterality). In only two of the 25 bilateral slips was the contralateral hip symptomatic. The authors do not recommend prophylactic pinning of a normal contralateral hip in patients with unilateral SCFE.

Kennedy JP, Weiner DS: Results of slipped capital femoral epiphysis in the black population. *J Pediatr Orthop* 1990;10:224–227.

This is a retrospective review of 44 slips in black children treated by either pin fixation or bone grafting. In 93.2%, excellent or good results were obtained. The authors conclude that blacks fair as well as whites with treatment for SCFE.

Loder RT, Aronson DD, Greenfield ML: The epidemiology of bilateral slipped capital femoral epiphysis: A study of children in Michigan. *J Bone Joint Surg* 1993;75A:1141–1147.

In this retrospective review of 224 children with SCFE without metabolic or endocrine abnormalities, 37% had a bilateral slip with one half of the bilateral slips occurring simultaneously and the other half sequentially, usually within 18 months of the initial slip. This study recommends radiographic follow-up until physeal closure of both hips.

Spero CR, Masciale JP, Tornetta P III, et al: Slipped capital femoral epiphysis in black children: Incidence of chondrolysis. *J Pediatr Orthop* 1992;12:444–448.

In this retrospective study of 29 black children (44 hips) treated by in situ pinning for SCFE, the overall rates of chondrolysis and osteonecrosis were 6.8% and 4.5%, respectively. Adherence to the technical details described in the article was believed to be able to reduce the complication rates even further. The authors conclude that blacks can expect results similar to whites.

Description: Imaging Studies

Kallio PE, Paterson DC, Foster BK, et al: Classification in slipped capital femoral epiphysis: Sonographic assessment of stability and remodeling. *Clin Orthop* 1993;294:196–203.

This paper proposes an ultrasonographic classification of SCFE. All unstable slips treated by reduction were associated with ultrasonographic hip joint effusions. Joint effusion represented physeal instability or recent progression, while ultrasonograpic remodeling was a sign of chronicity.

Kallio PE, Lequesne GW, Paterson DC, et al: Ultrasonography in slipped capital femoral epiphysis: Diagnosis and assessment of severity. *J Bone Joint Surg* 1991;73B: 884–889.

In recent-onset SCFE, ultrasound revealed a step at the anterior physeal outline, diminished distance between the anterior acetabular rim and femoral metaphysis, and hip joint effusion. As metaphyseal remodeling progressed, the physeal step decreased. Authors recommend ultrasound for diagnosis, staging, and follow-up care of SCFE.

Treatment: Stabilization Methods

Aronson DD, Carlson WE: Slipped capital femoral epiphysis: A prospective study of fixation with a single screw. *J Bone Joint Surg* 1992;74A:810–819.

Forty-four children (58 hips) with SCFE were treated with single screw fixation. Fifty-four (93%) were rated as having excellent or good results. Only one case of osteonecrosis was reported and no chondrolysis was noted. Results confirm the efficacy of single screw fixation.

Betz RR, Steel HH, Emper WD, et al: Treatment of slipped capital femoral epiphysis: Spica-cast immobilization. *J Bone Joint Surg* 1990;72A:587–600.

This is a retrospective study of 37 hips with acute on chronic or chronic SCFE treated with cast immobilization for 8 to 16 weeks. Casts were removed prior to closure of the physis. One slip progressed following cast removal. Chondrolysis was documented in five hips (14%) following treatment, and no osteonecrosis was seen. The authors conclude that cast treatment is as effective and safe as other treatment modalities.

Blanco JS, Taylor B, Johnston CE II: Comparison of single pin versus multiple pin fixation in treatment of slipped capital femoral epiphysis. *J Pediatr Orthop* 1992;12:384–389.

In this retrospective study comparing 43 single pin fixations with 71 multiple pin fixations for SCFE, there was no significant difference in the time to physeal closure for single screw fixation compared with multiple pin fixation. Complication and reoperation rates were significantly lower in the single pin fixation group.

Kibiloski LJ, Doane RM, Karol LA, et al: Biomechanical analysis of single- versus double-screw fixation in slipped capital femoral epiphysis at physiological load levels. *JPediatr Orthop* 1989;9:627–630.

Unstable SCFE was modeled in 12 pairs of bovine femora; one side was fixed with a single screw and the other with two screws. Specimens were then subjected to physiologic shear loads across the epiphysis. The rates of creep were not statistically significantly increased for either simulated slow or fast walking. Single screw fixation was recommended because of its satisfactory mechanics and association with decreased biologic complications.

Meier MC, Meyer LC, Ferguson RL: Treatment of slipped capital femoral epiphysis with a spica cast. *J Bone Joint Surg* 1992;74A:1522–1529.

Thirteen patients (17 hips) with SCFE were treated for an average of 3 months in cast. Further slipping after cast was

noticed in three hips and chondrolysis documented in nine hips, all of which developed degenerative changes. The authors advise the abandonment of spica cast treatment as an option for SCFE.

Ward WT, Stefko J, Wood KB, et al: Fixation with a single screw for slipped capital femoral epiphysis. *J Bone Joint Surg* 1992;74A:799–809.

This retrospective study of 53 hips treated with single screw fixation for SCFE demonstrated the efficacy of this treatment method. A longer time to physeal fusion was correlated with increasingly eccentric screw placement ($r = 0.44$) and inversely correlated to increasing slip severity ($r = -0.536$). Premature physeal closure was induced with a single screw. Complications of single screw fixation were minimal.

Treatment: Realignment Osteotomies

Abraham E, Garst J, Barmada R: Treatment of moderate to severe slipped capital femoral epiphysis with extracapsular base-of-neck osteotomy. *J Pediatr Orthop* 1993;13:294–302.

This is a retrospective review of 36 hips with moderate to severe SCFE that underwent base of femoral neck osteotomy. Ninety percent of the hips had good or excellent results by modified Southwick's criteria. Osteonecrosis did not occur. Limb length discrepancy greater than 1.5 cm did occur with large corrections.

Fish JB: Cuneiform osteotomy of the femoral neck in the treatment of slipped capital femoral epiphysis: A follow-up note. *J Bone Joint Surg* 1994;76A:46–59.

In this retrospective review of 61 patients (66 hips) that underwent subcapital cuneiform osteotomy, the results were rated excellent in 55 hips, good in six, fair in two, and poor in three. Six patients developed osteoarthritis and three demonstrated evidence of osteonecrosis. The authors conclude that subcapital osteotomy can be done safely if meticulous surgical technique is followed.

Complications

Krahn TH, Canale ST, Beaty JH, et al: Long-term follow-up of patients with avascular necrosis after treatment of slipped capital femoral epiphysis. *J Pediatr Orthop* 1993; 13:154–158.

This is a retrospective study of 264 slips in which 36 developed osteonecrosis. Twenty-four hips were reviewed at an average follow-up of 31 years. Nine hips had undergone reconstructive surgery. The 15 hips that did not undergo reconstruction all showed evidence of degenerative changes.

Vrettos BC, Hoffman EB: Chondrolysis in slipped upper femoral epiphysis: Long-term study of the aetiology and natural history. *J Bone Joint Surg* 1993;75B:956–961.

In this retrospective review of 55 slips, 14 developed chondrolysis: eight at time of slip diagnosis, and six following unrecognized persistent pin penetration into the joint. Chondrolysis did not develop in any of 11 hips with transient intraoperative pin penetration. At average follow-up of 13 years, no patient had pain but five hips were stiff.

Zionts LE, Simonian PT, Harvey JP Jr: Transient penetration of the hip joint during in situ cannulated-screw fixation of slipped capital femoral epiphysis. *J Bone Joint Surg* 1991;73A:1054–1060.

This is a retrospective study of 30 slips in which 14 had a transient intraoperative occurrence of joint penetration by a guide pin or screw, or both. Eleven hips were followed for at least 2 years with none demonstrating clinical or radiographic evidence of chondrolysis. The authors conclude that transient penetration of the hip joint did not lead to chondrolysis.

Long-Term Follow-Up

Carney BT, Weinstein SL, Noble J: Long-term follow-up of slipped capital femoral epiphysis. *J Bone Joint Surg* 1991;73A:667–674.

This is a retrospective review of 124 patients (155 hips) with SCFE seen at a mean follow-up of 41 years after the onset of symptoms. Multiple treatments were used for the slips. Iowa hip rating, osteonecrosis, chondrolysis, and degenerative joint disease all worsened with increasing slip severity and when reduction or realignment had been done. Authors stated that pinning in situ gave the best long-term results, regardless of the severity of the slip.

Siegel DB, Kasser JR, Sponseller P, et al: Slipped capital femoral epiphysis: A quantitative analysis of motion, gait, and femoral remodeling after in situ fixation. *J Bone Joint Surg* 1991;73A:659–666.

This is a prospective study quantifying motion, gait, and remodeling in 39 patients (57 hips) treated with in situ screw fixation and followed up for at least 2 years. Hip motion and gait improved significantly, but radiography and CT revealed no change in the femoral head–shaft alignment and minimal change in neck–shaft angle. Soft-tissue stretching and bone resorption in the anterolateral femoral neck were believed to be responsible for the increased motion seen at follow-up.

Wong-Chung J, Strong ML: Physeal remodeling after internal fixation of slipped capital femoral epiphyses. *J Pediatr Orthop* 1991;11:2–5.

Physeal remodeling led to a change in physeal shaft angle after internal fixation in one of 21 mild slips compared to 11 of 11 severe slips. Remodeling averaged 11.7°. The authors conclude that remodeling does occur and advise waiting at least 2 years before considering realignment osteotomy.

Miscellaneous

Cooperman DR, Charles LM, Pathria M, et al: Post-mortem description of slipped capital femoral epiphysis. *J Bone Joint Surg* 1992;74B:595–599.

Nine adult hips with untreated SCFE were identified from a museum skeleton collection. Seven of nine femora were retroverted beyond neutral. Osteoarthritis was present in eight of the hips. This study supports the association of SCFE and femoral retroversion.

Dietz FR: Traction reduction of acute and acute on chronic slipped capital femoral epiphysis. *Clin Orthop* 1994;302:101–110.

This is a retrospective review of 30 acute or acute on chronic slips. Thirteen hips underwent longitudinal traction in an attempt to obtain reduction, with successful reduction in only five hips. There was no significant difference in the rate of osteonecrosis between those hips undergoing reduction, not reducible, or fixed in situ without attempt at traction reduction. Authors conclude that longitudinal traction reduction appears to be a safe maneuver.

Loder RT, Richards BS, Shapiro PS, et al: Acute slipped capital femoral epiphysis: The importance of physeal stability. *J Bone Joint Surg* 1993;75A:1134–1140.

In this retrospective study, 30 slips were defined as stable (patient could bear weight, with or without crutches) and 25 as unstable (patient has such severe pain that weightbearing was not possible even with crutches). A reduction occurred in 26 of the unstable slips and in only two of the stable slips. Osteonecrosis developed in 47% of unstable slips but in none of the stable slips. The authors conclude that slip stability is the important correlation with osteonecrosis rather than occurrence of a reduction or duration of symptoms.

19

Legg-Calvé-Perthes Disease

Since the original independent descriptions in 1910, Legg-Calvé-Perthes disease (LCPD) has remained an enigma of both etiology and treatment. Although the sequence of femoral head fragmentation and repair is widely considered to represent the result of an idiopathic osteonecrosis, the process is considered by some to be part of a more generalized epiphyseal cartilage disorder.

For reasons unknown, LCPD occurs in a "susceptible child" generally between the ages of 4 and 8 years, although it can appear in children as young as 2 and as old as 12 years of age. It is four or five times more common in boys than in girls, and in 10% may be bilateral. There is no evidence for an inherited pattern; however, some social or environmental associations exist. These include older parental age, difficult birth presentations, a lower socioeconomic ranking, and an urban setting.

Clinical Picture

The typical presentation is a prolonged limp or waddling gait, usually with pain in the groin, thigh, or knee. Gluteal and thigh muscle atrophy may be noted if the condition has been present for an extended period of time. Although it is common for the child to have synovitis during the course of the disease, it is uncommon (less than 3%) for the child to be brought to the orthopaedist with acute synovitis and a normal radiograph, which later evolves into the fragmentation characteristic of LCPD. The majority of affected children (90%) have a delay in bone age (averaging 21 months) and short stature. Laboratory data are normal for children with LCPD.

Differential Diagnosis

The differential diagnosis should not be problematic unless the child has bilateral symmetric involvement in the capital femoral epiphysis. Avascular-like changes may appear in severe renal compromise, but in that situation the clinical appearance is one of an ill child. Bilateral symmetric involvement in a child with short stature should raise suspicion for hypothyroidism or for one of the generalized epiphyseal dysplasias, such as multiple epiphyseal dysplasia (MED) or spondyloepiphyseal dysplasia (SED). Other epiphyses, such as the knees, wrist, and spine, should be imaged to rule out a skeletal dysplasia. In bilateral LCPD, both hips usually do not become symptomatic at the same time. Instead, the contralateral hip becomes involved at a later date, or, if it is abnormal on the initial radiograph, is at a different stage of involvement.

Other Diagnostics

Because the prognosis in LCPD relates to age at presentation and the degree of involvement, radiographic assessment should include anteroposterior and lateral views of the hips, and a view of the wrist for determination of bone age. A radiograph of the pelvis with the hips abducted will help determine to what degree the femoral epiphysis centers or "contains" itself within the acetabulum. This information is important for treatment consideration.

In cases where the diagnosis is uncertain, a pin-hole collimated technetium 99 bone scan can be useful in demonstrating the extent of avascularity, especially early in the disease. Although magnetic resonance imaging (MRI) can show the involvement, there has been no direct correlation with later radiographic findings of collapse. Such abnormal findings may represent transient ischemic episodes and are not necessarily prognostic.

Etiology

The anterior and lateral portion of the femoral epiphysis most commonly is involved in the fragmentation process seen in LCPD. This area receives its circulation from the ascending lateral cervical vessels of the medial femoral circumflex artery. The typical timing of the clinical presentation is consistent with the fact that this circulation is less developed in the 3- to 10-year age group, particularly in boys. A double infarction theory states that a primary infarction in the circumflex system needs to be followed by a second infarction in order to produce the characteristic histologic LCPD changes that have been described in human specimens. Such ischemias may represent the primary pathologic event, yet no distinct cause of such ischemia has been clarified. However, there may be a secondary event occurring in abnormal cartilage of the epiphysis or growth plate. Abnormal somatomedin levels have been found in some LCPD patients. Presently, however, no definitive etiologic factor has been identified for this condition.

Classification

The extent of epiphyseal involvement has been shown by many to have prognostic significance and helps to define those patients who benefit most from treatment. The radiographic classification offered by Catterall (groups I to IV) is based on the degree of fragmentation of the epiphysis. In groups I and II, the fragmentation is anterior and

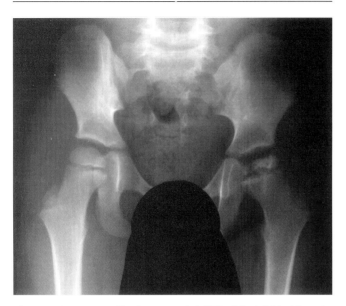

Fig. 1 Herring classification group A: LCPD of the left hip. There is clear demarcation between the normal lateral pillar and the area of fragmentation as seen in this anteroposterior radiograph.

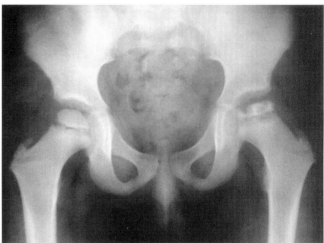

Fig. 2 Herring classification group B: LCPD of the left hip. The lateral pillar is sclerotic and, therefore, involved with the avascular process. However, the height remains more than 50% of that of the opposite normal hip.

superior, preserving the lateral portion (pillar) of the epiphysis. In Catterall groups III and IV disease, the lateral pillar is involved. The posterior portion of the epiphysis is preserved in group III, whereas the entire epiphysis fragments in group IV. Unfortunately, the Catterall classification has poor interobserver consistency, and because fragmentation may take 6 to 8 months to occur, its prognostic value may be limited.

Salter and Thompson attempted to simplify a prognostic classification by emphasizing the early-appearing subchondral fracture (crescent sign). Their group A hips (in which the crescent sign involved less than one half of the epiphysis) are characterized by no involvement of the lateral pillar. These correspond to Catterall I and II hips. Salter group B hips (Catterall III, IV) are more extensively involved and show pillar fragmentation. Recently, Herring and associates have proposed the more consistently applied "lateral pillar" classification in an effort to improve interobserver agreement and to provide more useful prognostic information. Their group A hips have no lateral pillar involvement, whereas groups B and C do have involvement (Figs. 1 through 3). In group B, greater than 50% of the epiphyseal height is maintained, compared to less than 50% in group C.

Prognostic Indicators

Catterall identified a number of "head-at-risk" findings that have been shown to correlate with long-term progno-

sis; the majority of patients with poor outcome have at least two. Lateral epiphyseal calcification as well as lateral subluxation may imply the development of a noncontained coxa magna. Gage's sign (a lateral epiphyseal-metaphyseal triangular lucency) and metaphyseal cysts are related to a greater degree of epiphyseal disruption. A horizontal appearance to the growth plate might imply abnormal growth of the lateral physis with later growth disturbance.

The clinical at risk signs of onset after the age of 8 years and loss of motion also correlate with poor outcome. Girls tend to have lateral pillar involvement and, therefore, may have a less favorable long-term prognosis.

Development of Deformity

When there is fragmentation of the lateral pillar, future head deformities commonly result. The reparative (revascularization) process is associated with collapse of the anterolateral epiphysis. The portion of the epiphyseal cartilage receiving nutrition through the synovium may enlarge, especially in the face of synovitis. Associated adductor spasm or contracture leads to an adducted position of the hip. Abduction beyond this position may force the weakened lateral area of the epiphysis under the lateral edge of the acetabulum leading to "hinge abduction" and resulting in further deformity of the femoral head (Fig. 4, *top* and *bottom left*). These flattened, ovoid, or saddle deformities of LCPD are seen mainly in the older population. The less frequently involved medial epiphysis, remaining contained within the acetabulum, generally pre-

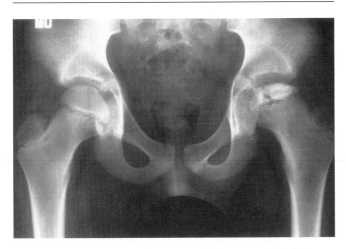

Fig. 3 Herring classification group C: LCPD of the left hip. The height of the lateral pillar is less than half that of the opposite normal hip.

serves a round, congruous shape that may be used in the late reconstruction of the saddle deformity by valgus osteotomy (Fig. 4, *bottom right*).

In addition to the deformity caused by mechanical compression of the weakened femoral head, secondary effects on the growth plate also lead to deformity. Partial disruption of the physis can be found in up to 70% of cases. If generalized throughout the physis, the result is a shortened femoral neck and relative trochanteric overgrowth.

A less common late deformity is an osteochondritis dissecans type lesion (less than 3%) that can result from failure of the epiphysis to heal fully. If symptomatic, this lesion can be drilled if the articular surface is intact or removed if it becomes a loose body.

Natural History

The literature concerning the natural history and treatment of LCPD is very difficult to interpret. Authors not uncommonly combined the entire spectrum of disease in their reports. Moreover, because the Catterall classification suffers from interobserver variability, the grouping found in the literature may vary from study to study. In addition, in many reported studies there was poor retrieval of involved patients and very short duration of follow-up. Given these significant shortcomings, the following factors still appear to be pertinent to the ultimate prognosis: the age of the patient when the disease begins, the degree of involvement of the epiphysis, the presence of head-at-risk signs, the age of the patient when treatment is begun, the stage of disease when treatment is instituted, and whether the hip is congruous at skeletal maturity.

A favorable prognosis exists for those in whom LCPD begins before 6 years of age and treatment begins before 8 years of age. When prognosis is based on epiphyseal involvement, more poor results (60% to 80%) are found with Catterall III and IV hips (Salter-Thompson B; Herring B and C), especially when two or more at risk signs are present. Hips graded as greater than 2 mm out of round or "aspherically congruent or incongruent" at skeletal maturity are at higher risk for poor results. Although most adolescents will function well clinically despite poor radiographs, long-term studies (greater than 35 years) reveal osteoarthritis in 70% to 90%.

Treatment

The goals of treatment are to reduce pain, improve function, and, for the long term, minimize femoral head deformity and, thereby, decrease the incidence of late osteoarthritis. Symptoms of synovitis and decreased range of motion merit treatment in any age patient with any grade LCPD. Available modalities include short-term bed rest, skin traction, abduction cylinder casting, protected weightbearing, anti-inflammatory medication, and physical therapy. Occasionally, adductor tenotomy followed by casting is useful in restoring abduction and achieving containment, especially in the older, more involved patient.

Containment treatment has not been shown to affect the outcome of children younger than 6 years of age at onset, and 50% to 70% in this age group will have a good outcome. The lateral pillar group A hips have a good outcome in all age groups and do not require treatment. Recent studies have shown that lateral pillar group B hips in children with a bone age of 6 years or less will do well without treatment, whereas group B hips in children with older bone ages have better results after containment treatment. The group C hips also have a better outcome if treated with containment.

Children 6 to 9 years of age should be followed carefully during the fragmentation stage, and failure to maintain range of motion heralds the need for containment. The Atlanta Scottish Rite Orthosis generally is used for brace containment, which continues for 8 to 12 months until the lateral pillar shows early ossification. However, recent publications cast doubt on the actual efficacy of brace treatment. The decision to operate to achieve containment rests with the treating orthopaedist and the patient's family; failure to maintain hip containment is also an indication for surgery.

If varus osteotomy is performed, resultant varus should not be less than 110° to 115° in the child with a skeletal age over 6 years, or neck–shaft angle recovery may not occur. Physeal damage secondary to the disease process may also perpetuate a varus neck. Minimal derotation is indicated; however, sufficient hip internal rotation should be maintained. If this is not done, internal rotation of the distal fragment is necessary.

Both femoral and innominate osteotomies have propo-

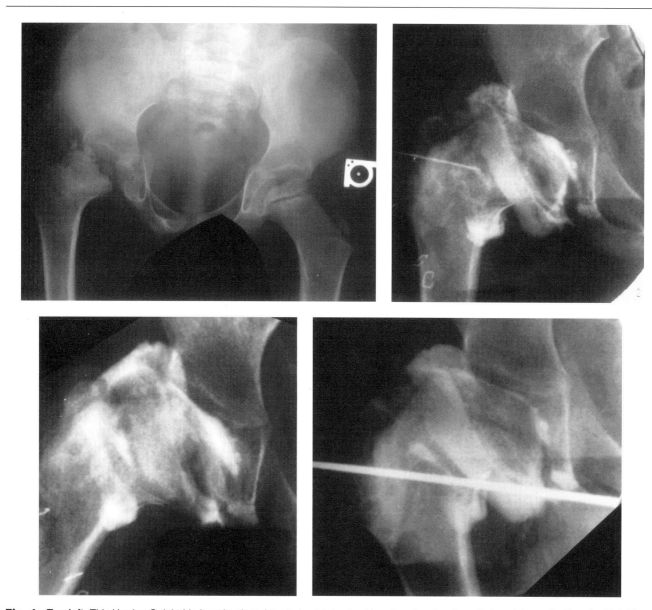

Fig. 4 Top left, This Herring C right hip has developed a proximal, lateral subluxation despite attempt at containment with a Scottish Rite abduction orthosis. The left hip is at the end of the reossification stage of an earlier Perthes process. **Top right,** Arthrogram of this hip confirms the presence of a lateral saddle deformity, as well as medial dye pooling. **Bottom left,** Attempt at abduction of this hip causes an increase in the medial dye pooling due to "hinge abduction" and an eccentric center of rotation. **Bottom right,** Adduction of the hip positions it in the most congruous state and minimizes the pooling of dye. Such a hip may benefit from a valgus osteotomy with a lateral shelf.

nents, and both require "near normal" range of motion as prerequisites. Preoperative traction and physical therapy may be necessary to meet this goal.

Treatment in the child older than 9 years of age remains controversial. Most of these children have extensive femoral head involvement but little hope for acetabular remodeling. Although surgery may be the better way to attempt containment, the results are frequently poor. In this age group, and whenever there is a question of whether a hip in any age group can truly be contained, dynamic hip arthrography is indicated. In the hip that cannot be contained, treatment is symptomatic. The patients in whom hinge abduction persists may later be candidates for valgus osteotomy to increase abduction and improve range of motion (Fig. 4). Cheilectomy is a less satisfactory option because this intra-articular surgery may increase hip stiffness. Hips that end up functioning as a hinge joint in the sagittal plane may benefit from the increased coverage and shared weight distribution achieved with a lateral shelf or Chiari osteotomy.

Late Sequelae

Difficulties other than late osteoarthritis can result from LCPD. If early growth cessation causes leg length inequality, serial orthoroentgenograms are indicated, and epiphysiodesis is an option.

Annotated Bibliography

Classification

Herring JA, Neustadt JB, Williams JJ, et al: The lateral pillar classification of Legg-Calve-Perthes disease. *J Pediatr Orthop* 1992;12:143–150.

Ninety-three hips with LCPD in 86 patients were classified during the fragmentation stage of disease into three groups based on radiolucency in the lateral pillar of the femoral head. The classification group was a stronger determinant than age of onset in predicting final outcome at maturity. Interobserver variability was better for the lateral pillar classification (0.78) than Catterall (0.42) or head-at-risk signs (0.35).

Ritterbusch JF, Shantharam SS, Gelinas C: Comparison of lateral pillar classification and Catterall classification of Legg-Calve-Perthes disease. *J Pediatr Orthop* 1993;13: 200–202.

Three independent observers reviewed 71 hips with radiographic follow-up to maturity. On classification of the early fragmentation stage films, the Herring classification was a significantly better predictor of Stulberg outcome than the Catterall classification.

Natural History

Schoenecker PL, Stone JW, Capelli AM: Legg-Perthes disease in children under 6 years old. *Orthop Rev* 1993; 22:201–208.

In a radiographic review of 109 patients with unilateral LCPD, all symptomatic before 6 years of age, 24% of patients with Catterall III and IV disease had a poor result at final follow-up (average, 12 years). These authors remind us that even young patients can do poorly and that degree of involvement is more prognostic than age.

Treatment

Crutcher JP, Staheli LT: Combined osteotomy as a salvage procedure for severe Legg-Calve-Perthes disease. *J Pediatr Orthop* 1992;12:151–156.

Salter innominate and femoral varus osteotomies were performed at a mean age of 8 years, 4 months on 14 patients with Catterall III (nine patients) and IV (five patients) LCPD. At an average 8-year follow-up, 11 had good clinical results (Ratliff), seven were spherically congruous. Epiphyseal extrusion index was less than 20% in 13 of 14 hips. However, 50% had poor Stulberg ratings.

Herring JA: The treatment of Legg-Calve-Perthes disease: A critical review of the literature. *J Bone Joint Surg* 1994; 76A:448–458.

This is a very critical and "must read" review of frequently quoted literature covering natural history, brace, and surgical treatment. Study weaknesses include the poor reliability of the Catterall classification, grouping of severe and nonsevere disease, variable protocols, small study groups with short-term follow-up. The preliminary results and recommendations of the prospective LCPD Study group are discussed.

Hoikka V, Poussa M, Yrjonen T, et al: Intertrochanteric varus osteotomy for Perthes' disease: Radiographic changes after 2–16-year follow-up of 126 hips. *Acta Orthop Scand* 1991;62:549–553.

The radiographic results of 126 intertrochanteric femoral varus osteotomies in 112 children with Catterall II to IV LCPD were analyzed 2 to 16 years postoperatively. There were very few good results over age 9 years; 50% of Catterall III and IV hips had good results. Catterall's grouping or head-at-risk phenomenon, bicompartmentalization of the acetabulum, and preoperative subluxation did not correlate with the result. The strongest prognostic factor was containment of the femoral head after osteotomy.

Kruse RW, Guille JT, Bowen JR: Shelf arthroplasty in patients who have Legg-Calvé-Perthes disease: A study of long-term results. *J Bone Joint Surg* 1991;73A:1338–1347.

In a retrospective review, 20 Catterall III and IV hips in 19 patients were treated at average age 11 years with traction, adductor tenotomy to reduce subluxation, and then shelf arthroplasty to improve femoral head coverage. Average follow-up was 19 years (2 to 47 years). Mose sphericity was significantly improved and the average Iowa hip score was 91 points. Hinge abduction was eliminated in 11 of 14 hips. Eighteen nonoperative hips in 17 patients followed up for 28 years (7 to 45) had inferior results with an average Iowa hip score of 81 points.

Martinez AG, Weinstein SL, Dietz FR: The weight-bearing abduction brace for the treatment of Legg-Perthes disease. *J Bone Joint Surg* 1992;74A:12–21.

Thirty-one patients (34 hips) with Catterall III (five) and IV (29) LCPD were treated at age 6 years (3 to 12) with the Atlanta Scottish Rite Orthosis and followed 7 years (2 to 13). By Mose criteria, no hip had a good result, 12 (35%) had a fair result, and 22 (65%) had a poor result. There were 14 (41%) class II, 18 (53%) class III and IV, and two (6%) class V Stulberg results.

This small series, excluding 30% of their treatment group, casts doubts on brace treatment. It shows that lateral column collapse is ominous, with 90% having Stulberg III to V results.

Meehan PL, Angel D, Nelson JM: The Scottish Rite abduction orthosis for the treatment of Legg-Perthes disease: A radiographic analysis. *J Bone Joint Surg* 1992; 74A:2–12.

Of 34 patients treated after age 6 years for Catterall III and IV LCPD using the Atlanta Scottish Rite Orthosis, 88% had Stulberg III and IV results. The patients were older, diagnosed at 8 years (6 years, 3 months to 11 years, 2 months), braced 14 months (4 to 33), and followed 6 years, 9 months to 15 years, 8 months. The group is small and not followed to maturity, yet raises doubts on the efficacy of this orthosis in the older patient.

Poussa M, Yrjonen T, Hoikka V, et al: Prognosis after conservative and operative treatment in Perthes' disease. *Clin Orthop* 1993;297:82–86.

The radiographic results in 112 patients (126 hips) at or near skeletal maturity after femoral varus osteotomy were good in 45%, fair in 21%, and poor in 34% of the hips. The figures after noncontainment treatment in 96 patients (106 hips) were 21%, 18%, and 61%, respectively. Surgery was performed at age 8, (5 to 13). The specifics on Catterall II to IV breakdown is not specified.

Yrjonen T: Prognosis in Perthes' disease after noncontainment treatment: 106 hips followed for 28–47 years. *Acta Orthop Scand* 1992;63:523–526.

The results in 96 patients (106 hips) with LCPD disease who had had conservative noncontainment treatment were studied after 35 (28 to 47) years. At skeletal maturity, the radiographic result was poor in 65 hips (61%), and at 43 years, arthrosis was found in 50%. The patient's age at diagnosis and the shape of the femoral head at skeletal maturity were the most reliable prognostic factors.

20

Developmental Dysplasia of the Hip

Introduction

Nomenclature

Developmental dysplasia of the hip (DDH) is the most common disorder affecting the hip in children. The term "developmental dysplasia" has recently supplanted "congenital dislocation" as the accepted name of this condition. It more accurately reflects the variable characteristics of this complex disorder, which is not always present at birth and does not always result in dislocation of the hip. DDH is a dynamic disorder; it includes some conditions that are clearly identifiable at birth (prenatal, teratologic dislocation); others that become apparent during the first year of life (postnatal instability); and yet others that are clinically silent during childhood but become symptomatic during adolescence or early adulthood (subluxation, acetabular dysplasia). The variants of this disorder are described in Table 1.

Incidence

The incidence of DDH varies depending on which definition of the condition is used. Reported rates of hip instability range from 2.7 to 17 per 1,000 live births. The incidence of established dislocation is much lower, approximately 1 per 1,000, and that of "late dislocation," subluxation, and acetabular dysplasia is lower yet (0.4 to 0.6 per 1,000). DDH is not a single entity; however, it may be overly simplistic to think of it merely as a continuum of pathology arising from neonatal hip instability that has a multitude of possible outcomes (resolution, frank dislocation, or dysplasia). Instead, it seems more accurate to consider DDH, with its many manifestations, a spectrum of diseases, which has differing etiologies, pathologies, and natural histories, and which affects both the proximal femur and acetabulum.

Etiology

The etiology of DDH is multifactorial (Outline 1). Physiologic, genetic, and mechanical factors have all been implicated. Ligamentous laxity, hormonally mediated by estrogen and/or relaxin in females or familial in nature (hyperlaxity syndrome) in either sex, is generally thought to play a role. Mechanical factors associated with abnormal intrauterine position and fetal crowding as well as postnatal practices such as swaddling also can adversely affect the hip. Breech position, oligohydramnios, birth order (first born), congenital recurvatum/dislocation of the knee, congenital muscular torticollis, and metatarsus adductus have long been considered risk factors for DDH.

The role of genetic influence is supported by family history, sibling, and twin studies in which the incidence of DDH has been observed to be as high as 34%.

Diagnosis

Screening

The value of early diagnosis and prompt treatment of DDH has generally been recognized. Although neonatal screening programs have resulted in improved early detection of unstable hips, the goal of completely eliminating "late" cases of dislocation, subluxation, and acetabular dysplasia has not been achieved. Most of the literature regarding hip screening indicates that all cases of DDH may not be detectable at birth; that late cases are not always previously misdiagnosed cases; and, most importantly,

Table 1. Variants of developmental dysplasia of the hip

Variant	Characteristics
Teratologic hip	Fixed dislocation that occurred prenatally and often is associated with neuromuscular disorders
Unstable hip	Femoral head is reduced in the true acetabulum but can be fully (dislocated) or partially (subluxated) removed
Dislocated hip	Femoral head does not articulate with any portion of the true acetabulum and may or may not be reducible
Subluxated hip	Femoral head contacts only a portion of the true acetabulum
Acetabular dysplasia	Acetabulum is shallow and femoral head is subluxated or normal

Outline 1. DDH etiology

Physiologic Factors
  Ligamentous laxity
    Hormonal (Estrogen, Relaxin): Females
    Familial hyperlaxity
Mechanical Factors
  Prenatal
    Breech position
    Oligohydramnios
    Primigravida
    Congenital knee recurvatum/dislocation
    Congenital muscular torticollis
    Metatarsus adductus
  Postnatal
    Swaddling
    Strapping
Genetic Factors
  Gender: Female
  Twin studies

that screening programs must be dynamic, with periodic examinations until walking age, if they are to be effective. In this context, clinical screening programs have been shown to favorably alter the short-term natural history of DDH, particularly in reducing the number of walking age children with missed dislocations, and to be economically beneficial.

Currently, the adjunctive use of ultrasonography in routine neonatal screening does not appear to be cost-effective or practical, and its utility in those with risk factors for DDH is controversial. Proponents of routine ultrasound screening argue that it is more effective than clinical examination alone in detecting cases of DDH in the early months of life when treatment is most effective and in detecting clinically silent cases of DDH that otherwise would have become evident late. Opponents of routine ultrasound screening have argued that sonography is too sensitive and leads to increased diagnostic and unnecessary therapeutic efforts while only marginally reducing the incidence of late cases when compared to clinical screening alone. Recently, it has been shown that the presence and severity of ultrasonographically diagnosed DDH in newborns with normal clinical examinations does not correlate with the ultimate status of the hip.

Given the variable nature of DDH, it may never be possible to predict outcome, in all cases, based on tests of the status of the hip joint at birth. However, "delayed" ultrasonographic screening for selected infants older than 6 weeks of age considered to be at-risk for DDH by virtue of historic (positive family history) and clinical parameters (breech presentation, foot deformity, a persistent "click") has shown promise. This approach would seem to be a rational and potentially more cost-effective alternative to global ultrasound screening but needs further study. It has also been suggested that radiographic imaging of the hip at 4 months of age may be a valuable adjunct to neonatal screening for infants at increased risk for DDH. However, it, too, requires further study.

Physical Examination

The clinical findings of DDH vary with age and reflect the underlying pathoanatomy of the condition (Table 2). Consequently, in the neonate up to the approximately 2- to 3-month-old infant in whom there is considerable soft-tissue laxity, the hip is often unstable and the diagnosis of DDH is based on the classic Barlow and Ortolani tests of hip instability and dislocation, respectively. The Barlow test actually involves two maneuvers. The first part is performed by gently adducting the flexed hip while applying downward pressure on the knee in line with the long axis of the femur, provoking the hip to dislocate or subluxate. The second part of the Barlow test is a reduction maneuver that is identical to that of the Ortolani test. Both are performed by abducting the femur while gently lifting the hip toward the socket and, when positive, are attended by the sensation of the hip relocating. Thus, a

Table 2. Clinical features of developmental dysplasia of the hip

Clinical Finding	Neonate	Infant	Toddler
Instability (Barlow/Ortolani)	+ +	+	−
Limited abduction	+	+ +	+ +
Shortening (Galeazzi)	+	+ +	+ +
Trendelenburg	−	−	+ +

+ + usually present
+ sometimes present
− absent

positive Barlow test demonstrates a hip that is reduced but dislocatable and a positive Ortolani test, a hip that is dislocated, but reducible.

In the older infant (> 2 to 3 months), the clinical findings reflect the changes of a more established dislocation. The hip may no longer be reducible with the Ortolani maneuver. The pelvic-femoral muscles adaptively shorten in response to the higher resting position of the hip, and limitation of hip abduction becomes the predominant finding. The thigh is foreshortened and there may be asymmetry of skin folds. The hip may "piston" owing to its unstable articulation with the pelvis. In the walking-age child, these changes are often accentuated, but the most obvious findings are of abnormal stance (excessive lordosis, pelvic obliquity) and gait owing to a combination of leg length inequality, hip flexion contracture, and abductor muscle insufficiency.

Imaging

Pelvic radiography generally is considered unreliable in diagnosing hip subluxation or dislocation in newborns and infants prior to the appearance of the proximal femoral ossific nucleus. The cartilaginous femoral epiphysis and acetabulum make it necessary to extrapolate information from immature osseous landmarks in an effort to interpret plain radiographs. As a consequence, traditional radiographic parameters, such as Shenton's, Perkins' and Hilgenreiner's lines and acetabular index, are subject to considerable variation. Moreover, important soft-tissue structures, such as the labrum and capsule, cannot be evaluated.

Ultrasonography is playing an increasingly prominent role in the early imaging of DDH although it is not recommended for general screening purposes because it may be overly sensitive in newborns with normal clinical examinations and no historic risk factors for DDH. However, when risk factors are present or the clinical examination is abnormal, ultrasound imaging has proven to be reliable for the diagnosis and follow-up of DDH compared to plain radiographs, particularly before the secondary ossification center appears. It is most useful in children under 6 months of age but can be used effectively until about 1 year of age. Ultrasonography is not invasive and does not expose the child to ionizing radiation. It allows visualization of the cartilaginous femoral head and the unossified

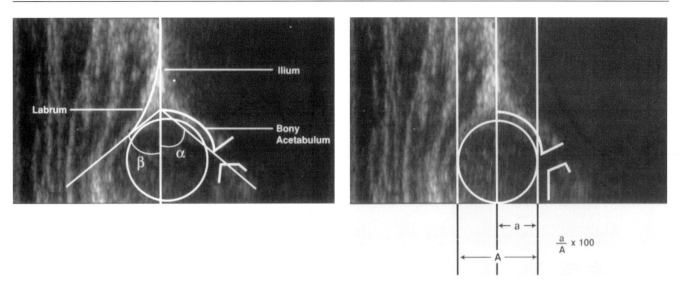

Fig. 1 **Left,** Ultrasound image of infant's hip, standard coronal projection with superimposition of baseline, inclination, and acetabular roof lines. Angle alpha (α) corresponds to the hard, bony roof of the acetabulum and angle beta (β), to the cartilaginous roof (normal infants: $\alpha > 60°$; $\beta < 50°$). **Right,** Method of determining femoral head size and percentage coverage. Percentage coverage = a/A x 100% (normal > 50%). (Reproduced with permission from Cheng JC, Chan YL, Huí PW, et al: Ultrasonographic hip morphometry in infants. *J Pediatr Orthop* 1994;14;24–28.)

portion of the acetabulum; early identification of the femoral ossific nucleus; and the ability to assess soft-tissue structures (labrum, capsule). As the femoral ossific nucleus matures, visualization of the acetabulum by sonography is progressively impaired. At this stage, plain radiographs are better to evaluate the hip.

Sonographic methods that emphasize both the morphology and the stability of the hip joint have evolved, although the techniques are currently more complementary than they are exclusive. Graf in 1981 was the first to report the use of ultrasound imaging of infant hips. His method emphasizes assessment of the morphology of the hip based on static measurements of the acetabulum in the coronal plane. In this technique, a reference line is drawn through the iliac bone and a second one from where the reference line crosses the osseous roof of the acetabulum to the bottom outer edge of that roof. The angle subtended by them, referred to as the alpha angle, represents the hard bony roof and reflects the depth of the acetabulum. A second angle, the beta angle, subtended by a line drawn through the labrum relative to the reference line represents the cartilaginous roof of the acetabulum and thus indirectly reflects the position of the femoral head (Fig. 1, *left*). Other morphologic parameters include femoral head size and coverage (Fig. 1, *right*). The dynamic method, proposed by Harcke, places greater emphasis on hip position and stability. With this technique, the joint is evaluated primarily in the transverse plane while being stressed with modified Barlow and Ortolani maneuvers. Instability of the hip

is measured by displacement of the femoral head from the acetabulum.

Contrast arthrography has been the gold standard for defining the pathoanatomy of DDH. Arthrography is invasive and requires general anesthesia, but it is capable of demonstrating soft-tissue impediments to reduction and the concentricity and stability of reduction with a fairly high degree of accuracy. Thus, this procedure can be used with closed or open reduction of the hip in order to assess quality of reduction. It can also provide useful information to guide surgical decision-making in more complicated cases of DDH when secondary reconstructive procedures are being contemplated.

Computed tomography (CT) can demonstrate positional relationships of the hip and acetabular morphology, and magnetic resonance imaging (MRI) allows direct visualization of the cartilage anlage of the femoral head and acetabulum. However, radiation exposure with CT is high; and both tests are expensive and require that the child be heavily sedated. Thus, neither modality plays a major role in the primary diagnosis of this disorder although both do have other uses. In the infant or toddler, low-dose CT (two or three axial projections) has been quite useful in assessing hip position in the spica cast following closed or open reduction (Fig. 2). In addition, CT and MRI data can be reformatted with software to produce three-dimensional (3-D) reconstructions of the hip joint that can help to characterize the complex pathoanatomy of residual hip dysplasia. By manipulating these 3-D images, the

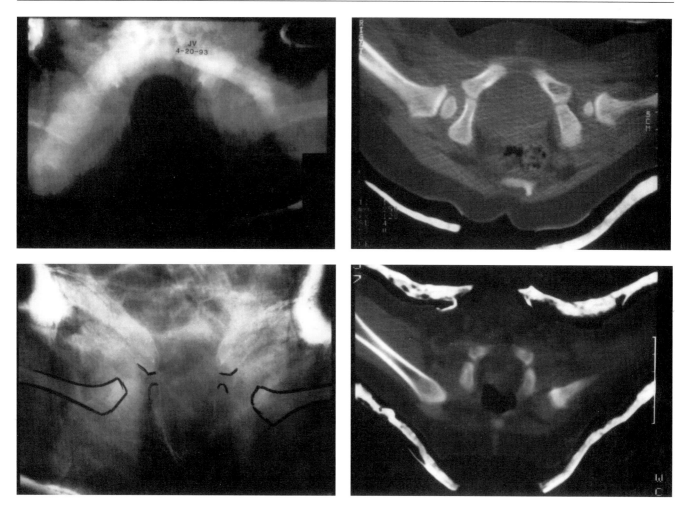

Fig. 2   Top left, Anteroposterior (AP) radiograph of the pelvis of a 15-month-old child following closed reduction of the left hip. Bone detail is obscured by the spica cast. **Top right,** Axial computed tomography (CT) scan of the same child confirming reduction. **Bottom left,** AP radiograph of the pelvis of an 8-month-old infant following reduction of bilateral dislocated hips, failing to show posterior displacement, which is readily evident on CT scan (**bottom right**).

effects of proposed reconstructive procedures can be simulated preoperatively. This simulation may be useful in the older child or adolescent.

Treatment

Although the methods of treatment for children with DDH have evolved, the principles remain unchanged. The goal is to obtain and maintain a concentric reduction of the hip so that normal development can resume and to do so in an atraumatic fashion without disrupting the blood supply. There is general agreement that treatment should begin at the time of diagnosis and that the best time to treat is in the newborn period. Under these circumstances, the goals of treatment can be accomplished by closed

methods in most instances. In the older child, particularly after walking age, surgical reduction may be necessary. However, individual circumstances may dictate the need for alternative methods at any age.

Closed Reduction

In infants up to 6 months of age, a gentle closed reduction can usually be achieved with the Pavlik harness. In this age group, the hip usually is either dislocatable, needing only to be stabilized, or dislocated, but capable of being reduced. Positioning the hip in flexion and abduction often achieves the desired stable reduction, and rigid immobilization in forced abduction is to be avoided. The Pavlik harness, which is a dynamic splint, allows a safe range of hip motion while maintaining the desired flexed-abducted

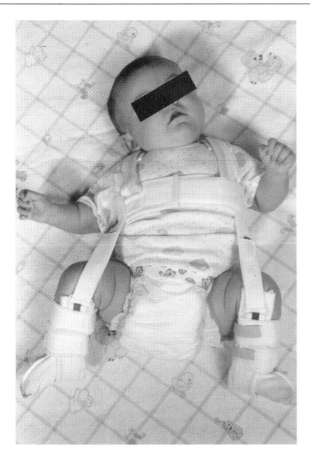

Fig. 3 Infant wearing the Pavlik harness. The hips are maintained in 100° of flexion by the anterior straps.

posture necessary to prevent redislocation. In addition to fulfilling the treatment prerequisites, it is easy to apply, adjustable, and relatively inexpensive. A number of other devices are available for positioning the hip; however, none are as universally applicable as the Pavlik harness and some risk rigid immobilization in extremes of abduction. The Pavlik harness can also be used in dislocated hips that are not reducible (Ortolani negative) provided the femoral head can be directed toward the acetabulum. In this situation, treatment should not continue beyond 3 weeks if the hip remains irreducible.

The harness is applied with the chest strap at or slightly below the nipple line. The anterior straps are located at the anterior axillary line and control hip flexion, which ideally should be from 100° to 110° (Fig. 3). The posterior straps, which attach at the tip of the scapula, restrict adduction of the hip by maintaining abduction of approximately 50°. Once the hip has been reduced, it is necessary to determine the range of flexion and abduction through which it is stable and to verify that this position does not result in excessive soft-tissue tension. Attention to these principles

of positioning is important because insufficient flexion or abduction can lead to loss of reduction. At the other extreme, excessive flexion can cause injury to the femoral nerve, and excessive abduction may lead to osteonecrosis.

Reduction of the hip should be confirmed radiographically or ultrasonographically by 3 weeks because continued use of the harness in the face of a nonconcentric reduction of the hip can potentiate dysplasia of the posterolateral portion of the acetabulum and complicate subsequent closed or open treatment. The harness should be worn continuously (particularly if the reduction is tenuous) until the hip stabilizes and should not be discontinued until the acetabulum normalizes. Weekly follow-up is recommended while the Pavlik is worn full time. Treatment with the Pavlik harness has been shown to be effective in achieving reduction more than 90% of the time. The incidence of osteonecrosis is low (less than 5%), particularly when treatment is initiated in the first 3 months of life. The most comon pitfall in treatment with the device is failure to obtain reduction, which is often compounded by a failure to recognize that fact. Risk factors for an adverse outcome with the harness are an inability to reduce the hip (negative Ortolani) prior to application of the device, bilaterality, and age (older than 7 weeks) when treatment is started.

Other methods are required for infants who fail dynamic abduction bracing and for infants over 6 months of age who are too large for the Pavlik harness treatment. In this group, there are significant adaptive, pathoanatomic obstacles to reduction that must be overcome to achieve a successful result. The typical impediments include constriction of the inferior capsule and contracture of the iliopsoas, which cause an "hourglass" narrowing of the isthmus to the acetabulum; infolding and hypertrophy of the labrum (neolimbus), which obstructs the superior boundary of the acetabulum; thickening and superior migration of the transverse acetabular ligament, which limits the inferior margin; and elongation of the ligamentum teres and proliferation of fibrofatty tissue (pulvinar) filling the depths of the acetabulum. Any or all of these findings may be present and usually become more pronounced as the child gets older.

Closed reduction is the preferred method of treatment in children up to 24 months of age provided stability and concentricity can be achieved without undue force. Perhaps the most controversial issue currently surrounding closed treatment is the need for preliminary traction. It has been widely held that traction, by stretching the contracted soft tissues around the hip, decreases the incidence of vascular injury to the femoral head and increases the likelihood of a successful reduction. Opponents argue that performing adductor tenotomy and immobilizing the hip in the "human" position effectively does the same thing as traction. Avoiding forced abduction protects the blood supply of the femoral head and flexing the hip and knee relaxes the muscles across the hip joint, thereby decreasing pressure on the femoral head.

Despite its widespread popularity among pediatric orthopaedic surgeons, no study has evaluated the effectiveness of traction as an isolated variable. Even among proponents, there is disagreement as to the most beneficial type of traction (skin versus skeletal), direction of pull (overhead versus longitudinal; divarication versus in-line), amount of weight, and duration of treatment. Moreover, several recent studies have shown no difference in the rates of osteonecrosis or of successful closed reduction in comparable groups of infants treated with and without traction.

Whether or not preliminary traction is used, closed reduction should be performed under general anesthesia with arthrographic guidance. This approach permits an objective visual and tactile assessment of the relocated hip that allows determination of the stability of reduction, not only in abduction–adduction (safe zone), but also in flexion–extension and internal–external rotation (stable cone). If the adductors are tight, percutaneous tenotomy of the adductor longus should be performed to effectively widen the safe zone. The quality of the reduction can be determined by arthrography and objectively defined by the width of the dye column between the femoral head and acetabulum and by the shape of the limbus. Hips with less than 5 mm of contrast between the femoral head and acetabulum and those with nonobstructive limbus patterns can reasonably be expected to have an acceptable outcome following closed treatment. Following reduction, the infant is immobilized in a spica cast with the hips in the human position, and reduction is documented by radiographs, sonography, or CT. Cast immobilization is usually continued for approximately 3 to 4 months with interim cast changes followed by nighttime abduction bracing until the acetabulum normalizes.

Open Reduction

Open reduction is indicated, at any age, whenever a concentric reduction cannot be obtained closed or when stability cannot be achieved without excessive positioning (safe zone is narrower than stable zone). It should be considered a primary option in "older children" in whom the disadvantages of closed reduction, including the need for prolonged casting and the higher rates of subluxation and osteonecrosis, outweigh the benefits of a nonsurgical approach. The purpose of open reduction is to remove the obstacles that prevent seating of the femoral head in the acetabulum and to make the hip stable. A variety of surgical approaches (medial, anterior, anterolateral, and lateral) to the hip have been described; the anterior and medial routes are used most commonly. Recognition of the characteristics of the dislocation (patient age, anticipated obstacles to reduction) and knowledge of the capabilities and limitations of the various surgical approaches are the keys to appropriate surgical decision-making.

The medial adductor approach of Ludloff allows direct access to all of the primary obstacles to reduction of the hip except the labrum. There are actually two routes to the hip via the medial approach; each is defined by the interval of dissection relative to the adductor brevis muscle. In the anteromedial approach, the interval is anterior to the adductor brevis and then either anterior or posterior to the pectineus, whereas in the posteromedial approach, the plane of dissection is deep to the adductor brevis. Both of these approaches have been used most effectively in children younger than walking age in whom release of the medial obstacles to reduction (tight adductors and iliopsoas tendon; the constricted, inferior portion of the capsule; and/or the transverse acetabular ligament) is sufficient to allow a concentric reduction of the hip. Cast immobilization is used to stabilize the hip until the capsule tightens because capsulorraphy is not possible once the femoral head has been relocated. The medial approach is ideally suited for dislocations in which the hip can be reduced but is not stable and for those in which the femoral head can be brought to the level of the acetabulum but not seated. This approach is generally not suited for hip dislocations in older children in whom the femoral head has migrated proximally, those in whom the labrum is a significant obstacle to reduction, and those in whom secondary skeletal deformity may dictate the need for concurrent pelvic or femoral osteotomy. In these situations, the anterior approach has proven to be much more effective.

In general, the anterior approach is the most versatile and commonly used method for surgical reduction of the dislocated hip. It is appropriate at any age and may be used in virtually all situations. It is preferred in children older than 18 months and generally is required in any dislocation in which the hip cannot be brought to the level of the acetabulum. The anatomic interval in this approach is between the sartorius and tensor fasciae latae muscles, and the dissection is more extensive than in either of the medial approaches. The procedure is technically demanding but provides excellent exposure of the acetabulum and access to all of the impediments to reduction. Capsulorraphy can be performed, providing immediate stabilization of the hip. If necessary, pelvic osteotomy may be done through the same incision.

Femoral Shortening

The trend away from the use of preoperative traction exists in open as well as closed reduction of the hip. Shortening the femur is now generally recognized to be an effective way to relieve soft-tissue contractures and reduce tension across the hip joint. It has been shown to be superior to traction in facilitating reduction of the hip and in reducing the risk of osteonecrosis, redislocation, and subluxation. Femoral shortening now is used routinely in children older than 2 years of age, but is also an appropriate adjunct to open reduction of the hip any time there is undue tension on the joint. From a technical standpoint, a lateral approach (separate from the anterior exposure needed for reduction) is made to the proximal femur and a subtrochanteric osteotomy is performed. Then, with the hip reduced, the amount of overlap of the proximal and distal ends of the osteotomy can be used to gauge the amount of shortening needed. Derotation and/or varus correction may be performed if necessary, and the osteotomy is fixed internally, usually with a plate and screws.

Secondary Procedures

Development of a normal joint following reduction of the hip is predicated on the ability of the acetabulum and proximal femur to remodel. Hip dislocation is often accompanied by increased femoral anteversion and anterolateral acetabular deficiency. These secondary skeletal deformities are typically more severe in children older than 2 years and may prevent maintenance of reduction of the hip or preclude biologic remodeling of the joint after a successful reduction. Depending on the predominant pathoanatomy, secondary surgical procedures (femoral osteotomy, pelvic osteotomy, or both) may be required to facilitate reduction of the hip, to address persistent subluxation or dysplasia of the proximal femur, or to correct residual acetabular dysplasia.

In children older than 3 years, simultaneous open reduction, femoral shortening, and redirectional osteotomy of the innominate bone usually are required to achieve concentric reduction, avoid osteonecrosis, and address the secondary acetabular pathology, which is often substantial. In younger children (18 months to 3 years), there is no consensus regarding the most appropriate site or choice of secondary procedure. Whether these secondary procedures (pelvic osteotomy in particular) should be done concurrently with open reduction or staged separately is controversial. Some surgeons are concerned that the risk of osteonecrosis may be higher when open reduction and pelvic osteotomy are performed simultaneously, although this combination of procedures continues to be used widely.

A rational approach to the management of these secondary skeletal deformities demands both an understanding of the anticipated development of the hip joint in response to reduction of the femoral head and knowledge of the remodeling potential of the acetabulum and proximal femur as the child grows. Development of a normal joint following reduction of the hip or redirectional osteotomy of the proximal femur is predicated on the ability of the acetabulum to remodel. Acetabular correction is indirect. The potential for improvement depends on the amount of acetabular growth remaining. It generally is recognized that remodeling of the acetabulum is most dramatic within the first 6 to 12 months after reduction of the hip. Remodeling is most predictable in children younger than 4 years of age, it may occur up to the age of 8 years, although far less reliably; and it is virtually nonexistent thereafter.

When excessive femoral anteversion is present, rotational femoral osteotomy is indicated at the time of open reduction and it usually is performed in conjunction with femoral shortening. Derotating the femur allows the hip to be reduced without having to position the lower extremity in extreme internal rotation to achieve stability. This procedure is consistent with the principle of a tension-free

reduction. Overcorrection of anteversion is to be avoided because this error can lead to posterior instability and dislocation of the hip, particularly if innominate osteotomy is done at the same time. In children younger than 4 or 5 years of age who have residual acetabular dysplasia following reduction, proximal femoral osteotomy may be performed as a staged procedure with the reasonable expectation that redirecting forces on the acetabulum will stimulate remodeling. Finally, osteotomy (varus, derotation) of the proximal femur may be performed at any age to correct persistent subluxation of the hip, provided a plain radiograph or arthrogram shows the femoral head to reduce in an abducted, internally-rotated position.

Osteotomy of the pelvis represents a more direct approach to the problem of acetabular dysplasia. In addition to its role in augmenting the stable zone of the acetabulum at the time of open reduction (discussed above), the primary indication for pelvic osteotomy in a child younger than 8 years of age is to correct residual acetabular dysplasia that fails to remodel over a 1- to 2-year period. In a child older than 8 years, any degree of dysplasia should probably be treated when discovered, given the negligible remodeling potential of the acetabulum at this stage. In adolescents and adults with residual subluxation and painful acetabular dysplasia, the rationale for treatment is to improve the biomechanical function of the hip in hopes of preventing, halting, or reversing deterioration of the hip joint.

Pelvic osteotomies are of two basic types: reconstructive procedures, which use hyaline cartilage to restore the articular surface, and salvage procedures, which use the joint capsule supported by bone or bone graft as the weight-bearing surface. In general, the goal should always be to cover the femoral head of the hip with articular cartilage. All of the reconstructive procedures are basically redirectional osteotomies of the innominate bone. They correct the existing deficiencies in the acetabulum by reorienting the articular surface and allowing weight to be borne on hyaline cartilage. In order for these to work, preoperative indications or prerequisites must be met. The hip must be concentrically reduced or it must be capable of being reduced, either by open reduction or femoral osteotomy, because an osteotomy performed over an unreduced hip will fail. The hip must have normal or near normal range of motion. The femoral head must be congruent with and adequately covered by the acetabulum in the simulated osteotomy position on plain radiograph or arthrogram. In adolescents and adults, a perfectly concentric reduction may not be possible because of the presence of more established, adaptive skeletal changes; however, there should be preservation of the joint space.

All of the reconstructive pelvic osteotomies effect improvement in the anterolateral deficiency of the acetabulum. They differ in design and execution and, therefore, in their capabilities and indications. A discussion of the nuances of the individual procedures is beyond the scope of this review. Briefly, though, the innominate osteotomy of Salter can be expected to provide about 25° to 30° of lateral coverage and roughly 10° to 15° of anterior coverage. In older patients, who may have limited mobility of the symphysis pubis or need additional coverage, the Steele triple innominate osteotomy or one of the technically demanding periacetabular osteotomies (Wagner, Eppright, or Ganz) may be more effective. The Pemberton and Dega procedures are pericapsular osteotomies that actually decrease the volume of the acetabulum and, thus, are appropriate for the severely misshapen, dysplastic acetabulum. When the hip cannot be reduced and does not meet the criteria for a reconstructive osteotomy, the shelf operation or Chiari osteotomy may be helpful. These are both salvage procedures that work by increasing the surface area in the hip joint over which forces are distributed.

Complications

Osteonecrosis

Osteonecrosis is the most common complication of treatment of DDH and is seen with every form of treatment for it, including the Pavlik harness. The causes of osteonecrosis are excessive pressure on the the femoral head or compression of the extrinsic blood supply of the femoral epiphysis. Treatment factors that have been associated with the occurrence of osteonecrosis include immobilization in excessive abduction, failure of prior closed treatment, and reoperation for failed reduction. There is no difference in the rate of osteonecrosis following open versus closed treatment.

Salter has provided the criteria for diagnosis of this condition. They include failure of appearance or growth of the ossific nucleus for a period of more than 1 year following reduction, broadening of the femoral neck over a similar period, increased radiographic density of the epiphysis followed by fragmentation, and residual deformity of the femoral head and neck after ossification is complete. Osteonecrosis has been classified by several authors as to the patterns of vascular injury. Although the classification systems are slightly different, they are conceptually similar in attempting to separate mild osteonecrosis, which affects only the epiphysis and rarely causes clinical problems, from more severe patterns of involvement, which affect the physis and often lead to severe deformity of the head and neck. Treatment is dictated by the pattern of involvement. Acetabular redirection should be considered in young children at the first sign of subluxation. Trochanteric epiphysiodesis (children younger than 8 years of age) or distal lateral transfer of the greater trochanter (children 8 years of age and older) may be necessary in the case of severe coxa breva (elevation of the greater trochanter) and abductor insufficiency. Contralateral distal femoral epiphysiodesis is occasionally needed to address limb length inequality.

Failed Reduction

Redislocation following closed reduction is not uncommon and usually can be managed by repeat closed methods or open reduction. However, redislocation following open reduction is a major problem. Factors predisposing to failure of the initial open reduction include failure to identify the true acetabulum, an inadequate inferior capsular release, inadequate capsulorraphy, and simultaneous femoral or pelvic osteotomy. Attempts to reduce the hip by closed methods are usually unsuccessful and repeat open reduction is virtually always necessary. There is a high rate of osteonecrosis and results of surgery generally are poor.

Annotated Bibliography

Introduction

Coleman SS: Editorial: Developmental dislocation of the hip: Evolutionary changes in diagnosis and treatment. *J Pediatr Orthop* 1994;14:1–2.

This editorial reviews the changes in the diagnosis and treatment of DDH over the past three decades. The rationale for the change in nomenclature from "congenital" to "developmental" dislocation or dysplasia of the hip is discussed. Classic articles documenting the major changes and advancements in the management of this condition are cited.

Hinderaker T, Daltveit AK, Irgens LM, et al: The impact of intra-uterine factors on neonatal hip instability: An analysis of 1,059,479 children in Norway. *Acta Orthop Scand* 1994;65:239–242.

The authors accessed birth records of 1,059,479 Norwegian children over an 18-year period and were able to analyze the interaction between birth order, sex, intrauterine position, and gestational age in occurrence of neonatal hip instability (NHI). Their data support the hypothesis that intrauterine mechanical factors, in combination with hormonal factors, are the cause of NHI. Prevalence (~12%) was highest in first born females carried in breech position to an older gestational age.

Diagnosis

Boeree NR, Clarke NM: Ultrasound imaging and secondary screening for congenital dislocation of the hip. *J Bone Joint Surg* 1994;76B:525–533.

The authors report preliminary results of delayed screening (2 weeks of age) for DDH using ultrasonography. Of 26,952 births, 1,894 infants with an abnormality on clinical examination or presence of a risk factor for DDH (breech presentation, foot deformity, positive family history) were referred for secondary screening. With this approach there was a reduction in the treatment rate (4.4/1000 births), a reduction in the late presentation rate (0.22/1000 births), and a decrease in need for surgical treatment (0.37/1000 births) compared to clinical screening alone.

Castelein RM, Sauter AJ, de Vlieger M, et al: Natural history of ultrasound hip abnormalities in clinically normal newborns. *J Pediatr Orthop* 1992;12:423–427.

In this study, 144 neonatal hips with sonographic abnormalities were identified from a population of 691 clinically normal hips (20.8% prevalence). Of these, 101 had morphologic ultrasound dysplasia (Graf) and 43 ultrasonic instability (Harcke). None were treated. At 6 months, radiographs showed only six of the former group and none of the latter group had any evidence of dysplasia. The severity of sonographic dysplasia (alpha angle) at birth was not related to ultimate development of the hip. However, five of the six with dysplasia had risk factors for DDH. The authors conclude that ultrasound should not be used as a general screening procedure in clinically normal newborns but suggest that infants with risk factors be followed.

Garvey M, Donoghue VB, Gorman WA, et al: Radiographic screening at four months of infants at risk for congenital hip dislocation. *J Bone Joint Surg* 1992;74B: 704–707.

From a population of 13,662 live births in a 2-year period, the authors identified 357 4-month-old infants at risk for DDH based on family history, breech presentation, or persistent click. Of this group, 46 had abnormal radiographs. Twelve required treatment, which resulted in normal hips, and 34 normalized while being observed. Of the 311 with normal radiographs, none examined after 15 months had any abnormalities.

Harcke HT: Imaging in congenital dislocation and dysplasia of the hip. *Clin Orthop* 1992;281:22–28.

This is an excellent review of imaging techniques and their indications in the diagnosis and management of DDH.

Hernandez RJ, Cornell RG, Hensinger RN: Ultrasound diagnosis of neonatal congenital dislocation of the hip: A decision analysis assessment. *J Bone Joint Surg* 1994; 76B:539–543.

Decision analysis was used to show that ultrasound is not the preferred screening strategy for DDH in neonates; its value in evaluating the high risk infant is good from an individual but not from a societal perspective and it is not reliable for follow-up. Their analysis shows physical examination is the preferred strategy in the neonate, and repeated physical examination during infancy, supplemented by radiographs at 3 to 4 months of age, is the superior strategy for patients at increased risk.

Millis MB, Murphy SB: Use of computed tomographic reconstruction in planning osteotomies of the hip. *Clin Orthop* 1992;274:154–159.

The use of 3-D CT reconstruction in the analysis of acetabular dysplasia and planning and simulation of pelvic and femoral osteotomies is discussed.

Rosendahl K, Markestad T, Lie RT, et al: Ultrasound screening for developmental dysplasia of the hip in the neonate: The effect on treatment rate and prevalence of late cases. *Pediatrics* 1994;94:47–52.

In this study, 11,925 neonates were randomized to receive general, selective, or no ultrasound screening in addition to clinical examination. The prevalence of late subluxation–dislocation was lower for the general ultrasound group than for the other two; however, the difference was not statistically

significant, and general ultrasound screening resulted in a higher treatment rate and a higher follow-up rate.

Stanton RP, Capecci R: Computed tomography for early evaluation of developmental dysplasia of the hip. *J Pediatr Orthop* 1992;12:727–730.

The authors reviewed 130 CT scans of the pelvis following closed reductions of 52 hips in 42 patients with DDH. They found it to be useful in confirming reduction of the hip after application of a spica cast but not otherwise predictive for development of osteonecrosis or acetabular dysplasia.

Treatment

Camp J, Herring JA, Dworezynski C: Comparison of inpatient and outpatient traction in developmental dislocation of the hip. *J Pediatr Orthop* 1994;14:9–12.

This study compares the effectiveness of inpatient to outpatient Bryant's skin traction prior to closed or open reduction in 72 patients (83 hips) with DDH. There was no difference between the two groups in the rate of closed (66%) versus open reduction (34%). There was a cost savings with home traction, and the rate of severe osteonecrosis was low (2.5%) despite the fact no attention was given to radiographic hip station. This study raises questions of the relative importance of prereduction traction in the treatment of DDH compared to safer reduction and casting techniques.

Chen IH, Kuo KN, Lubicky JP: Prognosticating factors in acetabular development following reduction of developmental dysplasia of the hip. *J Pediatr Orthop* 1994;14:3–8.

The factors predicting acetabular development following reduction in 75 hips with DDH were studied. The authors describe a new radiographic measurement, the center-head discrepancy distance (CHDD), which, when less than 6° was found to be the best predictor of success in unilateral cases. The study also confirms that younger age at reduction and significant improvement in the acetabular index (more than 10°) in the first year after reduction correlate with a favorable outcome.

Faciszewski T, Coleman SS, Biddulph G: Triple innominate osteotomy for acetabular dysplasia. *J Pediatr Orthop* 1993;13:426–430.

The results of triple innominate osteotomy in 44 patients (56 hips) were reviewed at average follow-up of 7 years (range 2 to 12 years). Improvement in pain and function was considered good in 53 hips. All but two patients (94%) reported that they would recommend the procedure.

Faciszewski T, Kiefer GN, Coleman SS: Pemberton osteotomy for residual acetabular dysplasia in children who have congenital dislocation of the hip. *J Bone Joint Surg* 1993;75A:643–649.

Results were reviewed for 52 hips in 42 patients who had a Pemberton osteotomy between 1968 and 1984 for residual acetabular dysplasia. The average duration was 10 years. Pemberton osteotomies are safe, effective procedures for treatment of acetabular dysplasia for DDH.

Fish DN, Herzenberg JE, Hensinger RN: Current practice in use of prereduction traction for congenital dislocation of the hip. *J Pediatr Orthop* 1991;11:149–153.

The authors surveyed 335 members of the Pediatric Orthopaedic Society of North America to define the use of preliminary traction for DDH. Only 5% of respondents stated they did not use traction. Seventy-five percent believed traction both decreases the risk of osteonecrosis and enables an easier reduction; 15% believed the only benefit is a decrease in the incidence of osteonecrosis; and 5% believed easier reduction is the only advantage. Home traction was favored by 31% of respondents. Although traction is commonly used, there is no concensus as to the benefits of such treatment.

Fleissner PR Jr, Ciccarelli CJ, Eilert RE, et al: The success of closed reduction in the treatment of complex developmental dislocation of the hip. *J Pediatr Orthop* 1994;14:631–635.

The authors review results of closed treatment of complex DDH in 68 patients (79 hips) whose mean age was 7.5 months (range, 0 to 36 months). Using arthrography and examination under anesthesia, they identified two factors, the limbus type (obstructive, nonobstructive) and the cone of stability (stable, unstable), that can be used as guidelines to select cases amenable to closed reduction and those likely to require open reduction.

Gabuzda GM, Renshaw TS: Reduction of congenital dislocation of the hip. *J Bone Joint Surg* 1992;74A:624–631.

This thorough review covers current concepts of closed and open treatment of DDH including use of the Pavlik harness, the controversy regarding prereduction traction, surgical approaches to the hip, the role and timing of secondary procedures (femoral and pelvic osteotomies), and classification and treatment of osteonecrosis.

Gulman B, Tuncay IC, Dabak N, et al: Salter's innominate osteotomy in the treatment of congenital hip dislocation: A long-term review. *J Pediatr Orthop* 1994;14:662–666.

The results of concomittant open reduction and innominate osteotomy (Salter) in 39 patients (52 hips) between 18 months and 8 years of age are presented. Mean follow-up was 13 years. Radiographic evidence of osteonecrosis (Bucholz-Ogden types 2,3,4) was seen in 34.6% of cases. Clinical and radiographic results were better when the operation was performed before the age of 4 years.

Malvitz TA, Weinstein SL: Closed reduction for congenital dysplasia of the hip: Functional and radiographic results after an average of thirty years. *J Bone Joint Surg* 1994;76A:1777–1792.

This study is a retrospective review, with long-term follow-up (mean, 30 years), of the functional and radiographic results of closed treatment of 152 developmentally dislocated hips in 119 children whose mean age at the time of reduction was 21 months (range: 1 to 96 months). In general, patients functioned well despite fairly high rates of proximal femoral growth disturbance (61%) and evidence of degenerative joint disease (43%). Subluxation was associated with poorer function. The younger the patient at the time of reduction, the better the clinical and radiographic results and the lower the rates of subluxation, degenerative joint disease, and proximal femoral growth disturbance.

Mankey MG, Arntz GT, Staheli LT: Open reduction through a medial approach for congenital dislocation of the hip. A critical review of the Ludloff approach in sixty-six hips. *J Bone Joint Surg* 1993;75A:1334–1345.

The authors report their results with open reduction via the medial approach in 66 developmentally dislocated hips (63 children). Osteonecrosis occurred in seven hips (11%), with an increased prevalence in reductions performed after 24 months of

age. One hip redislocated and two subluxated. The authors conclude that it is a safe and effective method of treating DDH in children under 24 months old who have failed closed treatment.

Millis MB, Poss R, Murphy SB: Osteotomies of the hip in the prevention and treatment of osteoarthritis, in Eilert RE (ed): *Instructional Course Lectures XLI.* Park Ridge, IL, American Academy of Orthopaedic Surgeons, 1992, pp 145–154.

Osteoarthritis of the hip is often due to residual deformity from DDH. Reconstructive and salvage osteotomies in the prevention and treatment of this problem are discussed.

Quinn RH, Renshaw TS, DeLuca PA: Preliminary traction in the treatment of developmental dislocation of the hip. *J Pediatr Orthop* 1994;14:636–642.

Seventy-two patients (90 dislocated hips) were treated with 3 weeks of traction; closed reduction was successful in 52 hips (58%) and open reduction was required in 38 (42%). Five patients developed significant osteonecrosis (Bucholz-Ogden types 2,3,4). Preliminary traction did not affect the rate of successful closed reduction or the incidence of osteonecrosis in this series compared to others in which traction was not used.

Tredwell SJ: Neonatal screening for hip joint instability: Its clinical and economic relevance. *Clin Orthop* 1992; 281:63–68.

This paper is a summary of three separate studies, dating to 1967, on the efficacy of neonatal hip screening. The retrospective study concluded that clinical screening is effective in identifying acetabular dysplasia. The prospective study established the effectiveness of early treatment with flexion–abduction splints for cases detected by screening. Economic analysis demonstrated a cost benefit of $15,000 Canadian per 1,000 infants screened.

Complications

Jones GT, Schoenecker PL, Dias LS: Developmental hip dysplasia potentiated by inappropriate use of the Pavlik harness. *J Pediatr Orthop* 1992;12:722–726.

The authors identified 19 patients with 28 dislocated hips who were treated unsuccessfully in the Pavlik harness for at least 8 weeks. Subsequent attempts at closed reduction failed in 17 hips that ultimately required surgical intervention. These hips had a deficiency of the posterolateral wall of the acetabulum, presumably due to prolonged positioning of the dislocated hip in flexion and abduction, which was thought to be the reason for the difficulties encountered with both closed and open treatment in these cases. The authors conclude that it is mandatory to confirm reduction of the hip during treatment with the Pavlik harness to avoid this complication and that Pavlik treatment should be discontinued if reduction cannot be obtained within 4 weeks.

Kershaw CJ, Ware HE, Pattinson R, et al: Revision of failed open reduction of congenital dislocation of the hip. *J Bone Joint Surg* 1993;75B:744–749.

Thirty-three hips (32 patients) requiring repeat open reduction for DDH were studied. Inadequate capsulorraphy, inadequate release of the inferior capsule, and simultaneous femoral or pelvic osteotomy were associated with failure of the initial open reduction. Over half had osteonecrosis at this stage prior to revision. Attempts to reduce these hips by closed means or by femoral or pelvic osteotomy were usually not successful. The results following repeat open reduction were dismal.

21

Tibial Deformity and Blount's Disease

Congenital Tibial Bowing

Congenital Anterolateral Bow

Congenital anterolateral tibial bow is the first physical sign of congenital pseudarthrosis of the tibia. Congenital pseudarthrosis is relatively rare, occurring in 1 in 190,000 to 1 in 250,000 live births. Its association with neurofibromatosis varies from 50% to 90%. Other physical signs of neurofibromatosis may be absent at birth, leaving the diagnosis in question for some time. Conversely, only approximately 10% of patients with neurofibromatosis have congenital pseudarthrosis of the tibia. Although rarely seen, congenital pseudarthrosis has also been associated with polyostotic fibrous dysplasia.

At birth the leg has anterolateral bowing and variable shortening and the foot and ankle may be in a dorsiflexed position. Other features of neurofibromatosis, such as café-au-lait spots, cutaneous neurofibromata, localized gigantism, or hemihypertrophy may or may not be present. The tibia may demonstrate a fracture at birth.

Isolated congenital fibular pseudarthrosis is extremely rare and most commonly is associated with the tibial condition. When present, with or without the tibial component, it may result in relative fibular shortening and secondary development of ankle valgus.

Although a number of classification systems exist for congenital pseudarthrosis of the tibia, Boyd's system is commonly used. Six types of pseudarthroses are described. Type I pseudarthrosis has anterior bowing and a tibial defect, which are present at birth. Type II has an associated hourglass constriction and a spontaneous fracture that usually occurs by the age of 2 years. This tibia classically has a sclerotic, obliterated medullary canal. It is the most common type, is associated with neurofibromatosis, and has a poor natural history with regard to fracture healing. Recurrent fracture is common if union is achieved. Type III has a cystic appearance (Fig. 1). The bowing may not be present before the tibia is fractured. Recurrent fracture is less common than in type II and successful healing occurs more frequently after a single operation. Type IV occurs through a sclerotic tibia of normal diameter (Fig. 2). The medullary canal is absent and often the fracture initially appears transverse and incomplete, like a stress fracture. Type V has an associated fibular pseudarthrosis or it can present as an isolated fibular pseudarthrosis, which, by itself, has a better prognosis. Type VI has an associated schwannoma or neurofibroma. It may be a factitious type of congenital pseudarthrosis. Very few cases of intraosseous neurofibromata have been documented; if it exists, this type is exceedingly rare.

Congenital pseudarthrosis that is not associated with neurofibromatosis or fibrous dysplasia often develops after a seemingly innocuous fracture in what appears to be reasonably normal bone. It usually occurs after the age of 5 years. Other radiographic abnormalities associated with this condition are a calcaneus hindfoot and diminished height of the lateral distal tibial epiphysis with variable limb shortening.

Treatment of the anterolaterally bowed prepseudarthrotic tibia initially consists of bracing. An ankle-foot orthosis with an anterior shell is used in an effort to prevent fractures from occurring. The role of onlay bone graft in infancy, in an attempt to widen the diameter or to "strengthen" the prepseudarthrotic tibia, remains unclear despite recent favorable reports. Osteotomy to correct the tibial deformity is contraindicated because it will most often precipitate the natural history of nonunion.

After the fracture has occurred, cast immobilization is generally unsuccessful and the established pseudarthrosis

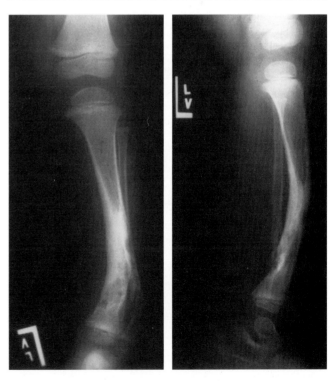

Fig. 1 Prepseudarthrotic tibia with medullary cystic changes, Boyd type III. Note the fibular pseudarthrosis.

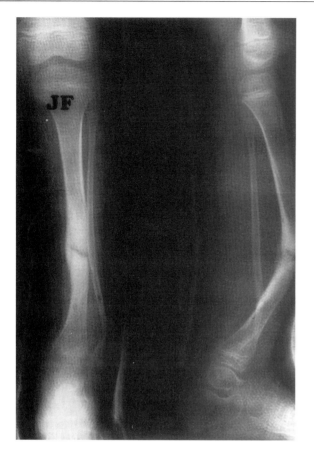

Fig. 2 Anteroposterior and lateral radiograph of a 4-year-old girl with neurofibromatosis and a congenital tibial pseudarthrosis in a cast following spontaneous fracture. Note the medullary sclerosis. Persistent nonunion led to treatment by bone transport using circular external fixation.

must be treated surgically. Conventional treatment, such as bone graft and plating, has a reported failure rate approaching 100% in patients with neurofibromatosis. Good results from intramedullary fixation were recently reported by Anderson using the Williams nail, bone grafting, and cast immobilization.

Newer treatment modalities, such as free fibular grafting and the Ilizarov technique, are able to achieve initial union in most cases. Although the refracture rate continues to be high, both of these procedures are promising. Weiland reported initial union in 18 of 19 patients by free fibular transfer. Unfortunately, this technique usually can be done only once by harvesting the contralateral normal fibula. As an alternative, another recent study reported success transferring the ipsilateral fibula with a vascular pedicle. Peroneal muscle weakness and a valgus ankle in the donor limb are possible complications with the free fibular transfer. Early reports of results using the Ilizarov technique

demonstrate union rates equal to that of free fibular grafting. The potential advantages of this technique include: full weightbearing during treatment, the ability to resect abnormal bone and periosteum and to transport "normal" bone into the defect, the equalization of limb lengths simultaneously, and the elimination of bony deformity.

Syme amputation, previously commonplace in those patients unable to achieve bony union, is not recommended as primary treatment except perhaps in extreme circumstances. Weightbearing without a prosthesis in those with persistent pseudarthrosis following Syme amputation is a problem. Below-knee amputation may be the ultimate solution in some of these patients once the risk of stump overgrowth has been eliminated.

After union has been achieved by any of the above techniques, continued total contact orthotic management is recommended until at least skeletal maturity. To date, no long-term studies that clarify the issue of bracing in adulthood are available in adults. Undoubtedly, continued use of the free fibular and/or Ilizarov technique will eventually provide sufficient mature patients to determine the most effective treatment programs for this condition.

Congenital Posteromedial Bow

Congenital posteromedial bow of the tibia is the more benign of the two congenital tibial deformities. The etiology of this condition is unknown and has been attributed to developmental circumstances, such as "uterine packing" and/or intrauterine fetal position.

The clinical findings in the newborn usually include a calcaneovalgus foot position with excessive ankle dorsiflexion. The dorsum of the foot often lies on the anterior surface of the leg with limited ability to plantarflex the foot. There is apparent or actual shortening of the leg and a posteromedial bow of the leg is present at the junction of the middle and distal third of the tibia. This condition is virtually always unilateral.

Radiographic findings include variable degrees of apex posterior bowing (ranging from 20° to 60°) and medial angulation of the tibia and fibula (Fig. 3). The bones are relatively normal with some thickening of the concave cortices, probably due to stress concentration.

The natural history of this condition demonstrates spontaneous correction of approximately 50% of the bony deformity within the first 2 years of life and slower improvement thereafter. Spontaneous correction of the foot position occurs within the first 9 to 12 months of life. In general, the severity of initial deformity is related to the amount of ultimate limb shortening. The discrepancy at maturity varies from 5% to 27% relative to the contralateral normal side.

The initial treatment for this condition consists of serial casting or stretching of the ankle deformity in infancy in order to eliminate the dorsiflexion contracture. Subsequently, careful clinical and radiographic follow-up is necessary to determine whether growth inhibition will require treatment to equalize leg lengths. Generally, the discrepancy, which rarely exceeds 4 to 5 cm, can be corrected by an epiphysiodesis of the normal tibia. If there is significant persistent deformity, however, limb lengthening with simultaneous correction of the tibial deformity could be considered. Early osteotomy with elimination of the bowed tibia appears to have no effect on the ultimate growth inhibition of the leg.

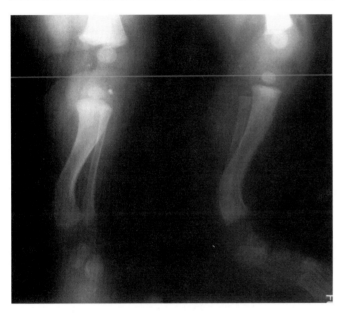

Fig. 3 Anteroposterior and lateral radiograph of an infant with congenital posteromedial tibial bow. Note the concave cortical thickening.

Blount's Disease

Blount's disease is considered to be a developmental condition, which affects the proximal medial tibial physis, resulting in a progressive varus deformity. The precise etiology is not known, although disordered endochondral ossification has been identified. There are two or three distinct forms of this condition, depending on age at presentation. Infantile Blount's affects those children younger than 3 years of age. The adolescent form affects those older than 8 years of age, and some authors describe a middle or juvenile group between these two.

The infantile form is often difficult to distinguish from physiologic bowing. This is particularly true before the age of 2 years, when bilateral involvement may be present. Nearly 60% of children with infantile Blount's disease are affected bilaterally. Mechanical factors, such as early walking age and increased weight, have been implicated in the etiology of this condition, although there is a lack of convincing evidence.

In general, the Langenskiöld classification of Blount's disease is relevant only to the infantile form and it may be difficult to apply accurately in the young child. This system has six stages, with progressively severe angulation of the medial proximal tibial physis (Fig. 4). Stage VI has a nearly vertical medial physis with evidence of growth arrest and, hence, the poorest prognosis. Because infantile Blount's has the potential to worsen progressively from an early stage, it should be treated early and aggressively in order to avoid permanent physeal damage and subsequent medial growth arrest.

Differentiation between very early infantile Blount's disease and physiologic bowing is often based on the radiographic metaphyseal-diaphyseal angle (Fig. 5). Radiographs must be obtained carefully to assure that long views of the limbs are obtained and that the patellae are pointing forward in order to avoid measuring rotated

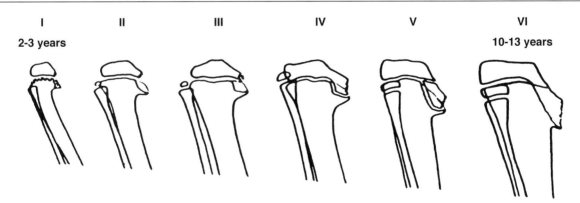

Fig. 4 Diagrammatic representation of Langenskiöld classification for infantile Blount's disease. (Reproduced with permission from Langenskiöld A: Tibia vara: A survey of 23 cases. *Acta Orthop Scand* 1952;103:1.)

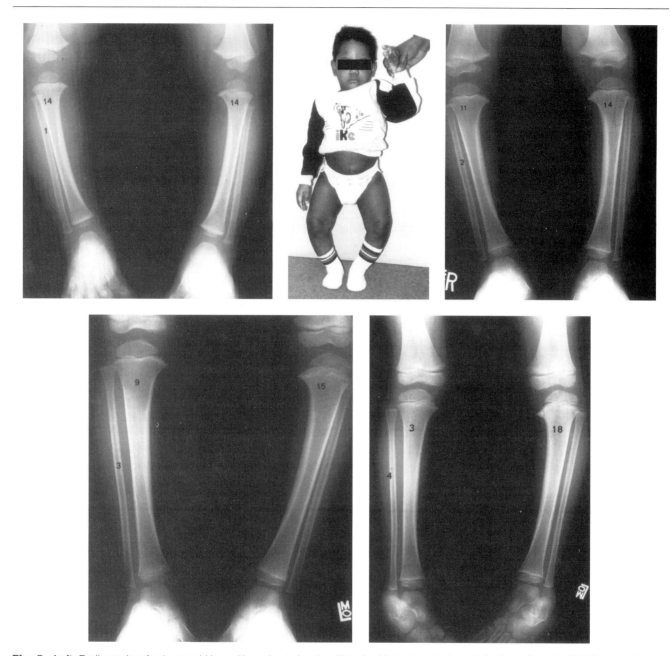

Fig. 5 **Left,** Radiographs of a 1-year-old boy with moderate bowing. Note the bilateral metaphyseal-diaphyseal angles (MDA) measuring 14°. **Top center** and **top right,** Photograph and standing radiographs of this patient at age 2 years. Note the subtle resolving deformity on the right but persistence of the 14° MDA on the left. **Bottom left** and **bottom right,** At ages 3 and 4 years it becomes clear that the physiologic bowing on the right has resolved, whereas the left leg is clearly affected by Blount's disease. (Reproduced with permission from Kasser JR (ed): *Orthopaedic Knowledge Update 5.* Rosemont, IL, American Academy of Orthopaedic Surgeons, 1996, pp 437–451.)

films. Once the patient is old enough (3 to 4 years of age), standing 3-foot radiographs should be taken. Recent reports have demonstrated inter- and intra-observer error inherent in measuring the metaphyseal-diaphyseal angle and have suggested that the previously recognized 11° threshold may be more reliably prognostic around 16°. However,

children with a metaphyseal-diaphyseal angle greater than 11° warrant close observation.

The diagnosis in the adolescent is usually easier and is accompanied by more obvious radiographic findings than in the young child. The varus deformity in the affected extremity varies markedly from normal, making it apparent

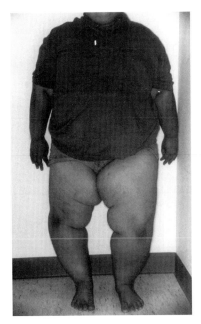 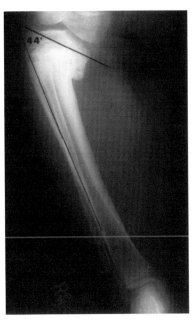 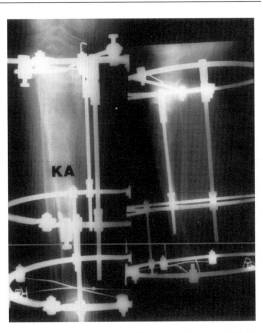

Fig. 6 **Left** and **center,** Clinical appearance and radiograph of an obese 11-year-old boy with unilateral Blount's disease and severe tibial deformity and a a 3-cm limb length inequality. **Right,** Circular external fixation achieved gradual correction of the deformity and restored equal limb lengths.

clinically. This form is more often unilateral than the infantile form and usually produces less severe deformity. Again, long radiographs of the affected extremity must be evaluated for the presence of potential concurrent femoral deformity, either varus or valgus.

The treatment of Blount's disease is determined by the age of the child and the severity of the condition. In the infantile form, certain authors have advocated bracing once the diagnosis is made and before there is significant deformity. The role of bracing remains unclear and may, in fact, be ineffective. If used, the brace must be a knee-ankle-foot orthosis (KAFO) and must be worn during weightbearing hours. If progressive deformity is identified, tibial osteotomy is indicated. The best results (least risk of recurrent deformity) have been demonstrated when surgery is performed before 4 years of age. Once the disease has progressed to a Langenskiöld stage V or VI, recurrent deformity and limb length inequality are predictable.

In those with Langenskiöld stage IV or greater, the medial tibial physis must be carefully evaluated for evidence of physeal bar formation. This can be done using computed tomography (CT), MRI, or conventional tomography. In those children with medial physeal closure, osteotomy must be combined with bar resection or, less commonly, with completion of the epiphysiodesis to try to eliminate the risk of recurrent deformity with continued skeletal growth.

For the treatment of adolescent Blount's disease, many osteotomy techniques are available. Current methods of rigid external fixation with acute or gradual correction allow for accurate alignment of the lower extremity. This may avoid overcorrection or undercorrection that can occur with osteotomy and internal fixation. The literature is replete with reports of poor results in the treatment of adolescent Blount's disease due to complications, such as nerve palsy, compartment syndrome, overcorrection, and undercorrection. External fixation, particularly with one of the gradual correction techniques now available, may prevent many of these potential complications (Fig. 6).

For those adolescent patients with significant growth remaining, one can consider selective lateral epiphysiodesis. Correction of mild deformities has been reported using this technique; however, its effectiveness is unpredictable. The assumption that the medial tibial physeal growth can accurately be predicted and can be expected to grow at a "normal" rate may be erroneous. This technique should only be considered in the adolescent with mild deformity.

If there is significant sloping of the proximal medial tibia, an epiphyseal-metaphyseal osteotomy or an intraarticular osteotomy, with elevation of the medial tibial plateau, can be performed. The need for either of these procedures can usually be ascertained by plain radiographs and/or arthrogram or MRI, demonstrating the contour of the medial tibial plateau.

Annotated Bibliography

Congenital Anterolateral Bow

Anderson DJ, Schoenecker PL, Sheridan JJ, et al: Use of an intramedullary rod for the treatment of congenital pseudarthrosis of the tibia. *J Bone Joint Surg* 1992;74A: 161–168.

Nine of 10 patients treated with a Williams rod and autogenous bone graft experienced fracture healing. The average time to union was 6 months. Five experienced refracture and required one or more additional surgical procedure(s). This method, used with an established pseudarthrosis, gives a straightforward approach to obtain union reliably in congenital tibial pseudarthroses.

Baker JK, Cain TE, Tullos HS: Intramedullary fixation for congenital pseudarthrosis of the tibia. *J Bone Joint Surg* 1992;74A:169–178.

Eighteen patients with congenital tibial pseudarthrosis were retrospectively reviewed. Ten had previous failed surgery. Union ultimately was achieved in 13 patients, ten of whom had intramedullary fixation with bone graft. Of these ten, seven had additional implantation of a bone stimulator with average time to union of 12 months. The remaining three required an average of 23 months to union. Despite intramedullary fixation, residual deformity was a problem in this group of patients with an average 12° sagittal plane and 5° coronal plane deformity.

Boyd HB: Pathology and natural history of congenital pseudarthrosis of the tibia. *Clin Orthop* 1982;166:5–13.

A complete description of Boyd's classification system is presented. Type II, characterized by an hourglass constriction of the tibia at birth, was the most commonly encountered fracture type.

Coleman SS, Coleman DA: Congenital pseudarthrosis of the tibia: Treatment by transfer of the ipsilateral fibula with vascular pedicle. *J Pediatr Orthop* 1994;14:156–160.

Five ipsilateral vascularized transfers combined with intra-medullary rodding and bone grafting were done for congenital tibial pseudarthrosis. All five united and hypertrophied with growth. The advantage of the procedure is that it avoids surgery in the contralateral normal extremity. The disadvantage is that many congenital pseudarthroses involve the fibula as well, making this procedure useful only in selected cases.

Paley D, Catagni M, Argnani F, et al: Treatment of congenital pseudoarthrosis of the tibia using the Ilizarov technique. *Clin Orthop* 1992;280:81–93.

This paper describes early results using the Ilizarov technique. The ability to obtain union appears equal or superior to that of free fibular transfer. The long-term prognosis is not clear.

Strong ML, Wong-Chung J: Prophylactic bypass grafting of the prepseudarthrotic tibia in neurofibromatosis. *J Pediatr Orthop* 1991;11:757–764.

Of nine tibiae with neurofibromatosis and congenital antero-lateral bow that underwent prophylactic bypass grafting at ages 0.9 to 9.2 years, six remained intact and three fractured and required further treatment. All allograft bone resorbed, whereas autograft healed. This procedure should be considered in an

attempt to "protect" the prepseudarthrosis tibia and/or to widen the diameter of the pathologic bone.

Tuncay IC, Johnston CE II, Birch JG: Spontaneous resolution of congenital anterolateral bowing of the tibia. *J Pediatr Orthop* 1994;14:599–602.

Forty-three patients with congenital anterolateral bow of the tibia were reviewed. At an average follow-up of 58 months, five had spontaneous resolution, with the exception of limb length discrepancy. These patients did not have neurofibromatosis. The most striking feature of these patients was the presence of subperiosteal callus on the concavity of the deformity. This finding is thought to be pathognomonic of the "benign" form of congenital anterolateral bow.

Weiland AJ, Weiss AP, Moore JR, et al: Vascularized fibular grafts in the treatment of congenital pseudarthrosis of the tibia. *J Bone Joint Surg* 1990;72A:654–662.

Union was obtained in 18 of 19 patients, with five patients requiring supplemented grafting procedures. Residual angulation was a common problem that may increase the likelihood of refracture.

Congenital Posteromedial Bow

Hoffman A, Wenger DR: Posteromedial bowing of the tibia. *J Bone Joint Surg* 1981;63A:384–388.

In the 13 children followed in this study, the mean limb length inequality was 3.1 cm. The degree of initial bowing correlated directly with the severity of ultimate leg length difference.

Pappas AM: Congenital posteromedial bowing of the tibia and fibula. *J Pediatr Orthop* 1984;4:525–531.

The author studied the growth and development of 33 patients with congenital posteromedial bow accompanied by an initial calcaneovalgus foot. The degree of initial bowing is correlated with ultimate limb length discrepancy.

Yadav SS, Thomas S: Congenital posteromedial bowing of the tibia. *Acta Orthop Scand* 1980;51:311–313.

The calcaneovalgus foot position can be corrected readily in most patients by serial casting. Conservative treatment was recommended.

Blount's Disease

Bell DF: Treatment of adolescent Blount's disease using the Ilizarov technique. *Oper Tech Orthop* 1993;3:149–155.

The author elucidates the step-by-step technique for correcting tibial deformity due to Blount's disease using circular external fixation. Proper application of the fixator and gradual angular correction can yield predictably good results with a relatively short treatment time. Those patients requiring lengthening will have proportionately longer treatment times.

Bradway JK, Klassen RA, Peterson HA: Blount disease: A review of the English literature. *J Pediatr Orthop* 1987;7:472–480.

This excellent article reviews the history, etiologic theories, classification systems, and treatment recommendations. The authors reiterate the need for early surgery in progressive infantile Blount's disease and the increased risk of progression with stages V and VI and in older children. This is a very thorough article with excellent bibliography although it is limited to conventional surgical techniques.

Feldman MD, Schoenecker PL: Use of the metaphyseal-diaphyseal angle in the evaluation of bowed legs. *J Bone Joint Surg* 1993;75A:1602–1609.

This study evaluates the accuracy of the metaphyseal-diaphyseal angle of the proximal tibia for the differentiation of physiologic bowing from infantile Blount's disease. If 11° is used as the point for differentiation, 33% false-positives and 9% false-negatives occur. More accuracy (5% error) is achieved when a 16° metaphyseal-diaphyseal threshold is used.

Greene WB: Infantile tibia vara. *J Bone Joint Surg* 1993;75A:130–143.

This article is a comprehensive review of infantile Blount's disease. Differentiations between tibia vara, physiologic bowing, and other causes of varus, such as hypophosphatemic rickets, are made. A clear approach to diagnosis and management options is presented. The specific surgical technique/option section is somewhat limited and does not discuss potential options of external fixation.

Henderson RC, Kemp GJ, Hayes PR: Prevalence of late-onset tibia vara. *J Pediatr Orthop* 1993;13:255–258.

A total of 1,117 adolescent boys were screened to determine the prevalence of late-onset tibia vara. Of the boys studied, 140 boys weighed more than 210 pounds and two of seven radiographed for genu varum demonstrated adolescent Blount's disease.

Henderson RC, Greene WB: Etiology of late-onset tibia vara: Is varus alignment a prerequisite? *J Pediatr Orthop* 1994;14:143–146.

The authors document two cases of neutrally aligned adolescent patients who subsequently developed late-onset tibia vara. This questions the theory that preexisting varus may lead to subsequent Blount's disease.

Johnston CE II: Infantile tibia vara. *Clin Orthop* 1990; 255:13–23.

Patients with advanced Langenskiöld (types IV and V) Blount's disease have a high incidence of recurrent deformity. Medial physeal resection with fat interposition may improve on the natural history of these children.

Kline SC, Bostrum M, Griffin PP: Femoral varus: An important component in late-onset Blount's disease. *J Pediatr Orthop* 1992;12:197–206.

The data in this article point to femoral varus as potentially contributing to the overall deformity in adolescents, but not infants, with Blount's disease. The femoral anatomic axis should be assessed carefully as well as the tibial in adolescent patients with tibia vara.

Kruse RW, Bowen JR, Heithoff S: Oblique tibial osteotomy in the correction of tibial deformity in children. *J Pediatr Orthop* 1989;9:476–482.

This article presents a technique previously introduced by Rab of oblique proximal osteotomy with the ability to effect multiplanar correction. Fourteen osteotomies for Blount's disease were performed with an average of 2 years follow-up and overall good results with few significant complications.

Levine AM, Drennan JC: Physiological bowing and tibia' vara: The metaphyseal-diaphyseal angle in the measurement of bowleg deformities. *J Bone Joint Surg* 1982;64A:1158–1163.

This article is the original description of the method of measuring the metaphyseal-diaphyseal angle. It was designed for use in infantile Blount's disease and was originated in an attempt to differentiate that disorder from physiologic bowing. It also points out that only 20% of the deformity in physiologic bowing is attributable to the proximal tibia as opposed to at least 60% in infantile Blount's disease.

Loder RT, Schaffer JJ, Bardenstein MB: Late-onset tibia vara. *J Pediatr Orthop* 1991;11:162–167.

Fifteen children (23 tibiae) with late-onset Blount's disease and moderate deformity (average tibiofemoral angle of 14°) were reviewed. Obesity was a common feature to all patients. Osteotomy was by conventional technique (dome or valgus wedge) with subsequent long leg cast application. There were 15 good results; two, fair; and six, poor. There are difficulties with conventional osteotomy and cast immobilization in this population of obese patients.

Martin SD, Moran MC, Martin TL, et al: Proximal tibial osteotomy with compression plate fixation for tibia vara. *J Pediatr Orthop* 1994;14:619–622.

The authors review 13 tibiae in nine patients with infantile and adolescent Blount's disease who underwent surgical correction of tibial deformity averaging 25° with A-O 3.5 DC plate fixation. Reoperations were required for recurrent deformity in one patient and for uncorrected internal rotation in a second. There were no other significant complications. Prebending of the plate with a template appears to allow accurate axial alignment of the extremity.

Price CT, Scott DS, Greenberg DA: Dynamic axial external fixation in the surgical treatment of tibia vara. *J Pediatr Orthop* 1995;15:236–243.

Thirty-one tibiae in 23 patients with Blount's disease underwent surgical correction using the Orthofix external fixator and proximal tibial osteotomy. Six patients required adjustment of the fixator position in the postsurgical period. There were two transient neurapraxia. Eighty-one percent of patients had a good result. The remainder had recurrence of deformity related to the severity of the Langenskiöld grade and/or residual varus.

Schoenecker PL, Meade WC, Pierron RL, et al: Blount's disease: A retrospective review and recommendations for treatment. *J Pediatr Orthop* 1985;5:181–186.

This is an excellent review article with attention to a grading system for results of treatment as well as treatment recommendations. Young children who were treated early had better results than those older than 5 years of age. A system for grading results is presented and should allow comparison of published results.

Schoenecker PL, Johnston R, Rich MM, et al: Elevation of the medial plateau of the tibia in the treatment of Blount disease. *J Bone Joint Surg* 1992;74A:351–358.

Seven children with severe depression of the medial tibial plateau were treated by elevation of the medial plateau. Other associated treatments included tibial osteotomy in all (three before, one after, and three at the same time as plateau elevation) and femoral osteotomy in four who had valgus deformity of the distal femur. Although the limb alignment was good in five of seven patients, four patients had limb length inequality requiring treatment and one required reosteotomy for residual varus.

Stricker SJ, Faustgen JP: Radiographic measurement of bowleg deformity: Variability due to method and limb rotation. *J Pediatr Orthop* 1994;14:147–151.

The authors point out the importance of neutral rotation in the measurement of angular deformity of the lower extremity. The intraobserver error was typically small; however, rotation affected the true angular measurements more significantly.

Thompson GH, Carter JR: Late-onset tibia vara (Blount's disease): Current concepts. *Clin Orthop* 1990;255:24–35.

The authors compare juvenile and adolescent forms of the disease. Except for the age of onset and patient weight, no significant pathophysiologic differences were found between the two groups. Recurrence of deformity after surgery is more common in younger patients.

Wenger DR, Mickelson M, Maynard JA: The evolution and histopathology of adolescent tibia vara. *J Pediatr Orthop* 1984;4:78–88.

The authors propose a mechanical basis for late-onset tibia vara, implicating obesity coupled with preexisting varus.

22

Limb Length Inequality

Limb length inequality in children is not an uncommon condition. There are numerous congenital and acquired causes. The need for treatment and the type of treatment are determined by the projected magnitude of the discrepancy at skeletal maturity. The long-held consensus remains that discrepancies of 2.0 cm or less do not require treatment or, at most, require only a small insole lift. Greater discrepancies, however, produce an increase in vertical pelvic motion with gait and thus a greater energy expenditure during walking. Furthermore, an uncompensated long leg stance results in a relative uncovering of the femoral head, a decrease in the center edge angle, and potentially the risk for long leg dysplasia of the hip. These risks, however, probably should be considered more potential than real. The amount of time spent in double leg stance during the normal gait cycle is extremely small. Furthermore, one would need to spend considerable time standing with shared weightbearing in order for these biomechanical considerations to come into effect. The literature suggests that there may be a significant relationship between uncompensated limb length inequality, compensatory scoliosis, and significant back pain, although the direct relationship to limb length equality remains somewhat anecdotal.

Etiology

Congenital Conditions

The most common congenital causes are the deficiencies, which include both proximal (femoral) and distal (tibial and/or fibular) abnormalities. The spectrum of femoral disorders include proximal femoral focal deficiency (PFFD; Fig. 1), the congenital short femur, and the hypoplastic femur. These three disorders have common elements that include variable hip dysplasia and proximal femoral deformity, shortening, external rotation (relative femoral retroversion), distal valgus, hypoplasia of the patella and lateral femoral condyle, and anteroposterior knee instability.

Congenital shortening of the femur is often accompanied by varying degrees of fibular hypoplasia or aplasia (Fig. 2). This shortening of the lower leg further compounds the overall limb length discrepancy. Various classification systems describe the severity of the fibular shortening, from those that are mild to those in which the fibula is absent (Fig. 3). With fibular hypoplasia, a mild anteromedial bow usually is present in the mid to distal third of the tibia. The foot is laterally displaced relative to the tibia and there is ankle and hindfoot valgus that may be mild, or, in cases with complete fibular absence, severe (Fig. 4). The foot may have absence of one or more of the hindfoot bones, tarsal coalition, and absent lateral rays. There is usually some degree of hindfoot equinus as well, with abnormal ankle motion.

Tibial hypoplasia or aplasia is much less common. Similar to fibular hemimelia, there may be a partial tibia with

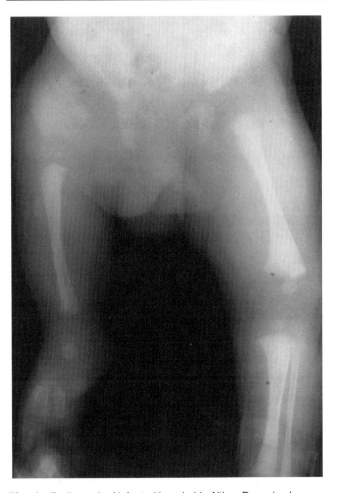

Fig. 1 Radiograph of infant with probable Aitken D proximal femoral focal deficiency. Note the subtotal absence of the femur with the ankle at the level of the contralateral knee.

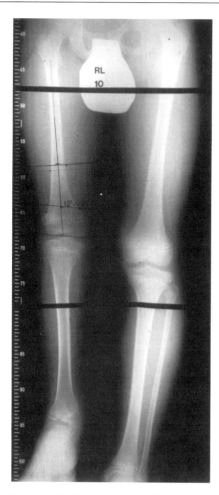

Fig. 2 Radiograph of a 10-year-old boy with right femoral hypoplasia and complete fibular hemimelia. Note the distal femoral valgus relative to the contralateral normal side.

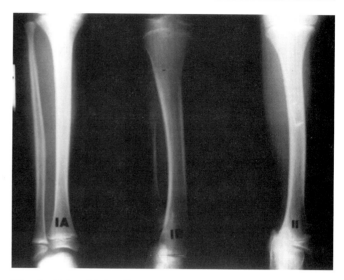

Fig. 3 Kalamchi classification of fibular hypoplasia. From left to right, type IA consists of mild shortening and a ball-and-socket ankle; type IB is a "miniature" fibula; type II has complete absence of the fibula. (Reproduced with permission from Kasser JR (ed): *Orthopaedic Knowledge Update 5.* Rosemont, IL, American Academy of Orthopaedic Surgeons, 1996, pp 437–451.)

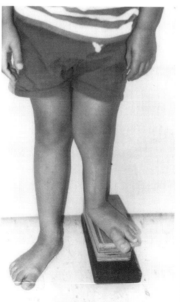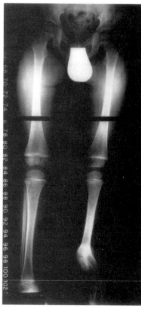

Fig. 4 Clinical **(left)** and radiographic **(right)** appearance of a patient with complete fibular hemimelia, a valgus four-ray foot, and mild femoral hypoplasia. (Reproduced with permission from Kasser JR (ed): *Orthopaedic Knowledge Update 5.* Rosemont, IL, American Academy of Orthopaedic Surgeons, 1996, pp 437–451.)

shortening or there may be complete absence of the tibia with loss of the quadriceps mechanism and "dislocation" of the knee (with the proximal fibula located adjacent to the distal lateral femoral condyle; Fig. 5). An apparent "clubfoot" is present; and the severity of the equinovarus deformity is related to the degree of tibial deficiency. This condition can be hereditary when accompanied by a lobster claw hand deformity (autosomal recessive).

Several conditions of hemihypertrophy or hemiatrophy exist, the most common of which is idiopathic, in which no apparent cause can be determined. In these cases, either the leg or the entire side of the body may be involved. In the infant or young child, it may be difficult to determine which is the abnormal side if the condition is mild. Because of the association between Wilms' tumor and hemihypertrophy, these infants should be screened yearly with abdominal ultrasound examinations until 5 or 6 years of age. Other conditions causing hemihypertrophy include

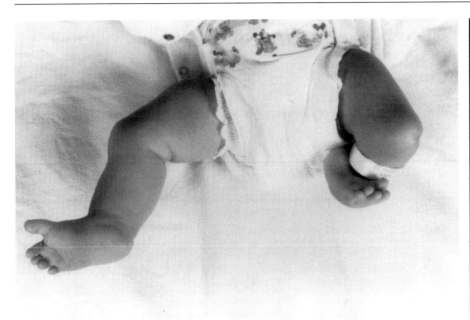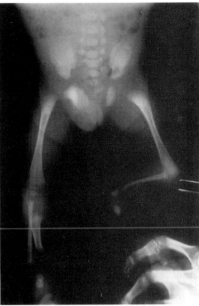

Fig. 5   Clinical **(left)** and radiographic **(right)** appearance of an infant with bilateral tibial hemimelia, complete on the left and incomplete on the right. (Reproduced with permission from Kasser JR (ed): *Orthopaedic Knowledge Update 5.* Rosemont, IL, American Academy of Orthopaedic Surgeons, 1996, pp 437–451.)

Klippel-Trénaunay-Weber syndrome, Proteus syndrome, and neurofibromatosis.

A variety of skeletal dysplasias are associated with limb length inequality. These include Ollier's disease, osteochondromatosis (multiple hereditary exostoses), fibrous dysplasia, and chondrodysplasia punctata (Conradi-Hünermann syndrome).

Acquired Conditions

Like congenital conditions, acquired causes of limb length inequality are extensive, and include inflammation, infection, trauma, or paralytic disorders. Inflammatory causes include juvenile rheumatoid arthritis and hemophilia, in which the joint inflammation stimulates growth. These inflammatory episodes will produce sporadic growth spurts that can be somewhat unpredictable and asymmetric, depending on the control of the primary inciting cause.

Infection remains a leading cause of physeal arrest, commonly as a sequel of neonatal sepsis or other systemic septic episodes in childhood. The most fulminant of these septic episodes can be seen with meningococcal septicemia, which often injures multiple physes and leads to severe bony deformities over time. Occult septic growth arrests are still common, particularly in premature infants who survive a long course in the neonatal intensive care unit.

The most common cause of trauma-related limb length inequality is the fracture involving a physis that leads to a growth arrest. Radiation and burns are other causes of traumatic growth arrest. Physeal closure may be complete or incomplete. Incomplete arrests are usually more problematic because of angular deformities that develop in addition to the limb length discrepancies.

Any asymmetric abnormality of the central or peripheral nervous systems in a growing child will have the potential to produce limb length inequality. Common causes include incompletely resolving birth palsies of the upper extremity and hemi- or monoplegia patterns that are congenital (cerebral palsy) or acquired (traumatic brain injury, tumor, polio, etc).

Assessment

The simplest method of clinically assessing lower limb length inequality is to place appropriate-sized blocks under the short leg until the pelvis is level. This block method is more accurate than using tape measurements from the anterosuperior iliac spine (ASIS) to the medial malleolus because measurements made using tape measures can be altered simply by abduction or adduction of the hip. One must examine the entire patient carefully to avoid errors from associated fixed pelvic obliquity, scoliosis, or knee and hip contractures. Furthermore, the standing height of the foot should be evaluated because it may be shorter in congenital causes of limb length inequality, particularly if there is a tarsal coalition.

Sequential radiographic assessments over extended periods of time are important in order to predict the ultimate limb length discrepancy and choose the correct treatment plan. The two most commonly used techniques for measuring limb length inequality are the scanogram and the orthoroentgenogram. Both involve the use of a radiopaque ruler under the limb. The scanogram uses an X-ray tube in linear motion with a slit diaphragm. Any movement by the patient will be detected by motion on the film. It includes all osseous structures so that any angular deformity can be detected. The orthoroentgenogram is a multiple exposure radiograph designed to obtain a straight projection through each joint of the extremity. It does not, however, show the entire extremity.

Both the scanogram and the orthoroentgenogram should be done with the patellae pointing forward to avoid any rotational alteration of limb alignment. Computed tomography (CT) scanogram is the most accurate technique, involves little radiation exposure, and can be done in the lateral projection to eliminate any errors induced by joint contracture. It is the most expensive technique, however, and may require special examination scheduling, thus making it awkward to use in the standard office/hospital setting on a daily basis.

The two widely used methods for predicting limb length inequality are the Green-Anderson Growth Remaining Chart and the Moseley Straight Line Graph method. With the latter technique, all of the patient's longitudinal data are recorded on a single sheet of paper, regardless of whether or not intervening procedures have been performed. In general, it is helpful to begin accumulating data within the first 4 or 5 years of life. Yearly visits with measurement radiographs and bone age radiographs are sufficient in the young child. Several precautionary points must be remembered. Bone age films, based on the Greulich and Pyle atlas, may have an inherent error of 12 to 18 months. In addition, neither the Moseley nor the Green-Anderson method will take into account the foot height and this must be added to the projected leg length discrepancy in order to achieve an accurate prediction. Finally, all limb length measurements should be done by the same method and ultimately measured by the same individual to reduce the likelihood of error.

Treatment

Several treatment options, used alone or in combination, are available for limb length equalization. These include nonsurgical methods (lifts, orthotics, prosthetics) and surgical methods (epiphysiodesis, shortening, lengthening, and physeal bar resection).

For small actual or projected discrepancies (less than 2 cm), no treatment is necessary or, if the patient desires and is more comfortable, a 1-cm insole shoe lift can be used. For larger discrepancies, a lift must be added to the sole of the shoe and should be tapered toward the toe to allow a more normal toe-off gait. Large lifts, exceeding 8 to 10 cm, are unsightly and may be unstable, requiring additional orthotic support (ankle-foot orthosis) to avoid "falling" off the lift. Extension prostheses are still used by those with severe leg length discrepancies in whom lengthening or amputation of the foot have been rejected. The extension prosthesis forces the child's foot into equinus in order to fit into a custom device that has a prosthetic foot attached distally. These should be discouraged in anyone who is likely to undergo attempts at limb lengthening because, over time, the ankle becomes fixed in plantarflexion and bony adaptive changes occur within the joint. This makes it extremely difficult to regain a plantigrade foot position with a mobile ankle joint.

Theoretically, epiphysiodesis is the appropriate option for children in whom predicted limb length inequality is less than 5 cm, axial alignment of the limb is normal, and adequate longitudinal data have been obtained in order to minimize error. Contraindications to this procedure include insufficient or inconsistent data, inadequate time remaining to equalize or nearly equalize limb lengths, and, perhaps, significant short stature. If there is a significant angular deformity in the short limb, epiphysiodesis may not be the best option because a second procedure will be required to correct the angular deformity.

The selected site of the epiphysiodesis should not result in significant knee height difference. Currently, a percutaneous technique using small (1.5 cm) medial and lateral incisions is preferred. A tissue protector can be used. The physis is drilled and curetted and the wounds are irrigated to eliminate any bony or cartilaginous debris. A soft bulky dressing is used and weightbearing as tolerated is allowed. Sports may be resumed after there is radiographic evidence of physeal closure. The older technique of Phemister epiphysiodesis is still used, with care being taken to avoid large unsightly scars. Physeal stapling is currently out of favor because of the need to remove intra-articular staples as well as the potential complications involved with their use.

In general, acute shortening should be performed only in the femur because of the reports of neurovascular compromise, compartment syndrome, and severe edema that occurs with acute tibial shortening. The indications for femoral shortening are essentially the same as for epiphysiodesis in those patients who are skeletally mature or in whom the existing data are inaccurate or confusing. Femoral shortening should be performed only at or close to skeletal maturity in order to assure the equalization of limb lengths.

The two basic techniques of femoral shortening are open subtrochanteric shortening with blade plate fixation and closed intramedullary shortening, as presented by Winquist and Hansen. The former has the advantage of being metaphyseal in location and potentially having less effect on the quadriceps mechanism. The latter requires the use of a specialized intramedullary saw and requires fixation with an intramedullary nail with both proximal and distal interlocking to avoid rotational malunion. All acute shortenings are accompanied by temporary loss of thigh muscle strength, which must be regained in order to assure normal limb function.

The indications for limb lengthening include limb length inequality greater than 5 cm and, potentially, limb length inequality less than 5 cm in a patient with significant short stature or coexistent limb deformity. Current methods use gradual incremental distraction techniques that avoid the use of bone graft and plate fixation. In general, percutaneous periosteal-sparing osteotomy techniques are preferred, with the optimal lengthening site being metaphyseal in location. This procedure promotes more rapid bone formation and healing. Lengthening in the diaphysis may also be achieved by these techniques should an associated deformity be in this location.

The two most popular current lengthening techniques include either monolateral or circular external fixation. The cantilever type fixators require half-pin fixation of the bone. The Orthofix slide lengthener is the most commonly used monolateral fixator in North America (Fig. 6). At least three half pins should be placed proximally and two or three are placed distally to the lengthening site. This avoids the potential for pin bending. The advantages of monolateral fixation is ease of application, fewer pin sites, less bulk than circular fixation, and more limited muscle fixation. The disadvantages are that it is impossible to gradually correct deformities and rotational deformity must be corrected acutely. The ball joint type fixator should not be used for lengthening because it is unstable to the forces encountered during limb lengthening.

The most commonly applied circular external fixation technique in North America is the Ilizarov technique. This technique traditionally uses small tensioned transosseous wires affixed to rings in order to achieve bony stability (Fig. 7). The advantages of this system are the simultaneous ability to correct multiplanar deformities, the control of adjacent joints to avoid subluxation or dislocation, no patient/bone size limitations, and the ability to correct any deformities that develop during lengthening without the need for anesthesia. The disadvantages of this system are its bulk, a steeper learning curve, more soft-tissue transfixion, and more pin sites.

A discussion of limb length equalization is not complete without mentioning physeal bar resection. The indications for resection are partial physeal arrest (less than 50% of the area of the physis) with significant longitudinal limb growth potential remaining. The physis must be assessed by polytomography or CT in both the anteroposterior and lateral planes (using 2-mm cuts). Magnetic resonance imaging (MRI) may be used, but is currently too sensitive and often shows a larger zone of abnormal physis than is actually involved in the bar.

Peripheral physeal bars can be addressed directly but tend to have a higher recurrence rate, probably due to periosteal damage. Central bar resection is more difficult and is accessed via a metaphyseal window. A dental mirror can be used for circumferential vision of the central bar. Fat interposition is used to avoid bar reformation and a marker is useful to monitor subsequent growth. In general, physeal bar resection is not useful in patients with less than 2 to 3 years of growth remaining. In addition, it may fail to achieve subsequent normal longitudinal growth.

Controversies in Limb Lengthening

Congenital Conditions

High grades of PFFD, such as Aitken C or D, are still difficult if not impossible to manage with current limb lengthening technology. One must be able to render the femoropelvic relationship stable in order to achieve significant lengthening. Certainly, Aitken A and B are salvageable but may require pelvic and/or femoral osteotomy prior to lengthening. Extension of circular fixation to the pelvis may be useful to protect the hip joint during lengthening. Staged lengthenings are required in order to minimize the complications associated with lengthenings.

With fibular hemimelia and femoral hypoplasia, large projected discrepancies are manageable if the foot is useful and has the potential to be made plantigrade. Discrepancies of over 18 to 20 cm are correctable through the use of two or three lengthening procedures with or without a contralateral epiphysiodesis. The lengthenings should be staged at least 3 to 5 years apart, leaving enough time for a contralateral epiphysiodesis to make up any remaining difference.

Most patients with tibial hemimelia, particularly with absent knee extension, are still best served by early through-knee amputation. If the proximal tibia is present and there is good active knee extension, differential lengthening of the tibia may be considered in an effort to match the fibular length. A formal ankle arthrodesis can stabilize the distal foot-leg relationship.

Lengthening for Stature

Limb lengthening for short stature remains controversial in North America. Contrary to popular belief, however, the issue is not simply one of cosmetic appearance. Activities of daily living, such as use of public transportation, toilet facilities, and drinking fountains, are compromised for individuals with significant short stature. Probably the best candidates for lengthening are those with normal joints and disproportionate short limb dwarfism (achondroplasia, hypochondroplasia, or mesomelic dysplasia). Patients with familial short stature may also benefit from limb lengthening, provided excessive lengthening (resulting in significant disproportion) is avoided. In these patients bilateral tibial lengthening may provide adequate increase in height and avoid the necessity for femoral lengthening.

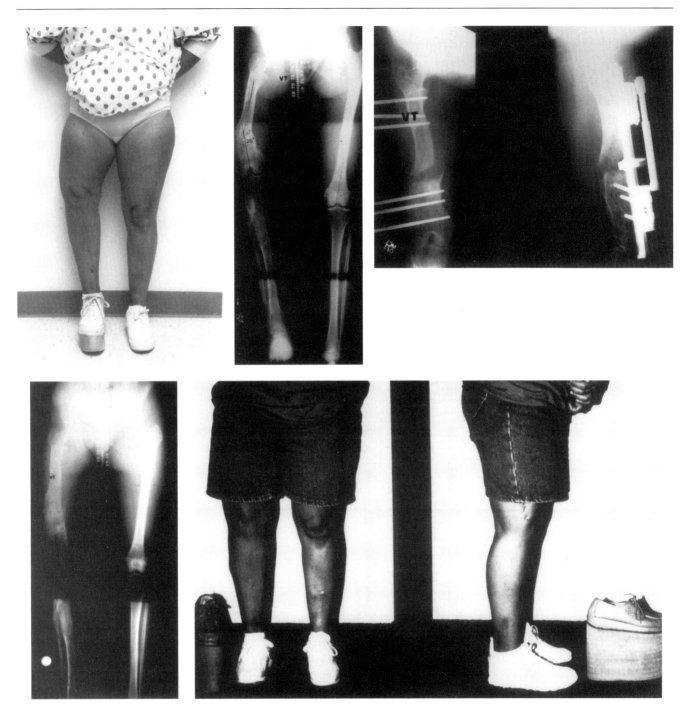

Fig. 6 Preoperative clinical **(top left)** and radiographic appearance **(top center)** of a patient with Ollier's disease and a 13-cm leg length discrepancy following tibial lengthening and prior to femoral lengthening. **Top right,** Radiograph of femur during distraction using an Orthofix slide lengthener. **Bottom left** and **bottom right,** Radiograph and clinical appearance at the end of treatment.

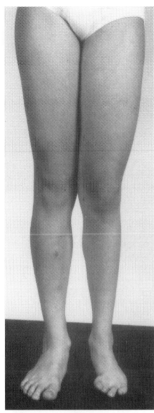
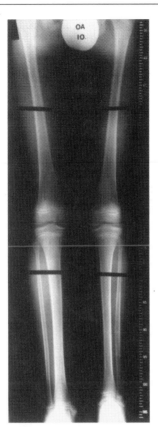
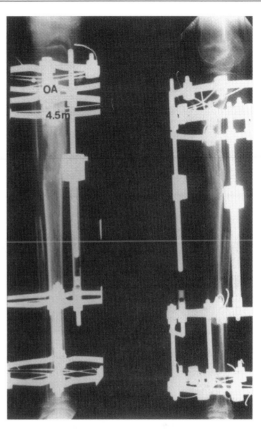
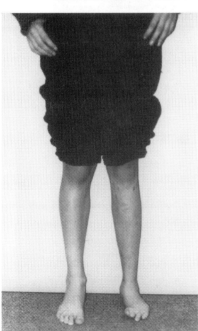
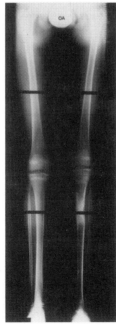

Fig. 7 **Top left** and **top center,** Preoperative photograph and radiograph of a boy with type IA fibular hemimelia and a projected 9-cm limb length discrepancy. **Top right,** Anteroposterior and lateral radiographs of the tibia during the consolidation phase. **Bottom left** and **bottom right,** Clinical appearance and radiograph at the conclusion of treatment. (Top center, top right, and bottom right. Reproduced with permission from Kasser JR (ed): *Orthopaedic Knowledge Update 5*. Rosemont, IL, American Academy of Orthopaedic Surgeons, 1996, pp 437–451.)

Particular care must be taken in those who have essentially normal limb function preoperatively and no limb length inequality. Lengthening for stature should be avoided in those patients with a natural history of early

degenerative joint disease and with grossly unstable joints, such as diastrophic dysplasia, pseudoachondroplasia, and, probably, the epiphyseal dysplasias.

Annotated Bibliography

Etiology

Achterman C, Kalamchi A: Congenital deficiency of the fibula. *J Bone Joint Surg* 1979;61B:133–137.

The authors present a good review of the spectrum of fibular hypoplasia through aplasia and the associated anomalies, with presentation of a simple, easily applicable classification system.

Pirani S, Beauchamp RD, Li D, et al: Soft tissue anatomy of proximal femoral focal deficiency. *J Pediatr Orthop* 1991;11:563–570.

A consistent pattern of soft-tissue anatomy in PFFD is elucidated using biplanar MRI. All muscles are present (although in abnormal orientation), accounting for the externally rotated, abducted position of the limbs; these muscles may serve a role in hip stability in PFFD.

Schoenecker PL, Capelli AM, Millar EA, et al: Congenital longitudinal deficiency of the tibia. *J Bone Joint Surg* 1989;71A:278–287.

This is an extensive review of all types of longitudinal tibial deficiency with recommendations for treatment based on type. The most common procedures were knee disarticulation and Syme amputation with limb lengthening being used in the least severe deficiencies.

Shapiro F: Developmental patterns in lower-extremity length discrepancies. *J Bone Joint Surg* 1982;64A:639–651.

The author describes five patterns of limb growth inhibition and points out potential limitations of limb length discrepancy prediction.

Assessment

Moseley CF: Assessment and prediction in leg-length discrepancy, in Barr JS Jr (ed): *Instructional Course Lectures XXXVIII.* Park Ridge, IL, American Academy of Orthopaedic Surgeons, 1989, pp 325–330.

The author describes in detail the three principal methods used to predict leg length discrepancy. A clear article on "how to do it."

Treatment

Choi IH, Kumar SJ, Bowen JR, et al: Amputation or limb-lengthening for partial or total absence of the fibula. *J Bone Joint Surg* 1990;72A:1391–1399.

Thirty-two patients with fibular hemimelia are reported and results of Wagner-type limb lengthening are compared with early amputation and prosthetic fitting. Potential limitations of the study are the inclusion of patients with significant proximal deficiencies and use of rapid distraction type of limb lengthening.

Gabriel KR, Crawford AH, Roy DR, et al: Percutaneous epiphyseodesis. *J Pediatr Orthop* 1994;14:358–362.

Fifty-six physeal obliterations by percutaneous technique showed no angular deformities or infections. This procedure produces reliable results with low morbidity and excellent cosmesis.

Hope PG, Crawfurd EJ, Catterall A: Bone growth following lengthening for congenital shortening of the lower limb. *J Pediatr Orthop* 1994;14:339–342.

Twelve patients were reviewed who had undergone femoral or tibial lengthening for congenital shortening of the leg. None of the patients exhibited significant stimulation or reduction in their growth velocity rate in lengthenings performed after the age of 9 years.

Loder RT, Herring JA: Fibular transfer for congenital absence of the tibia: A reassessment. *J Pediatr Orthop* 1987;7:8–13.

The results of the Brown procedure in six children are presented. Despite adequate knee extensor mechanisms in three children, long-term follow-up revealed significant instability and poor active range of motion. Knee disarticulation is recommended as the initial procedure of choice.

Miller LS, Bell DF: Management of congenital fibular deficiency by Ilizarov technique. *J Pediatr Orthop* 1992;12:651–657.

This paper reviews results obtained by current methods of gradual distraction limb lengthening for patients with fibular hemimelia. The results suggest that many patients who previously would have required amputation and prosthetic fitting may be suitable candidates for limb salvage surgery.

Paley D: Current techniques of limb lengthening. *J Pediatr Orthop* 1988;8:73–92.

The article provides an exhaustive review of current limb lengthening techniques and an extensive bibliography.

Sasso RC, Urquhart BA, Cain TE: Closed femoral shortening. *J Pediatr Orthop* 1993;13:51–56.

Eighteen femoral shortenings averaging 4.4 cm (range 3 cm to 5 cm) were reviewed. Complications included acute respiratory distress syndrome (ARDS) (one) and loss of fixation (three). The authors discussed technical details and reiterated that proximal and distal locking should be performed to avoid rotational malunion.

Snyder M, Harcke HT, Bowen JR, et al: Evaluation of physeal behavior in response to epiphyseodesis with the use of serial magnetic resonance imaging. *J Bone Joint Surg* 1994;76A:224–229.

Limb Length Inequality** 193

Sequential MRI evaluations of patients following percutaneous distal femoral and proximal tibial epiphysiodesis were performed at 1 week, 4 months, and 8 months, and 1 year following surgery. A mature bone bridge was evident by 8 months following surgery. This method is sensitive and potentially useful in assessing physeal cartilage injury.

Stanitski DF, Bullard M, Armstrong P, et al: Results of femoral lengthening using the Ilizarov technique. *J Pediatr Orthop* 1995;15:224–231.

This paper describes the results of 30 femoral Ilizarov lengthenings in 30 patients. The majority had a congenital etiology of shortening. The average lengthening was 8.3 cm. Although the complication rate was significant (premature consolidation in four, malunion in two, knee subluxation in two), this technique is a major improvement over rapid distraction methods of lengthening.

Steel HH, Lin PS, Betz RR, et al: Iliofemoral fusion for proximal femoral focal deficiency. *J Bone Joint Surg* 1987;69A:837–843.

This article describes the technique of iliofemoral fusion for patients with severe PFFD. The existing knee joint functions as a hip. Distal management of rotationplasty versus Syme amputation is discussed, with preference for the latter procedure.

Suzuki S, Kasahara Y, Seto Y, et al: Dislocation and subluxation during femoral lengthening. *J Pediatr Orthop* 1994;14:343–346.

Twenty-six femoral lengthenings by callous distraction for various disorders were reviewed. In the 12 patients with preoperative center edge (CE) angles of 20° or smaller, one dislocated the hip and four exhibited a decrease in CE angle. Of the 14 hips with CE angles of more than 20° preoperatively, none demonstrated subluxation, dislocation, or deterioration in the CE angle following femoral lengthening. In the uncovered hip, coverage of the femoral head should be obtained prior to femoral lengthening.

Timperlake RW, Bowen JR, Guille JT, et al: Prospective evaluation of fifty-three consecutive percutaneous epiphysiodeses of the distal femur and proximal tibia and fibula. *J Pediatr Orthop* 1991;11:350–357.

The authors describe the technique and results, which indicate excellent outcomes with minimal complications.

Winquist RA: Closed intramedullary osteotomies of the femur. *Clin Orthop* 1986;212:155–164.

The author reviews the results of femoral shortening in 154 patients with discrepancies of 2 cm to 12 cm. The technique and complications are discussed.

23

Knee Disorders

Basic Considerations

The knee attains its adult form by the completion of the embryonic period (8 weeks). Active motion has begun and the quadriceps-patella-femoral complex is well developed. The distal femoral epiphysis is present radiographically at birth in the full-term infant. The patella ossifies at 3 to 5 years.

A multitude of congenital abnormalities may occur and include such conditions as congenital patellar or knee dislocations, discoid menisci formation, variances of patellar morphology and anterior cruciate absence, either isolated (rare) or associated with femoral, tibial, or fibular anomalies. Various syndromes have knee (primarily patellar) components, eg, nail-patella, Down syndrome, multiple epiphyseal dysplasia, and arthrogryposis.

Congenital Knee Dislocation

Congenital knee dislocation presents as recurvatum and is evident at birth. It may be an isolated entity or may occur with associated problems, eg, dislocated hips, clubfoot, myelodysplasia, Larsen's syndrome, or arthrogryposis. A spectrum of involvement is seen from mild (type I) to severe (type III). Routine lateral radiographs identify the femoral/tibial relationship (Fig. 1). A knee ultrasound or magnetic resonance imaging (MRI) define the magnitude of joint incongruency and associated problems such as quadriceps fibrosis. Most type I (hyperextended knee) and type II (knee subluxation) cases respond rapidly to a serial casting program. A Pavlik harness may be used to provide further stability once 90° of flexion is reached. In patients unresponsive to nonsurgical treatment and in most type III (knee dislocation) cases, early open reduction and quadricepsplasty is required. Knee dislocation must be resolved prior to treatment of concurrent hip instability.

Congenital Patellar Dislocation

Congenital patellar dislocation is irreducible at birth. Hypoplasia of the patella, the lateral femoral condyle, and the quadriceps mechanism are seen along with lateral displacement and fixation of the patella. Flexion contracture, genu valgum, and external tibial rotation deformities are also present. Surgical correction is required in infancy and includes a complete lateral quadriceps mechanism and iliotibial band release, medial stabilization of the quadriceps mechanism (vastus medialis advancement and possible medial hamstring transfer), and patellar tendon centralization.

Discoid Meniscus

A discoid lateral meniscus is seen in 1% to 3% of patients, with a higher frequency in Asian populations. Medial discoid menisci are extremely rare. At no time is a discoid-shaped meniscus found in normal human knee development and, therefore, it does not result from arrested development. Classification is into three types: types I and II are stable, thick, and of varying amounts of disk configuration, ie, complete or incomplete. Type III is unstable and normally crescent-shaped, except for a thickened posterior horn. Its instability is due to congenital absence of the meniscotibial ligament (Fig. 2).

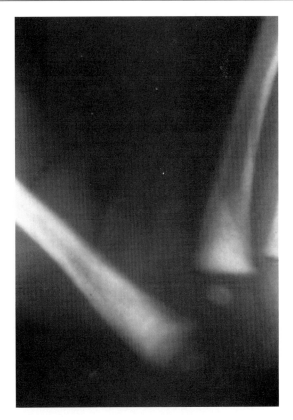

Fig. 1 Congenital knee dislocation type I: hyperextended knee that rapidly responded to a serial casting program.

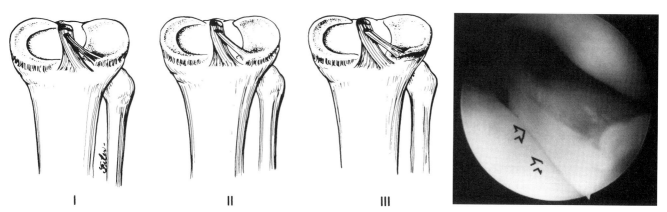

Fig. 2 **Left,** Watanabe classification of discoid menisci. Type I: stable, complete; type II: stable, incomplete; type III: unstable due to lack of meniscotibial ligament continuity. (Reproduced with permission from Stanitski CL, DeLee AB, Drez CD (eds): *Pediatric and Adolescent Sports Medicine.* Philadelphia, PA, WB Saunders, 1994, p 383.) **Right,** Arthroscopic view of a discoid lateral meniscus noted at time of anterior cruciate ligament reconstruction. The patient was asymptomatic regarding the meniscus.

Symptoms of snapping and popping usually occur between the ages of 6 and 12 years. Patients with type III discoid menisci may present with complaints of instability. Physical examination documents snapping in mid to full flexion in types I and II. With type III menisci, symptoms are reproduced in full flexion or in extension. Routine radiographs may show a widened lateral joint space and tibial eminence flattening. MRI will confirm the diagnosis. Treatment is indicated only when the patient is symptomatic; ie, secondary to instability or tears. Treatment depends on the type of meniscus. Sculpting of the meniscus to a normal configuration is attempted for types I and II. If an unstable tear is present, the meniscus is sculpted and meniscal repair is attempted. Type III menisci should be stabilized using a capsular suture. Most discoid meniscal surgery is performed by arthroscopic techniques. Complete meniscectomy should be avoided.

Multipartite Patella

Multipartite patellae are often asymptomatic radiographic curiosities and noted incidentally. The reported prevalence is between 1% and 6% of the general population. Bilaterality is common. Boys are more frequently involved than girls (8:1).

The etiology is not known. The Saupe classification is based on fragment location: type I, inferior patella (5%); type II, lateral border (20%); type III, superior lateral corner (75%) (Fig. 3).

Symptoms may occur at the patella-fragment junction due to acute trauma or repetitive microtrauma causing separation. In acute trauma, a fracture is ruled out by focal tenderness at the fracture and radiographic evidence of fragment margin irregularity. In a chronic symptomatic bipartite patella, the patient complains of localized pain at the junction and has tenderness at that site. The patella

is larger than normal. Radiographs reflect the type and junctional morphology. Type I may be confused with a patellar sleeve fracture or Sinding-Larsen-Johansson disease.

Acute injuries are treated by immobilization if the fragment is undisplaced. Patients with chronic complaints are treated by activity modification if overuse is a factor or by brief periods of immobilization. If symptoms persist, fragment excision produces excellent results.

Adolescent Anterior Knee Pain

During adolescence, the knee is a common site of complaints resulting from acute trauma and/or repetitive minor trauma. Knee pain in the skeletally immature patient must be considered referred hip pain until proven otherwise, and a thorough hip examination must be part of the evaluation of knee complaints.

The term chondromalacia patella has evolved from describing gross pathologic change of the articular surface of the patella (noted at autopsy or surgery) to an ill-defined, nonspecific, clinical entity. Theories on causes of anterior knee pain include retinacular neuronal changes and minor tracking abnormalities of the patella that cause increased lateral pressure. Few long-term studies of the natural history of adolescent anterior knee pain exist. There is little evidence that anterior knee pain is associated with premature aging of the patellofemoral joint.

The nonspecific term, chondromalacia, must be avoided and efforts should be focused on identifying more precise causes of pain. Identifiable sources of anterior knee pain include patellar instability, pathologic plica, osteochondritis dissecans, saphenous nerve entrapment, patellar tendinitis, Sinding-Larsen-Johansson disease, or reflex sympathetic dystrophy. Diagnosis usually can be made by history and physical examination.

Patients with nonspecific anterior knee symptoms com-

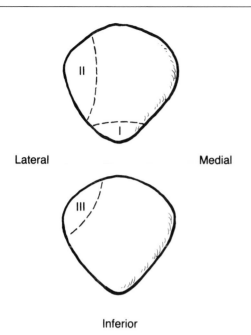

Fig. 3 Saupe classification of bipartite patella. (Reproduced with permission from Stanitski CL, DeLee AB, Drez CD (eds): *Pediatric and Adolescent Sports Medicine*. Philadelphia, PA, WB Saunders, 1994, p 312.)

plain of poorly localized pain, which may or may not be related to activity. When asked to point out the site of the pain, the patient often grasps the entire anterior knee (grab sign) instead of indicating a specific area. The pain may be aggravated by sitting and stair climbing and be associated with pseudolocking. In athletes, overuse factors associated with training must be considered. Because of the volatile psyche during the teenage years, one must be cautious of the teenage patient whose parent complains more about the child's condition than the child does.

Physical examination should include assessment of gait; lower extremity alignment; range of motion of hips, knees, ankles, and feet; knee stability; and patellar tracking. Patellar glide and tilt are frequently discussed, but there are no normative values for children and adolescents. Flexibility and strength of the quadriceps and hamstrings should be evaluated. Patella alta is often seen during the adolescent growth spurt when soft-tissue adjustment has not kept pace with the osseous growth rate. It is also seen in patients with neurologic compromise; eg, those with cerebral palsy or myelodysplasia who have a crouched gait. Tenderness over the patella, patellar tendon, and joint lines may be present. Anterior joint line tenderness is more common with patellar complaints than with meniscal pathology in which the discomfort is located at the mid to posterior joint line.

Routine four-view radiographic images (anteroposterior, lateral, tunnel, skyline) are usually normal. These static images of a dynamic process often are not helpful unless gross patellar instability or malformation are present. A multitude of radiographic measurements of the patella-femoral relationship exist, but these are often based on nondynamic, nonweightbearing positions. Nonossified areas of the tibial tubercle and patella make radiographic ratios unreliable in children. Computed tomography (CT) is helpful when assessing patellar instability by evaluating patellar tilt, translation, or combination of tilt plus translation. Radiographs may be taken, beginning with the quadriceps relaxed and then contracted from 25° of flexion and progressing to full extension. A bone scan may be helpful when reflex sympathetic dystrophy is suspected, but it is dependent on the stage of the disease. MRI is useful to assess patellar osteochondritis dissecans.

Once other sources of the anterior knee pain are ruled out, nearly 80% of patients with this idiopathic condition respond well to nonsurgical (and often nonspecific) treatment programs that emphasize normalization of quadriceps flexibility, hamstring flexibility, and quadriceps/hamstring strength ratios. Minor lower extremity malalignments may require shoe orthotic correction. A variety of patellar stabilizing braces have been advocated, but none have had any controlled, documented, objective data relative to their mechanism of action or outcome. Placebo effect and possible proprioceptive feedback by these devices or by taping techniques may account for their reported effectiveness. If the pain persists despite the patient's compliance with a well-monitored rehabilitation program, one must question the accuracy of the diagnosis and search for other causes of the pain, including nonorthopaedic and psychosocial causes.

Parental and patient reassurance is a major part of the treatment program to allay concerns of a perceived serious problem. Arthroscopy should be avoided for nonspecific knee pain. Patellofemoral joint surgery has the highest arthroscopic complication rates.

Overuse Disorders

The patellofemoral joint is a site of numerous junctional tissues, including the patellar-quadriceps retinaculum, patella-patellar tendon junction and the patellar tendon-tibial-tubercle junction.

Overuse symptoms occur when abnormal demands are made on normal tissue without adequate time for repair. Persistent submaximal trauma leads to a secondary inflammatory response at these junctional areas. Efforts should be made to identify causative factors such as anatomic malalignment, environmental problems (training surfaces, equipment), and overzealous training programs, or a combination of any of these factors. Causative factors are often identified by history and physical examination. A five-step treatment protocol includes factor identification, factor modification, control of pain (after diagnosis), progressive rehabilitation, and a maintenance program to prevent recurrence.

Osgood-Schlatter Disease

Osgood-Schlatter disease involving the tibial tubercle is seen in adolescent boys, and less frequently girls, who undergo rapid growth. It is becoming more common in girls because of the increased number of girls participating in athletics. Twenty percent of affected patients have bilateral symptoms but it is not unusual to see bilateral tibial tubercle enlargement with only one side being symptomatic. Nonathletic individuals rarely have symptoms. The lesion in Osgood-Schlatter disease is considered secondary to unresolved, submaximal avulsion fractures at the patellar ligament–tibial tubercle junction. The classic presentation of a preteen with swelling at the anterior knee and intermittent, activity-related symptoms makes the diagnosis rather straightforward. Patient and parent are often concerned of the presence of a tumor because of the increased size of the tibial tubercle. Physical examination shows varying degrees of tibial tubercle prominence and exquisite tenderness at the site. Radiographs are used to rule out other rare conditions such as tumors or infections. The symptoms gradually resolve as the child matures. Symptoms rarely persist into adulthood despite the persistence of the prominent tubercle. Ossicle formation occurs within the patellar ligament in nearly 40% of patients. Treatment is usually symptomatic and consists of ice massage, anti-inflammatory medication, quadriceps and hamstrings flexibility exercises, and the use of knee pads. The patient and family must understand the undulating pattern of symptoms and that discomfort may persist for 18 to 24 months. Activities involving squatting and kneeling should be avoided. Resting the knee in an immobilizer or cylinder cast for brief periods is not commonly needed but may be used when pain interferes with routine daily activity. Ossicle excision is required only if symptoms persist at that site. Skeletal maturity does not have to be reached before the ossicle is enucleated. Debulking of the tibial tubercle may be done at the time of ossicle excision in patients who are skeletally mature.

Sinding-Larsen-Johansson Disease

Sinding-Larsen-Johansson disease is the proximal counterpart of Osgood-Schlatter disease; ie, it occurs at the inferior patellar pole-superior patellar ligament junction and represents a sequelae of chronic tensile stresses at that site. The disease is most common in boys aged 9 to 11 years old and symptoms are related to activity. Tenderness is present at the inferior patellar pole. In the adolescent, signs and symptoms occur at the proximal patellar ligament, the so-called "jumper's knee." In Sinding-Larsen-Johansson disease, lateral radiographs show variable changes in distal patellar pole ossification. The differential diagnosis includes a Saupe type I (inferior fragment) bipartite patella and patellar sleeve fracture. Treatment consists of ice massage, anti-inflammatory medication, and

use of knee pads, as well as counseling regarding the 6 to 18 months required for spontaneous physiologic resolution.

Synovial Plica

Plicae are normal synovial folds. Pathologic changes within a plica may occur from direct or indirect trauma with subsequent hemorrhage, hyalinization, and fibrosis. The patients complain of snapping in mid-flexion and have localized tenderness over the plica, usually medially. Treatment begins with identification of causative factors and modification of them, if overuse is the etiology. In unresponsive cases, arthroscopic resection may be required. Indiscriminate resection of normal plicae should be avoided. The appropriate history and findings on physical examination should correlate with a thickened, fibrotic plica and concomitant articular erosion seen at arthroscopy.

Reflex Sympathetic Dystrophy

Reflex sympathetic dystrophy (RSD) is being seen with increasing frequency in children. RSD is often not considered in the differential diagnosis of knee pain in children, leading to long delays in making a correct diagnosis. Secondary negative effects of disuse (atrophy, loss of motion, and loss of strength) may be advanced. The hallmark of RSD diagnosis is pain that is out of proportion to the precipitating injury. Extreme complaints of pain accompany the slightest touch. Autonomic dysfunction, such as skin color and sweat changes (absent in the early period), may occur as the condition progresses. It is essential to rule out underlying psychosocial and familial problems (divorce, loss of a parent or sibling, family illness, school difficulties) that trigger this conversion type response. Routine radiographs are usually normal but effects of disuse, such as osteoporosis, become apparent as the disease progresses. Bone scan will reflect varying stages of the disease. Treatment consists of nonsteroidal anti-inflammatory medications, an active, functional rehabilitation program, and psychological services, where required. If these aspects of treatment are unsuccessful, sympathetic nerve blocks may be required. In general, the prognosis of RSD is better in children than in adults.

Complaints of anterior knee pain in the adolescent are extremely common as sequelae of acute trauma and overuse situations. The correct diagnosis must be established in order to prescribe appropriate specific treatment. Most chronic painful knee conditions are managed nonsurgically and are appropriately diagnosed by history and physical examination rather than by MRI or arthroscopy. Modification, but not elimination, of activity is usually possible with encouragement for continued participation.

Patellar Instability

The patella normally follows a toroidal path; ie, flexion/ extension, rotation, and translation in three axes through the femoral sulcus. This normal motion is a result of complex interaction of static and dynamic stabilizers producing a four-quadrant equilibrium in three planes. The term patellar instability covers a wide spectrum of patterns that range from mild tracking abnormalities to subluxation to total dislocation.

Unfortunately, the definition of instability has been clouded by the interchangeable use of the terms malalignment, maltracking, and instability. Malalignment, an abnormal static relationship between the patella and femur, may be the result of congenital, developmental, or traumatic causes. Maltracking refers to dynamic aberrations of normal patellar tracking and can range from mild to severe and may or may not be symptomatic. Maltracking may be related to malalignment. Subluxation and dislocation are the classic instabilities with loss of articular continuity during a phase of patellar excursion, usually at 0° to 25° of flexion. Instability may be produced by direct contact or, more commonly, by noncontact mechanisms (deceleration, rotation). In recurrent patellar instability, the frequency and magnitude of precipitating events and any previous treatment need to be assessed. Physical examination must include evaluation of lower extremity alignment, joint motion, patella alta, ligamentous laxity, muscle strength, and the quadriceps retinacular competence. The quadriceps complex, patella, and femur must be thought of as a unit. Patellofemoral sulcus incongruity, if present, may be the result of anatomic maldevelopment. Anything that limits motion (particularly flexion) may cause patellar instability; eg, quadriceps fibrosis from multiple injections. A multifactorial etiology is usually present.

When obtaining the history, it is important to evaluate the mechanism of injury, acuity, previous treatment, and status of the opposite knee. In addition to those factors mentioned earlier, physical examination also assesses lower extremity alignment, including Q angle; the presence of an effusion or hemarthrosis (particularly any that has fat present within it); tenderness; and attenuation or gap in the quadriceps retinaculum (at either the immediate peripatellar zone or the adductor-quadriceps junction). The integrity of the anterior cruciate ligament (ACL) should also be evaluated because similar derotation, deceleration mechanisms that cause patellar instability can cause ACL injury. Four-view knee radiographs should be obtained. Oblique radiographs are occasionally helpful to identify an occult osteochondral fracture. Patellar marginal avulsions are usually seen on the medial aspect in acute as well as long-term recurrent cases. In reported series, 20% to 40% of chondral and osteochondral injuries are not visualized with plain radiographs. In patients with chronic patellar instability, CT is helpful in assessing the relationship of the patellofemoral joint in terms of tilt or translation, or both.

Treatment is individualized and is based on the patient's lower extremity alignment, joint motion, ligamentous laxity, muscle strength, and quadriceps competence. The goal of treatment is to prevent recurrence. In the absence of intra-articular injury, nonsurgical management, consisting of limb immobilization for 7 to 10 days, a rehabilitation program to restore motion, and quadriceps and hamstring strengthening is indicated. A multitude (over 100) of surgical reconstructions have been proposed for treatment of patellar instability. These procedures include one of three basic techniques, or some combination of them: lateral retinacular release, medial vector augmentation, and patellar ligament alignment. Commonly, surgical treatment includes arthroscopic evaluation of articular surface injury with removal or replacement of osteochondral fragments, lateral retinacular release for patients with CT evidence of tilt, and direct medial retinacular repair in acute dislocations. Quadriceps transfers, particularly the vastus medialis obliquus are used to restore medial vector balance. Medial hamstring transfer (Galeazzi technique) may be required to provide a tenodesis effect in troublesome cases. Distal realignment using tibial tubercle medial transposition is done in the skeletally mature patient. Distal and posterior transfer fixation of the tubercle with creation of patella baja must be avoided. The Hauser procedure has been associated with significant recurrence, patellofemoral pain (because of patella baja), and compartment syndrome. Tibial tubercle rotational realignment, described by Elmslie and Trillat, has proven to be successful without drastically altering patellar realignment. A combination of tibial tubercle transfer, proximal lateral release, medial capsulorrhaphy and tendon transfer may be required to establish appropriate alignment. Patellar instability associated with abnormal ligamentous laxity; eg, Down syndrome and Ehlers-Danlos syndrome, presents a significant challenge. These patients must be advised of the abnormal nature of their collagen biology and should recognize that surgical reconstruction may not overcome this genetic predisposition for instability. In general, patients with Down syndrome function quite well, despite chronic patellar displacement due to a combination of increased laxity, genu valgum, and hypotonia.

Osteochondritis Dissecans

Osteochondritis dissecans (OCD) is a lesion of subchondral bone and articular cartilage that may result in instability of the subchondral bone, articular cartilage, or both. Its etiology is unknown. Following acute trauma, an acute osteochondral fracture must be considered if a radiographic lesion is seen. The condition is most common in adolescent males (in a male to female ratio of 4:1). The incidence of bilaterality is 20% to 30%. Previous reports have combined data from juvenile and adult types of OCD. This has led to some confusion in the expected outcome and treatment requirements in adolescents because

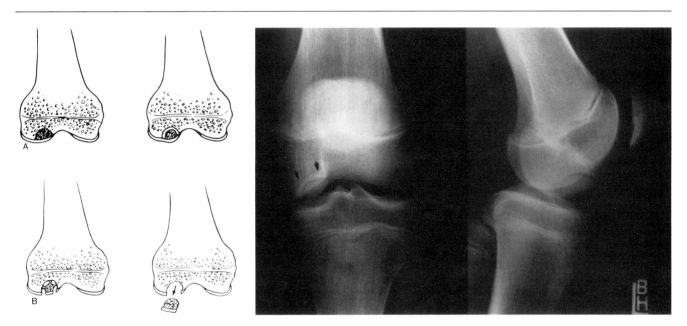

Fig. 4 Left, Osteochondritis dissecans classification based on articular cartilage continuity and subchondral stability. (Reproduced with permission from Stanitski CL, DeLee AB, Drez CD (eds): *Pediatric and Adolescent Sports Medicine.* Philadelphia, PA, WB Saunders, 1994, p 396.) **Right,** Symptomatic osteochondritis dissecans in a 15-year-old boy. Note classic location at lateral portion of medial femoral condyle.

of the markedly different nature of the natural history and prognosis for each type. Patient symptoms are related to the condition's acuity, may be present only with activity, and may be associated with recurrent effusions. Locking is rare. Physical examination is usually nonspecific; ie, effusion and generalized tenderness. Local tenderness may be present with direct pressure at the lesion if it is unstable.

Standard radiographs, particularly the tunnel view, demonstrate the lesion. The classic site of the condition (70% of all cases) is in the nonweightbearing, posterior lateral aspect of the medial femoral condyle. Twenty percent involve the lateral femoral condyle and 10%, the patella. MRI is used to assess the fragment's articular cartilage continuity and the size and viability of its subchondral bone. A dynamic, computerized bone scan can assess the circulation between the fragment and its bed. If increased flow is present, the prognosis for healing is good. None of the techniques assesses the subchondral-articular composite stability. Lesions are classified based on articular cartilage integrity (open or closed) and the stability of the underlying subchondral bone and its bed (stable or unstable). A loose body is an example of an open, unstable lesion (Fig. 4).

The natural history is directly dependent on age. In the juvenile type (patients with completely open distal femoral physis), the prognosis is excellent if the lesion is a closed, stable one. In the adolescent with partial physeal closure, the prognosis is unknown because the lesion may act as either the juvenile or adult type. The adult type (closed physis) has a poorer prognosis because of the limited heal-

ing potential of the lesion. Previous series reporting excellent results using prolonged treatment with casting and immobilization have confused the treatment issue because they included patients with normal ossific variances with spontaneous resolution. Treatment recommendations are based on the patient's age and status of the fragment. If lesions are closed and stable, the healing potential is high. Conversely, instability and/or loss of continuity of the articular surface compromise healing. Nonsurgical management is recommended for those with closed, stable lesions. Activity modification may be required and immobilization is occasionally necessary for episodes of discomfort or effusion. In skeletally mature patients whose subchondral junction is unstable, surgical management is suggested for closed lesions. Fragment fixation allows subchondral union to occur and prevent conversion to an open, unstable lesion. In lesions that are open and stable, curettage and grafting of the subchondral bed with fragment fixation is helpful. In an open, unstable lesion (loose body), restitution is recommended if the fragment is able to be replaced anatomically, has a satisfactory amount of subchondral base, and has a congruent articular surface following replantation. If minimal or no subchondral bone is present on the fragment, or if the fit is incongruous, then fragment excision is advised. Osteochondral grafting should be considered for irreparable lesions in the weight-bearing zone, often on the lateral femoral condyle. Associated meniscal and/or tibial articular surface damage must be assessed. Meniscal repair or partial meniscectomy may be required.

Patellar OCD is uncommon and presents as mechanical knee pain during adolescence. The lesion occurs in the distal half of the patella. Twenty percent to 30% of the lesions are bilateral. The differential diagnosis should include dorsal patellar defect, infection, or tumor. The prognosis for patellar OCD is even less clear than it is for femoral OCD. Subchondral bed sclerosis denotes a poor prognosis, similar to femoral lesions. Treatment principles are similar to those for femoral OCD.

Annotated Bibliography

Congenital Knee Dislocation

Parsch K, Schulz R: Ultrasonography in congenital dislocation of the knee. *J Pediatr Orthop* 1994;3:76–81.

Ten congenitally hyperextended knees in seven patients had ultrasound evaluations shortly postpartum and through the first year. Two knees had hyperextension (type I), five had subluxation (type II), and three had dislocation (type III). Ultrasound avoids use of ionizing radiation (radiographs, arthrograms) or need for sedation/anesthesia (MRI). Popliteal ultrasound approach is needed for type III knees. Ultrasonographic verification of progress allowed continued nonsurgical management with objective documentation.

Roy DR, Crawford AH: Percutaneous quadriceps recession: A technique for management of congenital hyperextension deformities of the knee in the neonate. *J Pediatr Orthop* 1989;9:717–719.

Six infants with knee hyperextension deformity due to myelodysplasia (three), arthrogryposis (one), and Larsen's syndrome (two) were surgically treated in the newborn period. Three had formal open quadricepsplasty and three had percutaneous quadriceps mechanism release. All gained and maintained knee flexion and restored normal extension. Aggressive management of these complex disorders allow early treatment to coexistent lower extremity problems (developmental dysplasia of the hip, clubfeet). If the percutaneous technique is inadequate, femoral open quadricepsplasty can be done. The role of the procedures in the management of isolated (nonsyndromic) types II or III congenital knee dislocations has yet to be defined.

Congenital Patellar Dislocation

Gao GX, Lee EH, Bose K: Surgical management of congenital and habitual dislocation of the patella. *J Pediatr Orthop* 1990;10:255–260.

Twelve patients with congenital patellar dislocation were evaluated at an average 5 years after surgery. Average age at diagnosis was 5 years. Ten patellae remained centralized and full knee flexion was gained in 88%. Early surgical intervention was recommended. Extensor lag took 3 to 6 months to recover. Patellar and quadriceps mechanism development appeared normal at follow-up in the majority of patients.

Discoid Meniscus

Fujikawa K, Iskei F, Mikura Y: Partial resection of the discoid meniscus in the child's knee. *J Bone Joint Surg* 1981;63B:391–395.

The authors reviewed 32 patients 3 to 15 years of age who had discoid menisci. Seven patients had arthroscopically sculpted Watanabe types I or II discoid menisci. Excellent results were reported at follow-up 1 to 2 years later. The authors recommend meniscal sculpting instead of excision if the symptomatic meniscus is not excessively thick, shows no degeneration, and is not hypermobile.

Multipartite Patella

Bourne MH, Bianco AJ Jr: Bipartite patella in the adolescent: Results of surgical excision. *J Pediatr Orthop* 1990;10:69–73.

Sixteen adolescent patients were evaluated at an average follow-up of 7 years following excision of a symptomatic bipartite patellar fragment. All had Saupe type III lesions. None were improved with nonsurgical treatment. Fifteen of 16 were completely asymptomatic at follow-up.

Adolescent Anterior Knee Pain

Fulkerson JP, Shea KP: Disorders of patellofemoral alignment. *J Bone Joint Surg* 1990;72A:1424–1429.

This review article emphasizes the correlation of patellar alignment between the clinical examination and imaging studies. Tangential patellar radiographs at 15° to 30° of flexion (routine and/or CT) are use to evaluate patellar tilt and translation, or a combination of both. If nonsurgical management fails, lateral release is helpful in patients with patellar tilt. Patients with translation (subluxation/dislocation) alone or translation plus tilt require individualized extensor mechanism reconstruction.

Guzzanti V, Gigante A, DiLazzaro A, et al: Patello-femoral malalignment in adolescents: Computerized tomographic assessment with or without quadriceps contraction. *Am J Sports Med* 1994;22:55–60.

The authors reviewed CT results of 27 adolescents with knee pain with and without minor patellar instability. Objective measurement of various patellofemoral relationships were made with the knee in 15° of flexion and the quadriceps relaxed or contracted. Changes in type and severity of patellofemoral malalignment was seen in 52% of cases with quadriceps contraction (more evident tilt and lateralization). Use of this dynamic component is a helpful adjunct in difficult diagnostic circumstances and as an aid in decision making for surgical procedures.

Sandow MJ, Goodfellow JW: The natural history of anterior knee pain in adolescents. *J Bone Joint Surg* 1985;67B:36–38.

Fifty-four adolescent girls were reviewed by questionnaire 2 to 12 years following diagnosis of idiopathic anterior knee pain. Treatment was mainly reassurance of the benign nature of the condition, occasional physical therapy, and, rarely, a brief period of immobilization. At follow-up, all had occasional, nondisabling pain, 15% had enough discomfort that sports were discontinued.

The authors emphasized that the symptoms improved with time and rarely caused a serious disability. Indications for surgery would appear quite limited.

Stanitski CL: Anterior knee pain syndromes in the adolescent, in Schafer M (ed): *Instructional Course Lectures 43.* Rosemont, IL, American Academy of Orthopaedic Surgeons, 1994, pp 211–220.

This article reviews the potential causes of anterior knee pain in adolescents, including Osgood-Schlatter disease, Sinding-Larsen-Johansson disease, multipartite patella, pathologic plica, and reflex sympathetic dystrophy. Emphasis was placed on the need for specific diagnosis in idiopathic anterior knee pain. Patellar instability, overuse conditions, and patellar lesions must be ruled out. The term chondromalacia applied to this condition is a misnomer and its use should be eliminated.

Synovial Plica

Broom MJ, Fulkerson JP: The plica syndrome: A new perspective. *Orthop Clin North Am* 1986;17:279–281.

The authors reviewed 28 patients (including adolescents) with clinical and arthroscopically documented pathologic plicae. They noted that a high (76%) number of patients were involved with team athletics. Fifty-five percent had a preoperative diagnosis of a torn medial meniscus. Direct trauma as well as overuse associated with extensor mechanism malalignment may cause pathologic changes in this otherwise normal synovial fold. Plica excision resolved the symptoms in 25 of 28 cases. The authors emphasized that the diagnosis of pathologic plica is specific, and normal (nonfibrotic, noninflamed) synovial folds should not be excised.

Reflex Sympathetic Dystrophy

Dietz FR, Matthews KD, Montgomery WJ: Reflex sympathetic dystrophy in children. *Clin Orthop* 1990; 258:225–231.

The authors reported on five new cases and reviewed 80 reported cases of RSD in children 3 to 17 years of age. They emphasized its increasing recognition in children and adolescents. Diagnosis is based on prolonged pain out of proportion to injury/surgery and hypersensitivity to touch. In contrast to adults, lower extremity involvement predominates. Noninvasive, functional treatment usually results in symptom resolution without recurrence.

Wilder RT, Berde CB, Wolohan M, et al: Reflex sympathetic dystrophy in children: Clinical characteristics and follow-up of seventy patients. *J Bone Joint Surg* 1992;74A:910–919.

The authors reported a series of 70 patients with RSD whose average delay in diagnosis from the time of injury was 1 year. A

management algorithm is presented, which includes functional clinical management with cognitive behavioral pain management techniques. Outcome in children is more favorable than it is in adults.

Osteochondritis Dissecans

Crawfurd EJ, Emery RJ, Aichroth PM: Stable osteochondritis dissecans: Does the lesion unite? *J Bone Joint Surg* 1990;72B:320.

The authors reviewed 31 knees (28 patients) with radiographically and arthroscopically documented osteochondritis dissecans to see if stable lesions spontaneously united. They reported that 21 of 31 lesions were stable; 13 of 21 had healed, but only three of 10 in the classic (lateral portion of the medial femoral condyle) position healed. Healing was independent of lesion size, age of onset, or gender.

Desai SS, Patel MR, Michelli LJ, et al: Osteochondritis dissecans of the patella. *J Bone Joint Surg* 1987;69B: 320–325.

Eleven athletes were reviewed in a multicenter study. Seven were between 10 and 15 years of age. Two patients treated nonsurgically with decreased activity had excellent results in two of three knees. Marginal sclerosis or clinical or radiologic evidence of a loose body were indications for surgery. In 11 of 14 knees treated surgically (fragment excision or curettage and drilling), six had excellent results; four good; and one, fair. Patients with 5- to 10-mm lesions did well.

Linden B: Osteochondritis dissecans of the femoral condyles: A long-term follow-up study. *J Bone Joint Surg* 1977;59A:769–776.

The authors report on 28 patients who developed juvenile OCD before the age of 13 years. They report the results after an average follow-up of 33 years and at an average age of 45.5 years. In these untreated patients, no complications associated with the OCD could be found, in contrast to a comparison group of adult-onset OCD who showed significant progression to early degenerative joint disease. Skeletal maturity and lesion stability in the juvenile group were not discussed.

Litchman HM, McCullough RW, Gandsman EJ, et al: Computerized blood flow analysis for decision making in the treatment of osteochondritis dissecans. *J Pediatr Orthop* 1988;8:208–212.

The authors report on 13 patients (six between 11 and 18 years of age) with radiographic evidence of OCD. Dynamic bone scanning was used to assess its value in predicting healing of the lesion. Patients with absent or persistently diminished flow were found to have nonviable subchondral zones at surgery. In patients with increased flow, the lesion healed.

24

Congenital Clubfoot

Introduction

The goal of treatment for clubfoot (talipes equinovarus) is a plantigrade foot that is functional, painless, and stable over time. The original standard of care for clubfoot was serial manipulation and casting. The most articulate proponent of this nonsurgical treatment, Hiram Kite, MD, stated that "with manipulation and prolonged casting, clubfoot was correctable with only a 12% recurrence rate." Although many surgeons have treated clubfoot conservatively, few have been able to achieve Kite's level of success or exceed the excellent results that current surgical treatments provide.

Congenital clubfoot occurs in approximately one of every 1,000 live births, and 65% of those affected are male. The incidence is even higher in stillbirths. The incidence of bilaterality is as high as 30% to 40%. The etiology is multifactorial, although many of these factors are speculative. Some of these factors are abnormal intrauterine forces; arrested fetal development; abnormal muscle and tendon insertions, with a question of imbalance between fast twitch and slow twitch muscle fiber groups; abnormal rotation of the talus in the mortise; and germ plasm defects. Some of the pathologic conditions associated with clubfoot include proximal femoral focal deficiencies, congenital bifurcation of the femur, Pierre Robin syndrome, Larsen's syndrome, amniotic band syndrome, neuromuscular problems such as myelodysplasia, arthrogryposis multiplex congenita, and diastrophic dwarfism.

The morphologic features of the lower limb in patients with a clubfoot usually will include a dimple over the anterior lateral aspect of the talus, forefoot adduction, heel varus, and ankle equinus. A controversy remains as to whether there is internal or external rotation of the talus within the mortise. A three-dimensional computer analysis of one clubfoot revealed the talus to be externally rotated. A similar controversy exists over whether there is internal rotation of the tibia. The extremity with a clubfoot is usually somewhat shorter than one without a clubfoot, the calf is invariably smaller, and the foot is smaller and shorter.

Radiologic Assessment

The most common radiographic manifestation of a clubfoot is an abnormal Kite angle. The Kite angle is formed by an intersection of lines drawn through the axis of the talus and os calcis on an anteroposterior (AP) radiograph of the foot. The normal angle is usually 20° to 40°. An angle of less than 20° implies varus. A true clubfoot always demonstrates a varus Kite angle, with relative parallelism between the talus and calcaneus. Although the navicular is known to be medially subluxated on the talus in clubfoot, it does not ossify before 5 or 6 years of age, and is therefore not helpful in the initial radiographic evaluation. The calcaneocuboid joint is medial to the tibiofibular interosseous space on an AP view of the foot and ankle. One of the more helpful radiographic views is the lateral maximum dorsiflexion view. In the normal foot, a straight lateral view with forced dorsiflexion shows that the os calcis tends to tilt dorsally and the talus retains its relative position in the mortise. As a result of the dorsal angulation of the calcaneus, there is convergence of the anterior talocalcaneal joint on the lateral view. This complete convergence does not occur in the clubfoot, and the os calcis and talus remain parallel on the forced dorsiflexion radiograph, ie, the calcaneus tends to be in equinus and almost parallel to the lateral axis of the talus. Locked or stacked are frequently used terms for this condition that denote superimposition of the talus and calcaneus upon each other in addition to their failure to rotate.

Treatment

There are three general classes of clubfoot. Postural clubfoot probably arises from simple intrauterine positioning and responds to simple stretching and casting treatment. Congenital clubfoot occurs typically in an otherwise normal child and varies in rigidity from a clubfoot that responds quickly to serial casting to a clubfoot with a short first ray, deep medial skin creases, and marked cavus, which nearly always requires surgery. Syndromic clubfoot is associated with, but is not limited to, arthrogryposis, myelomeningocele, diastrophic dwarfism, and Larsen's syndrome. The vast majority of clubfeet are classified as congenital clubfeet, and the remainder of this chapter discusses only this entity. The incidence of surgical treatment of congenital clubfoot seems to be increasing as new studies and reports are published. In addition, surgery is being performed on younger patients, perhaps because of the favorable results being presented. The congenital clubfoot with a rigid small heel and severe midfoot crease tends to have fewer good to excellent results, when compared with the less rigid congenital clubfoot.

In the past 20 years, successful surgical reconstruction has been widely reported. A review of the *Cumulative Index Medicus* and the *Annual Bibliography of Orthopaedic Surgery* from 1971 to 1989 encountered 215 articles that addressed the treatment of clubfoot. Among these articles, 108 (50%) dealt with surgery and 12 (6%) dealt with nonsurgical treatment. The current trend toward aggressive surgery began in 1971 when Turco introduced the one-stage posteromedial release with internal fixation. The subsequent good and excellent results reported with one-stage posterior and medial releases in the later 1980s marked a turning point in the approach to treatment of the clubfoot. Surgical releases became more radical, such as the posteromedial lateral and complete subtalar releases, but, former problems of stiffness, scarring, and undercorrection with persistent deformity were replaced by overcorrection and valgus.

Nonsurgical Treatment

The treatment of clubfoot should begin shortly after birth. Gentle manipulation should be used and retention casts applied. A sincere effort to correct the majority of deformity should be made during the first 3 months of life. Although early aggressive daily manipulation and cast application have been advocated in some centers, this approach is extremely impractical, difficult for families, expensive, and has shown no demonstrable benefit over traditional weekly cast changes. Serial stretching and taping of the clubfoot is an alternative procedure for the hospitalized neonate. Careful attention must be paid to the skin to prevent skin slough.

Manipulation and cast changes are typically performed weekly for the first 6 to 12 weeks of life. Whether to attempt correction of all components of the deformity simultaneously, or to correct the adducted forefoot first, followed by correction of the hindfoot varus, and finally, the hindfoot equinus is a controversial issue. There is also controversy surrounding the use of below knee or above knee casts. Although below knee casts are easier for the patients' families to maintain, they are prone to fall off. Above knee casts are more difficult to take care of, but have the theoretical advantage of controlling rotational correction better than below knee casts. The casts themselves are only holding devices; all of the correction occurs during the stretching sessions immediately prior to cast application. The position of the foot in the first few casts remains in some equinus until the deformity becomes partially corrected and allows the foot to be placed in a more plantigrade position (Fig. 1).

An assessment must be made regarding the response of the foot during initial nonsurgical treatment and, if necessary, a decision whether to abandon nonsurgical treatment in favor of surgical treatment must be reached. Radiographs of the forced dorsiflexion lateral and simulated weightbearing AP views are quite useful to help determine whether nonsurgical treatment has been successful. A convergence of the talocalcaneal angle in the lateral view and a hindfoot that is in neutral plantigrade position on both views means that a successful result has been achieved. Casting can be discontinued and other holding devices can be used. Other holding devices include reverse last shoes, bivalved casts, and polypropylene ankle-foot orthoses. These holding devices are typically used until the child is a well-established walker. An iatrogenic rocker bottom foot should be avoided at all costs. If the patient develops this condition all casting treatment should be abandoned in favor of surgery.

Limited percutaneous soft-tissue releases (Achilles tendon lengthening ± plantar fascial releases) are sometimes performed at approximately 3 months of age in the patient with a very severe clubfoot, as part of a continuum in nonsurgical treatment. The criterion for percutaneous release, as cited by proponents of this approach, is persistent radiographic equinus on a forced lateral maximum dorsiflexion radiograph at 3 months of age or following 3 months of manipulation and retentive casting. After a percutaneous release, serial stretching and casting is continued for an additional 2 months. When stretching and casting, with or without the percutaneous releases, do not provide adequate correction, definitive surgery is needed.

Surgical Treatment

Surgery should be viewed as an integral component of successful management of the deformity and the need for surgery should not be interpreted as a failure of nonsurgical treatment. Most authors recommend that surgery should be performed when the child is between 6 and 12 months of age, although some controversy exists about correct timing of surgery. The surgery performed should address all components of the deformity at one time, rather than having the patient undergo several surgical procedures over a span of several years. With current surgical management of the congenital clubfoot, the need for repeat surgery is uncommon.

Controversies exist surrounding the type and extent of release, pin fixation, duration of postsurgical immobilization, and type of incision used. The one-stage release (posteromedial release) that was first described by Turco has been expanded and modified in the past 15 years. McKay has extended the posteromedial release to include the posteromedial lateral release in an effort to address the contracted posterior talofibular and calcaneofibular ligaments, which are believed to cause medial spin and hindfoot varus. Simons has proposed the complete subtalar release, which often includes the talocalcaneal interosseous ligament, to address the tethering forces in the lateral complex, including release of the calcaneocuboid joint in more severe deformities. Talocalcaneal interosseous ligament release is still controversial. In addition to its vascular contribution, the talocalcaneal interosseous ligament acts as a tether and restraint to valgus overcorrection and possible translocation of the talocalcaneal joint. To date, no conclusive study has been done that identifies overcorrection or vascular problems following complete release of the interosseous ligament. A complete talocalcaneal capsular release adequately allows correction of subtalar subluxation and achieves hindfoot realignment. Goldner and others avoid releasing the subtalar joint, yet still obtain correc-

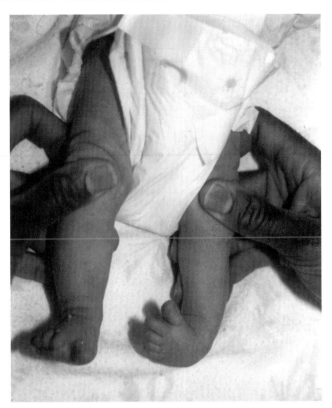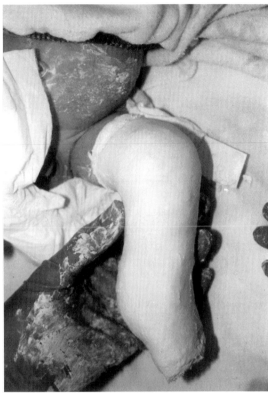

Fig. 1   **Left,** Five-day-old infant's left foot with severe equinovarus position. Note that it is smaller than the right foot. **Right,** Position of the foot in a cast after manipulation. No attempt was made to correct equinus with the initial manipulation. (Reproduced with permission from Crawford AH, Jaglan SS, McDougall P: Cincinnati surgical approach to idiopathic clubfoot. *J Pediatr Orthop,* in press.)

tion of hindfoot varus by releasing the deltoid ligament. These various surgical procedures reflect the complexity and difficulty of interpreting the pathoanatomy in three-dimensional congenital deformities. Future research may shed more light on our knowledge of clubfoot pathoanatomy and surgical approaches.

If postsurgical pin fixation is elected, the surgeon must determine how many pins are needed and which joints need fixation. The pins are typically smooth and cross the talonavicular joint, talocalcaneal joint, calcaneocuboid joint, or any combination of these joints. The use of intraoperative radiographs to document adequate correction remains controversial. The duration of postsurgical casting varies from short-term hinged casts to several months of fixed above knee casting.

The incision proposed by Turco was a single posteromedial incision, which made it difficult to reach the posterolateral complex. This problem can be circumvented by using either the transverse Cincinnati incision or the two-incision approach of Carroll. Proponents of the Cincinnati incision, which extends around the heel to the lateral malleolus or even to the calcaneocuboid joint, note that it affords a wide exposure that facilitates an appropriate soft-tissue release. No portion of the surgical anatomy is excluded. The vessels, nerves, tendons, and immature articular surfaces are seen and easily protected. Direct visualization of the bony alignment of the foot in all planes is achieved, especially for pin placement. Skin closure is usually obtained with minimum tension of the suture line. Some surgeons allow the wound to remain partially open and granulate without any tension and they report excellent cosmetic results. The Cincinnati incision has been made perpendicular to previous vertical scars and has healed uneventfully. Achilles tendon lengthening can be achieved without difficulty using the Cincinnati incision. Finally, the exposure achieved by the Cincinnati incision facilitates teaching by allowing the student unrestricted visualization of the pathology and anatomy of the foot.

Critics of the Cincinnati incision discuss potential skin necrosis or slough as a major concern. In addition, they feel posterior soft-tissue scarring may limit the range of motion and contribute to recurrence of the deformity. The two-incision approach of Carroll avoids the potential skin necrosis, and because of a more limited exposure, may also reduce the amount of postsurgical scarring and subsequent recurrence of the deformity.

Table 1. Results of clubfoot treatment

Series	Surgery	Satisfactory Results
Main et al, 1977	PMR*	74%
Turco, 1979	PMR	84%
McKay, 1983	PMLR†	70%
Simons, 1985	PMLR	72%
Derosa, 1986	PMLR	95%
Yamamoto, 1988	PMLR	70%
Franke, 1988	PMLR	94%

*Posteromedial release
†Posteromedial lateral release

Treatment Results

Clubfoot treatment will not result in a completely normal foot. Careful scrutiny will show calf atrophy, asymmetry of foot size, limitation of subtalar mobility, pes planus, metatarsus adductus, or a toe-in gait. The goal of surgery should be to produce a near anatomically normal, pain-free plantigrade foot that has reasonable mobility, fits into a normal shoe, and maintains lasting correction. A cosmetically pleasing appearance is also an important goal sought by the patient's surgeon and family.

The inherent difficulty when comparing results of clubfoot treatment is that no two clubfeet are the same before treatment, and the lack of a universally accepted rating system for assessment of results after treatment hinders comparison of nonsurgical and surgical techniques. Results of most studies are evaluated based on clinical, radiologic, or functional criteria, or some combination of these criteria. Since 1966, at least 46 articles evaluating surgical treatment of clubfoot in the English language literature have appeared, each one espousing its own system for the evaluation of postsurgical results.

There is no satisfactory standardized method of documenting the severity of the presurgical clubfoot deformity and results can be skewed in favor of either a successful or poor outcome by inclusion of mild or severe cases, respectively. The various parameters of evaluation suffer from inter- and intraobserver error. The highly subjective description of the appearance of a treated clubfoot, in addition to inaccurate range of motion measurements in young children with small joints, cause an elaborate grading system to be difficult to interpret. Radiographic studies are more objective, but still suffer from potential positioning inaccuracies of the small foot without a standard holding device. These limitations are acknowledged in Table 1, where the clubfoot treatment results of various authors are presented.

Recently, the results of three different approaches to clubfoot treatment, by Turco, McKay, and Carroll, were studied and found to be clinically similar. Therefore, it may not be necessary to discuss the superiority of one technique over another from a clinical perspective.

Another recent study compared the radiographic, rather than clinical, results in clubfeet that were treated by three different approaches. Thirty-one patients (43 feet) underwent either a posteromedial release as developed by Turco,

a two-incision posteromedial and lateral release, or complete subtalar release with Cincinnati incision. A wedge-shaped navicular and avascularity were noted in 37% of patients in the two-incision release group and 6% of patients in the posteromedial release group; none were noted in patients in the complete subtalar release group. No statistically significant difference between groups was noted with regard to sclerosis of the navicular. Flattening of the talar head was most prominent in patients in the two-incision release group, whereas flat-top talus and a short talar neck were equally common in all three groups. Irregularity and narrowing of the talonavicular joint occurred more frequently in the two-incision release group, but did not occur at all in the complete subtalar release group. Dorsal subluxation of the navicular occurred in approximately 40% of patients in each group. The complete subtalar release group developed less osteonecrosis, fewer changes in the navicular, and less cavus and adductus. The highest rate of radiographic abnormalities occured in the two-incision release group. These abnormalities may have occurred because a more blind release technique was used.

The most frequent residual clinical deformity is metatarsus adductus, which occurs in up to 21% of clubfeet. The metatarsus adductus is usually not a functional problem and in some feet may correct spontaneously. Its clinical appearance may be unacceptable to patients and families. Indeed, residual forefoot adduction was found to be the main indication for repeat surgery in one series of 159 feet that underwent 210 repeat surgeries. Failure to recognize residual forefoot adduction on the intraoperative radiographs at the time of the primary surgery was identified as the cause of the problem. The majority of the cases did not undergo calcaneocuboid release during the first surgery. If intraoperative AP radiographs are to be used to assess forefoot adduction, it is extremely important that the foot be properly positioned plantigrade on the cassette in order to prevent inaccurate interpretation. Releasing the dorsal and medial calcaneocuboid joint during the primary surgery may prevent residual metatarsus adductus from occurring.

Radiographic analysis, as noted above, adds more objectivity to any study on clubfoot treatment. AP and lateral views of the talocalcaneal angle, tibiocalcaneal angles, forefoot subluxation, metatarsus adductus, and the talar deformities can all be radiographically assessed. Improvements in angular measurements can be documented and the deformities described clinically can be corroborated radiographically. The most persistent radiographic deformity seen is metatarsus adductus, with up to 33% of feet having a positive talar–first metatarsal angle on the AP view.

A flat top talus may be present in nearly 20% of feet after surgery and will be seen on the lateral radiograph. The question of relative versus absolute talar flattening based on the projection of a true transmalleolar radiograph of the ankle always exists. A true lateral radiograph of the ankle will show the fibula superimposed on the tibia, not located behind the tibia. The presence of a flat top talus could impede ankle range of motion and subsequent function of the foot.

Dorsal subluxation of the forefoot may occur following surgical correction and denotes a cavus component with persistent shortening of the medial column. It is very important to avoid dorsal malreduction of the navicular on the talus during surgery. Excessive lateral displacement of the navicular and forefoot must also be avoided in order to prevent overcorrection.

Overcorrection and poor functional results have been reported in patients younger than 6 months who have undergone surgical release. Although some surgeons have recommended surgical release within the first few days or weeks of life, the results are not superior, and the procedure is technically difficult. Because of the difficulty of working with the small bones and cartilaginous structures in this patient group, occurrences of both overcorrection and undercorrection have been reported, signifying that this early approach may not be advisable. It has been recommended that surgery be delayed until the child is at least 6 months old, and, in some cases, until the child is 9 to 12 months old. Although the optimum age for surgical intervention remains debatable, it is agreed that treatment should ideally be completed by the time the child is ready to walk.

Residual deformities following initial surgical management of clubfeet may be addressed by soft-tissue or osseous techniques. The adduction/supination deformity is often treated by anterior tibialis tendon transfer, most often to the midportion of the foot, or by splitting the anterior tibialis tendon and placing one limb on the lateral aspect of the foot. The Heyman-Herndon-Strong tarsal metatarsal capsulotomy may also be used to correct forefoot adduction; however, the procedure has recently been criticized because of late complications associated with it. Other procedures to correct residual deformities include the Dwyer os calcis osteotomy, for retained heel varus; metatarsal osteotomies for uncorrected adduction of the forefoot; calcaneal distal resection or cuboid resection to shorten the lateral column; cuneiform lengthening osteotomy with bone grafting from the cuboid fragment to lengthen the medial column; and the Dilwyn-Evans procedure, which includes a calcaneal cuboid fusion in addition to a posterior medial release. A triple arthrodesis may be indicated at a later date for severe unrelenting resistant cases.

Annotated Bibliography

Crawford AH, Jaglan SS, McDougall P: Cincinnati surgical approach to idiopathic clubfoot. *J Pediatr Orthop,* in press.

Resistant clubfoot deformities in 58 children (79 feet) were treated with posteromedial lateral release (PMLR) with the Cincinnati incision and investigated retrospectively. Early percutaneous soft-tissue releases were performed at 3 to 4 months in 31 feet. One-stage PMLR only was performed in 48 feet. Asymptomatic metatarsus adductus was the most common residual deformity, followed by nonclinical flat-top talus, dorsal forefoot subluxation, and hindfoot varus/valgus. A 95% satisfaction rate by parents and physicians was reported, and only four feet (5%) required further surgery.

Del Bello: Abstract: A radiographic analysis of the congenital clubfoot: A comparative study of three reconstructive procedures. *J Pediatr Orthop* 1993;13:806.

The author retrospectively reviewed charts and radiographs of 31 patients (43 feet) who underwent either a posteromedial and lateral release (Turco), a two-incision posteromedial and lateral release, or a complete subtalar release with Cincinnati incision. A wedge-shaped navicular and osteonecrosis of the navicular were noted in 37% of patients in the two-incision group and 6% of patients in the posteromedial group, but were not noted in the complete subtalar release group. Patients in the two-incision group had the highest rate of radiographic abnormalities, which may be related to a more blind release technique.

DeRosa GP, Stepro D: Results of posteromedial release for the resistant clubfoot. *J Pediatr Orthop* 1986;6:590–595.

Downey DJ, Drennan JC, Garcia JF: Magnetic resonance image findings in congenital talipes equinovarus. *J Pediatr Orthop* 1992;12:224–228.

The authors used magnetic resonance imaging (MRI) to evaluate the feet of 10 infants with congenital talipes equinovarus. They were able to identify the articular cartilages of all the bones using the T2 imaging sequence because of the high signal intensity at the articular surfaces. The authors' principal observations were medial angulation of the talar neck and rotation of the calcaneus with the anterior portion shifting medially and the posterior portion shifting laterally. They concluded that the primary clubfoot problem is talar head and neck deformity with the anterior calcaneus following the deformed anterior talus and causing a pivot about the interosseous ligament so that the posterior calcaneus is forced laterally.

Franke J, Hein G: Our experiences with the early operative treatment of congenital clubfoot. *J Pediatr Orthop* 1988;8:26–30.

Howard CB, Benson MK: Clubfoot: Its pathological anatomy. *J Pediatr Orthop* 1993;13:654–659.

The authors discuss the dissection of three clubfeet, including the shape, orientation, and alignment of the bones. Particular attention is paid to the medial tie and its etiologic role. The bony abnormality of the talus is identified. The authors highlight the abnormal soft-tissue medial tie that is identified as a dense, fibrous knot at the inferior medial aspect of the foot. They also stress that entering the subtalar joint surgically in the immature foot may be difficult, in part because of the fibrous knot at the middle facet. The orientation of the joint compounds the problem; supination of the calcaneus dictates that the joint is sagittally rather than coronally oriented. It is important not to inadvertently excise the calcaneal facet: damage to the middle facet may compromise the results of surgery.

Ikeda K: Conservative treatment of idiopathic clubfoot. *J Pediatr Orthop* 1992;12:217–223.

The author treated 25 patients (36 feet) and followed them for 4 to 16 years. In 95% of the patients, the outcome was either excellent or good. Treatment was started on the second to 64th day of life, except for two patients who were believed initially to have had postural foot deformities. In addition to initial strapping and casting, followed by short leg brace, some patients underwent late sequential casting with re-treatment. This was followed by corrective shoeing. It was the author's opinion that all clubfoot deformities could be treated with strapping and sequential casting. Only one child underwent surgery (Morita's leverage wire correction) in this series. The author did not believe surgery was indicated for those patients who had obvious clubfoot malposition without rigidity, who walked on the lateral border of the foot with the heel in varus that was not rigid, and those who walked with intoeing that was passively correctable. In those cases, he stated that all clubfeet could be controlled by waiting for natural development of better muscle balance or by late sequential casting.

Magone JB, Torch MA, Clark RN, et al: Comparative review of surgical treatment of the idiopathic clubfoot by three different procedures at Columbus Children's Hospital. *J Pediatr Orthop* 1989;9:49–58.

A new rating system that places emphasis on dynamic functional results was used to compare results in 99 feet in 54 children who were both clinically and radiographically evaluated following one of three different procedures of soft-tissue clubfoot release. Radiographic complications included both over- and undercorrection at the talonavicular articulation; avascular necrosis of the talus, navicular, and calcaneus; and talar dome flattening. Recommendations concerning technical aspects of surgical approach to clubfeet include more physiologic orientation of bimalleolar axis, anatomic alignment at the talonavicular joint, and use of the hinged ankle cast brace to increase final ankle range of motion.

Main BJ, Crider RJ, Polk M, et al: The results of early operation in talipes equino-varus: A preliminary report. *J Bone Joint Surg* 1977;59B:337–341.

McKay DW: New concept of and approach to clubfoot treatment: Section III. Evaluation and results. *J Pediatr Orthop* 1983;3:141–148.

Ponseti IV: Treatment of congenital club foot. *J Bone Joint Surg* 1992;74A:448–454.

The author presents his view on nonsurgical management of clubfoot deformity. This treatment has stood the test of time and has resulted in excellent clinical appearance of clubfeet that are extremely functional. He strongly advocates clinical management because radiographs may not show anatomic alignment. The process consists of manipulative correction of the forefoot adduction, midfoot cavus, and hindfoot varus. He feels the foot can be maintained in external rotation only if the talus, ankle, and leg are stabilized by a plaster cast that extends from the toes to the groin, with the knee flexed at 90°. A below-the-knee cast cannot immobilize the foot in firm external rotation under the talus. If the equinus becomes a problem, a percutaneous Achilles tenotomy is performed and continued manipulation and retentive cast applied. The author strongly believes in remanipulation and

casting for 4 to 8 weeks any time there appears to be a relapse or recurrence of the deformity rather than an immediate approach of radical surgery.

When the child is ambulating and the foot appears to be supinated or in an in-toe position, an anterior tibialis tendon transfer is recommended. Surgical correction of a clubfoot is indicated when the deformity has not been treated successfully with proper manipulation and serial application of a cast. Even though extensive surgery achieves better anatomic and radiologic correction, the pinning and immobilization required to maintain position creates a stiffer foot. The author believes that deformities of the bones and joints are rarely, if ever, corrected completely. Some persistent medial displacement of the navicular bone and talocalcaneal index that is outside of the normal range are compatible with a fully functional, normal looking, pain-free plantigrade foot.

Simons GW: Complete subtalar release in club feet: Part II. Comparison with less extensive procedures. *J Bone Joint Surg* 1985;67A:1056–1065.

Spero CR, Simon GS, Tornetta P III: Clubfeet and tarsal coalition. *J Pediatr Orthop* 1994;14:372–376.

The authors noted tarsal coalition in 18 cases of rigid equinovarus deformity. Of the 14 patients in this series, six had associated pathologic conditions that were deemed teratologic that might have caused their clubfeet, whereas eight did not have teratologic associated pathologic conditions and were considered to have congenital clubfeet. Four patients in this series had bilateral coalitions. Presurgical radiographs demonstrated the coalition in only one case and a presurgical MRI clearly showed the coalition in another case. The authors state that the association between tarsal coalition and peroneal spastic flatfoot is well documented and well recognized; however, less commonly reported is the occurrence of tarsal coalition in clubfeet. There were 17 talocalcaneal navicular coalitions and one calcaneal navicular coalition in the series. The authors state that because of the distortion of the anatomy in clubfeet, the joints involved may be abnormal. Intraoperatively, it may be challenging to differentiate a coalition from a malformed joint. Tarsal coalition adds another degree of variability to the difficulty of treatment and the spectrum of surgical results in clubfeet.

Stanitski CL, Ward WT, Grossman W: Noninvasive vascular studies in clubfoot. *J Pediatr Orthop* 1992; 12:514–517.

The authors designed a two-phase study to investigate vascularity in idiopathic clubfeet undergoing a comprehensive soft-tissue release by the Cincinnati incision. Oxygen (O_2) saturation of the great toe was measured by pulse oximetry and Doppler ultrasound studies and measurements were done in three positions: in feet at rest; in maximum passive correction; and immediately after surgery. In five feet in three patients, passive correction immediately before surgery caused O_2 saturation diminution to less than 94%. Oxygen saturation values in four of five feet immediately after surgery were 97% to 100% with similar O_2 saturations at cast change 3 weeks later. There were no problems with O_2 saturation. At postsurgical cast change, all 32 feet (100%) demonstrated great toe pulse oxygenation measurements of 97% to 100%. Doppler studies were carried out on the posterior tibial dorsalis pedis and peroneal pulses. The dorsalis pedis pulse was present in 37 of 38 feet, and peroneal pulses were noted in 20 of 30 feet (67%). Posterior tibial artery and radial artery controls were equal in all specimens studied in the premanipulated state. The authors question the recently suggested clinical problem regarding why there is no overwhelming incidence of minor and major vascular complications after manipulation and surgical procedures if vascular dysplasia is so prevalent. Their study presents the reader with a noninvasive method of evaluating vasculature and perfusion in talipes equinovarus.

Tarraf YN, Carroll NC: Analysis of the components of residual deformity in clubfeet presenting for reoperation. *J Pediatr Orthop* 1992;12:207–216.

The authors reviewed the records and radiographs of 125 children with 159 clubfeet re-operated on for residual deformity after surgical repair (210 re-operations). They concluded that residual forefoot adduction and supination were the most common persistent deformities (present in 95% of the feet) and that these deformities resulted from undercorrection at the time of primary surgery. The authors advocated closer scrutiny of the intraoperative radiograph to pursue proper alignment. They believed that the fate of the clubfoot was determined by three factors: the calcaneocuboid joint alignment; the plantar fascia tightness; and the surgeon's failure to recognize residual forefoot adduction on intraoperative radiographs, in addition to failure to address the calcaneocuboid joints specifically.

Thometz JG, Simons GW: Deformity of the calcaneo-cuboid joint in patients who have talipes equinovarus. *J Bone Joint Surg* 1993;75A:190–195.

The authors conducted a retrospective analysis of the records and radiographs of 100 consecutive clubfeet that had been surgically treated and describe a method of evaluating calcaneocuboid joint alignment. When the calcaneocuboid is in normal alignment, the central point of the cuboid ossification center lies on the midlongitudinal axis of the calcaneus. When there is a grade I deformity, the midpoint of the cuboid ossification center lies lateral to the medial tangent but medial to the longitudinal axis of the calcaneus. When there is a grade II deformity, the central point of the cuboid lies on or medial to the medial tangent of the calcaneus. The grade I deformity did not require correction. A grade II deformity was present in 26% of the feet. After soft-tissue release (specifically, release of the talonavicular and subtalar joints), the navicula, cuboid, and calcaneus move as a unit. If the calcaneal cuboid joint is markedly displaced, the navicula will force the cuboid laterally when reduced, in turn forcing the anterior aspect of the calcaneus in a lateral direction and leading to an increased talocalcaneal angle with malalignment of the calcaneal cuboid joint on the AP radiograph. Only when the abnormality of the calcaneocuboid joint, as well as the adduction of the forefoot, are corrected, does the lateral side of the foot appear to be straight clinically. The authors state that in their experience approximately 25% of clubfeet that need surgical treatment also need surgical correction of the calcaneocuboid joint.

Turco VJ: Resistant congenital club foot: One stage posteromedial release with internal fixation. A follow-up report of a fifteen-year experience *J Bone Joint Surg* 1979;61A:805–814.

Yamamoto II, Furaya K: One-stage posteromedial release of congenital clubfoot. *J Pediatr Orthop* 1988;8:590.

25

Flexible Flatfoot and Tarsal Coalition

Flexible Flatfoot

The flexible flatfoot is a variation from the normal foot shape and rarely causes disability, but nevertheless, has engendered much controversy and speculation. Indications for treatment of the flexible flatfoot have not been clearly defined, and many of the treatment methods that have been proposed are unnecessary, unproven, and potentially unsafe. There are several reasons why the indications for surgical treatment have not been well defined. First, flatfeet, other than the flexible variety, often cause pain and disability. Second, no long-term prospective studies have been done on the natural history of the untreated flexible flatfoot. Third, no controlled prospective studies that document avoidance of long-term pain or disability by prophylactic surgical or nonsurgical treatment exist.

A basic problem with our understanding of the flexible flatfoot is the lack of a universally accepted clinical or radiographic definition of a flatfoot. Nomenclature is confusing and inconsistent in the literature. Flatfoot is the term applied to a foot shape that results from a number of altered relationships between several bones of the foot; it is not a single deformity at a single joint. A reasonable description that characterizes a weightbearing flatfoot includes: plantarflexion of the talus and calcaneus; excessive eversion of the subtalar complex; valgus, external rotation, and dorsiflexion of the calcaneus in relation to the talus; abduction and dorsiflexion of the navicular on the head of a plantarflexed talus; resultant midfoot sag with lowering of the longitudinal arch; short lateral column (or border) of the foot relative to the medial column; and supination of the forefoot on the hindfoot (Fig. 1). It is important to recognize that an isolated valgus deformity of the hindfoot or isolated excessive eversion of the subtalar joint is not synonymous with a flatfoot, but either of these may be a component of that deformity. If excessive eversion of the subtalar complex is combined with a talonavicular joint dislocation, the deformity is known as a vertical talus. When the same hindfoot deformity is associated with adduction and plantarflexion of the forefoot on the midfoot, it is called a skewfoot.

The height of the longitudinal arch, like all measurable physiologic quantities, has an average value and a range of normal values. The shape of the footprint has been used as a clinical means to assess the height of the longitudinal arch, but there are no reliable and widely agreed upon parameters that indicate when a low normal arch becomes a flatfoot. In addition, no studies that correlate the appearance of the footprint with radiographic measurements have been done. Only one radiographic study in adults and

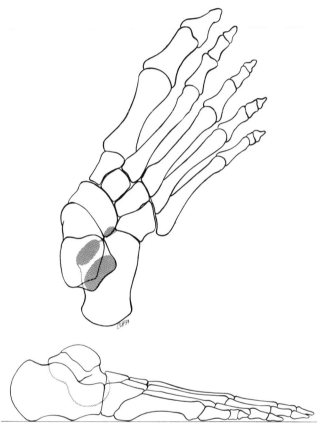

Fig. 1 Flatfoot. **Top,** A flatfoot is characterized by excessive eversion of the subtalar complex, which includes external rotation of the calcaneus in relation to the talus and abduction of the navicular on the head of the talus. The lateral column of the foot is short relative to the medial column. **Bottom,** Although the calcaneus is dorsiflexed in relation to the talus (increased lateral talocalcaneal angle), the calcaneus and talus are both plantarflexed in relation to the tibia. The navicular is dorsiflexed on the head of the talus, creating a sag at the talonavicular joint with lowering of the longitudinal arch. The hindfoot is in valgus, yet all metatarsal heads touch the ground. The forefoot, therefore, must be supinated in relation to the hindfoot. (Reproduced with permission from Mosca VS: Calcaneal lengthening for valgus deformity of the hindfoot: Results in children who had severe, symptomatic flatfoot and skewfoot. *J Bone Joint Surg* 1995;77A:500–512.)

one study in children report the average values and normal ranges for various interosseous angular measurements of the foot. In both studies, the authors clearly state that ra-

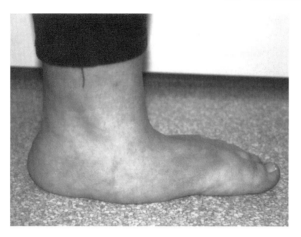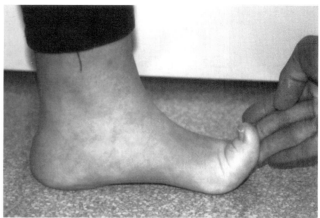

Fig. 2   The Jack toe-raising test for flexibility of a flatfoot. **Left,** Medial view of a flatfoot that is bearing full weight. **Right,** The hallux is dorsiflexed and the longitudinal arch is elevated by the windlass effect of the plantar fascia. The subtalar complex must be mobile (or flexible) for elevation to occur. (Reproduced with permission from Mosca VS: Flexible flatfoot and skewfoot, in Drennan JC (ed): *The Child's Foot and Ankle.* New York, NY, Raven Press, 1992, pp 355–376.)

diographic values should not determine clinical management even if the values are beyond the normal range.

Despite the lack of strict, consensual criteria for the definition of a flatfoot, there is no question that certain feet have excessive flattening of the longitudinal arch. In 1947, a 22.5% incidence of flatfeet was reported in the general adult population; almost two thirds of the flatfeet were flexible. They defined a flexible flatfoot as a foot with depression of the longitudinal arch that occurs with weightbearing, good mobility of the subtalar complex, and normal length of the Achilles tendon. Mobility of the subtalar complex is determined by manual testing and is confirmed by creating the longitudinal arch with toe standing or with the Jack toe-raising test (Fig. 2). The Achilles tendon is considered to be of normal length when it allows at least 10° of ankle dorsiflexion when tested with the subtalar joint held in neutral alignment and the knee fully extended. Flexible flatfeet are present from birth and are accompanied by normal muscle function and good joint mobility. The shape of the longitudinal arch is determined by the laxity of the ligaments and the shapes of the bones. Muscles are necessary for function and balance, but not for the structural alignment of the foot. Harris and Beath pointed out that the flatness of the arch in weightbearing was of less importance as a cause of disability than the mobility of the joints and tendons. Flexible flatfeet are rarely a cause of disability. Two other less common types of flatfeet, flexible flatfeet with short Achilles tendons and rigid flatfeet, such as those seen in tarsal coalitions, more commonly cause pain and disability.

It has clearly been established by both clinical and radiographic studies that the average arch height is lower in the child than in the adult, that the height of the longitudinal arch increases spontaneously during the first decade of life in most children, and that there is a wide range of normal arch heights at all ages, particularly in young children (Fig. 3). In fact, in young children, most normal arch heights are considered to be flat (Fig. 4).

Authors of several uncontrolled studies have reported that a longitudinal arch can be created in children's feet by using certain shoes and shoe inserts. This information must be considered dubious given the known natural history of arch development in children. Two recently published, well-controlled, prospective studies were not able to show any benefit from shoe modifications or inserts over spontaneous natural improvement in the development of the longitudinal arch in children with normal feet who were followed for 3 to 5 years.

Some children with flexible flatfeet have activity-related pain in the leg or foot that is relieved by shoe inserts. Shoe inserts may also increase the useful life of shoes that would otherwise be worn unevenly by children with severe flatfeet. Soft-, firm-, and hard-molded arch supports that are fabricated from foam, leather, cork, Plastazote, compressed felt, and plastic have all been found useful for achieving these beneficial effects. Simultaneous permanent improvement in the height of the longitudinal arch, however, should not be expected from the use of shoe inserts.

Some children with flexible flatfeet develop pain with weightbearing and/or the presence of calluses under the head of the plantarflexed talus. Contracture of the Achilles tendon is often present in these symptomatic flatfeet, a finding that defines these as flexible flatfeet with short Achilles tendon. A contracted Achilles tendon prevents normal ankle dorsiflexion during the midstance phase of the gait cycle. The dorsiflexion stress is shifted to the talonavicular joint, where the soft tissues under the head of the plantarflexed talus experience excessive direct axial

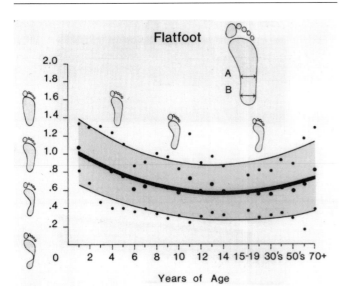

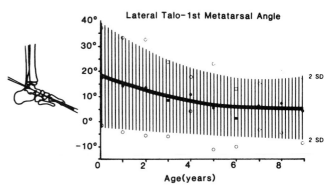

Fig. 4 The lateral talo–first metatarsal angle plotted against age in untreated individuals. A larger angle signifies a greater sag of the midfoot and a flatter longitudinal arch. (Reproduced with permission from Vanderwilde R, Staheli LT, Chew DE, et al: Measurements on radiographs of the foot in normal infants and children. *J Bone Joint Surg* 1988;70A:407–415.)

Fig. 3 The height of the longitudinal arch as determined by evaluation of the footprint. The ratio of midfoot-to-heel width (A/B) is plotted against age in untreated individuals. The average value and two standard deviation ranges change spontaneously with age. A higher ratio, which is higher on the graph, represents a flatter foot. (Reproduced with permission from Staheli LT, Chew DE, Corbett M: The longitudinal arch: A survey of eight hundred and eighty-two feet in normal children and adults. *J Bone Joint Surg* 1987;69A:426–428).

loading and shear stress. These pressures may be exaggerated by firm arch supports, resulting in the formation of painful calluses. An aggressive Achilles tendon stretching program may relieve these symptoms.

Surgery is rarely, if ever, indicated for the flexible flatfoot with an Achilles tendon of normal length. More commonly, it is the flexible flatfoot with a short Achilles tendon that requires surgical intervention because of the failure of nonsurgical management to relieve the pain and callus formation under the head of the plantarflexed talus. Numerous surgical procedures have been proposed during the last century to correct the flatfoot. These include osseous excisions, osteotomies, arthrodesis of one or more joints, and interposition of bone or Silastic plugs into the sinus tarsi. Most of these procedures have been abandoned because of the failure to relieve symptoms or to achieve or maintain correction of the deformity. Reports of all long-term studies reviewing arthrodeses of the midtarsal joints, such as those performed in the modifications of the Hoke procedure, have shown degenerative arthrosis at adjacent unfused joints. The technique of Silastic plug interposition in the sinus tarsi has never been embraced by most orthopaedic surgeons, whose usual experiences consist of implant removal because of infection or pain. The posterior calcaneal displacement osteotomy can improve the clinical appearance of the valgus hindfoot, but it does not correct the subtalar complex deformity. The calcaneal lengthening osteotomy (Fig. 5), originally described by Evans, has

been shown to correct all components of the subtalar complex deformity in the valgus hindfoot, restore function of the subtalar complex, relieve symptoms, and theoretically protect the ankle and midtarsal joints from early degenerative arthrosis by avoiding arthrodesis. Indications for the calcaneal lengthening osteotomy, or for any surgical procedure for flatfoot, should be limited to those patients who fail prolonged conservative management, and who experience pain, callosity, and/or ulceration under the fixed plantar flexed talus. These patients always have accompanying contracture of the Achilles tendon, which should be lengthened simultaneously. Rigid forefoot supination deformity, if present, must be recognized and managed as a second deformity. A medial column osteotomy is often effective treatment in these cases.

Tarsal Coalition

Tarsal coalition is a fibrous, cartilaginous, or bony connection between two or more tarsal bones that results from a congenital failure of differentiation and segmentation of primitive mesenchyme. Some tarsal coalitions are associated with other congenital disorders, such as fibular hemimelia, Apert's syndrome, or Nievergelt-Pearlman syndrome. The focus of this review is the autosomal dominant variety of tarsal coalition (with nearly full penetrance) that affects less than 1% of the general population and causes progressively rigid flatfeet.

Tarsal coalitions were first recognized in 1750. Although the first detailed clinical description of a peroneal spastic flatfoot was presented by Jones in 1897, it was not until 1921 that Slomann linked peroneal spastic flatfoot with calcaneonavicular coalition, and not until 1948 that Harris and Beath linked peroneal spastic flatfoot with talocalcaneal coalition. Since 1965, tarsal coalition has also been

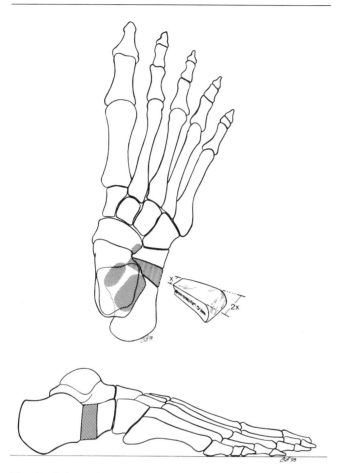

Fig. 5 Calcaneal lengthening osteotomy. All components of the subtalar complex deformity have been corrected by insertion of a trapezoid-shaped, tricortical iliac crest graft into the osteotomy that was made between the anterior and middle facets of the calcaneus. (Reproduced with permission from Mosca VS: Calcaneal lengthening for valgus deformity of the hindfoot: Results in children who had severe, symptomatic flatfoot and skewfoot. *J Bone Joint Surg* 1995;77A:500–512).

linked with the infrequently occurring tibialis spastic varus foot.

The most common types of tarsal coalitions are calcaneonavicular and talocalcaneal coalitions. Based on a review of the literature, calcaneonavicular and talocalcaneal coalitions occur with about equal frequency and, together, account for approximately 90% of the total number of coalitions. The true relative incidence of the different types of coalitions, like the true incidence of tarsal coalitions in general, is unknown because many asymptomatic individuals are never evaluated. The incidence of bilaterality is also unknown, but it is most likely greater than 50% and perhaps as high as 80%.

Only about 25% of individuals with tarsal coalitions become symptomatic. The onset of symptoms usually coincides with metaplasia of the coalition from cartilage to bone. This generally occurs between 8 and 12 years of age for those children with calcaneonavicular coalitions, and between 12 and 16 years of age for those with talocalcaneal coalitions. Ossification of the coalition also coincides with the occurrence of progressive valgus deformity of the hindfoot, flattening of the longitudinal arch, and restriction of subtalar motion. All of these findings are more severe in feet with talocalcaneal coalitions.

The onset of pain is often insidious, but may be precipitated by some unusual activity or trauma. Pain is frequently aggravated by activity and relieved by rest. Mild to moderate deep aching pain is usually experienced in the sinus tarsi area, particularly with calcaneonavicular coalitions. The pain from talocalcaneal coalitions may be localized to the same area, but may also be experienced in the anterior or lateral ankle and has been described as recurrent "ankle sprains." Pain with weightbearing under the head of the plantarflexed talus, such as pain that occurs in a flexible flatfoot with a short Achilles tendon, is also reported in feet with the most severe valgus deformities.

The normal subtalar complex is the shock absorber of the foot and has both gliding and rotatory motions during walking. When these subtalar motions are restricted, excessive stress is applied to other joints of the foot. The talar beak, which often forms on the dorsal surface of the head of the talus in feet with tarsal coalitions, most likely represents a traction spur created by stress on the dorsal talonavicular ligament. The talar beak likely does not signify early degenerative arthrosis of the talonavicular joint, although a talar beak will be present eventually when actual degeneration of the articular surfaces occurs. Flattening and broadening of the lateral talar process, as seen on the lateral radiograph, are other indications of unusual stresses created by restricted subtalar motion and result from impingement of the talus on the lateral aspect of the calcaneal sulcus.

What appears to be spasm of the peroneal muscles is often present in feet with tarsal coalitions. The whole concept of peroneal spasm, however, has been questioned. There certainly appears to be adaptive shortening of the peroneal tendons associated with tarsal coalitions, but most authors question whether the muscles are actually in spasm.

The described pathomechanics clearly relate to symptoms, but the exact etiology of the pain is unknown. Pain has been attributed to ligament strain, peroneal muscle spasm, sinus tarsi irritation, subtalar joint irritation, and, ultimately, degenerative arthrosis. The severity of pain seems to be correlated with the severity of hindfoot valgus deformity.

The diagnosis of tarsal coalition must be considered when a child between 8 and 16 years of age presents with diffuse, activity-related pain in the sinus tarsi region of a progressively flattening foot. This foot shape matches the clinical description of the flatfoot presented in Figure 1. Rigidity of the subtalar complex differentiates a tarsal coalition from a flexible flatfoot, however. A longitudinal arch is not created with toe standing (Fig. 6) or by the Jack

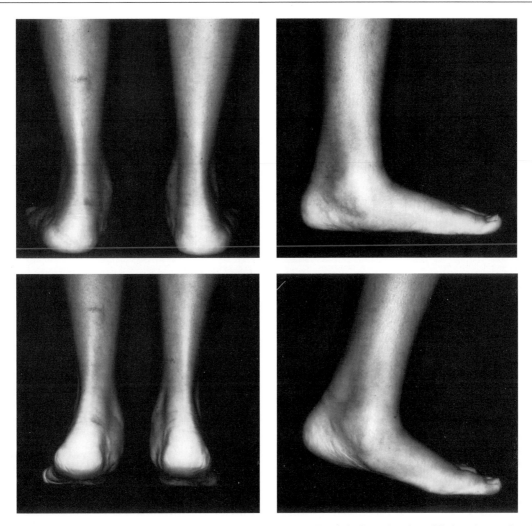

Fig. 6 Rigid flatfoot. There is no mobility (or flexibility) of the subtalar complex. **Top left,** Posterior view of flatfeet that are bearing full weight. **Top right,** Medial view of a flatfoot that is bearing full weight. **Bottom left** and **right,** There is no change in the appearance of the hindfoot or the longitudinal arch when standing on the toes because the subtalar complex is immobilized by a talocalcaneal coalition.

toe-raising test, particularly in the foot with a talocalcaneal coalition. There may be tenderness over the calcaneonavicular or talocalcaneal coalitions.

Proper radiographic evaluation includes standing anteroposterior, lateral, oblique, and axial (Harris) views. A calcaneonavicular coalition can best be seen on the oblique view (Fig. 7). A talocalcaneal coalition may be seen on the axial view, although proper orientation of the X-ray beam to produce a diagnostic image is often more a matter of luck than skill. Computed tomography (CT) images in the coronal plane, ie, perpendicular to the plantar aspect of the foot, will reliably demonstrate a talocalcaneal coalition (Fig. 8). Occasionally, a coalition will become symptomatic while it is still in the fibrous stage. In this situation, bone scintigraphy or magnetic resonance imaging (MRI) can be used to help confirm the diagnosis.

Treatment is indicated only for the symptomatic tarsal coalition. The first line of treatment is to try to convert the symptomatic coalition to an asymptomatic coalition, which is the type that exists in three of four people with this anatomic variation. Lasting pain relief has been reported in 30% to 68% of patients with talocalcaneal coalitions and in 58% of patients with calcaneonavicular coalitions who were treated by nonsurgical means, such as shoe inserts and one or sometimes two below-the-knee walking casts for 4 to 6 weeks each.

Surgical management is indicated for the symptomatic tarsal coalition that has failed legitimate attempts at nonsurgical treatment. The surgical options include resection of the coalition, osteotomy, and triple arthrodesis. Resection of calcaneonavicular coalitions was first reported in 1967, and extensor digitorum brevis interposition was

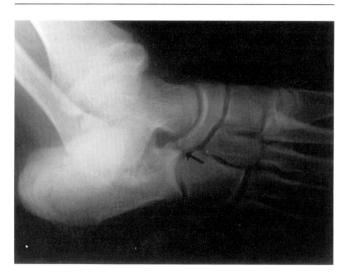

Fig. 7   Oblique radiograph of a foot with a cartilaginous calcaneonavicular coalition (arrow).

added to the procedure and reported on in 1970. The addition of extensor digitorum brevis interposition decreased the incidence of recurrence of the coalition and increased the incidence of long-term pain relief to 77% of patients. Presently, resection of a calcaneonavicular coalition with muscle interposition is indicated in a patient younger than 16 years of age who has a cartilaginous bar with no other coalitions present and no degenerative arthrosis, and who has undergone unsuccessful nonsurgical treatment. The presence of a talar beak is not indicative of degenerative

arthrosis and is not, by itself, a contraindication for resection.

The role of surgical resection of a talocalcaneal coalition remains less clear than that of a calcaneonavicular coalition. The talocalcaneal coalition is located on the tension side of the foot deformity, and progressive flattening of the arch may occur following resection. The foot with the talocalcaneal coalition also tends to be stiffer and flatter than the foot with a calcaneonavicular coalition. Nevertheless, more and more clinical studies on resection of a talocalcaneal coalition are appearing in the literature, with good-to-excellent short-term results reported in over 80% of feet. Surgical indications are similar to those for a calcaneonavicular coalition. A frequently quoted, but unproven, statement in the literature that a talocalcaneal coalition should not be resected if it occupies greater than one half of the width of the talocalcaneal joint surface has only recently been investigated. Wilde and associates reported unsatisfactory results of resection in feet in which the ratio of the surface area of the coalition to the surface area of the posterior facet was greater than 50%, as determined by CT scan mapping of the entire joint. All feet in the series in which the the ratio was greater than 50% also had excessive heel valgus, and many had mild narrowing of the posterior talocalcaneal joint and impingement of the lateral talar process on the calcaneus. Therefore, the independent influence of the size of the coalition remains unknown.

Documented degenerative arthrosis, particularly in adults, or persistent pain following resection of a coalition represent reasonable indications for a triple arthrodesis.

There are two additional surgical techniques that have been shown to relieve symptoms in feet with tarsal coalitions. These techniques are the medial closing wedge oste-

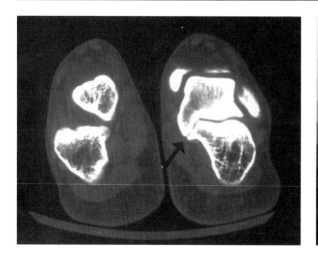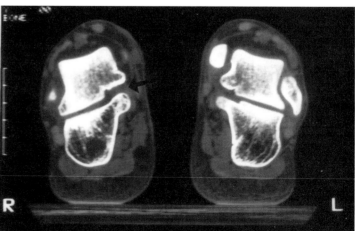

Fig. 8   **Left,** CT image of a foot with a talocalcaneal coalition of the middle facet of the subtalar joint (arrow). The facet joint is narrow, irregular, and down-sloping. **Right,** Appearance of a normal middle facet of a subtalar joint as seen on CT scan (arrow).

otomy of the posterior portion of the calcaneus, which improves the clinical alignment of the hindfoot, and the calcaneal lengthening osteotomy described by Evans, which corrects the valgus deformity of the subtalar complex. The respective roles of these procedures in the management of tarsal coalitions remains uncertain. These two procedures could be considered for the rigid flatfoot with severe valgus deformity, minimal degenerative arthrosis, and complete or nearly complete ossification of the coalition.

Annotated Bibliography

Flexible Flatfoot

Gould N, Moreland M, Alvarez R, et al: Development of the child's arch. *Foot Ankle* 1989;9:241–245.

This was a prospective, controlled clinical and radiographic study on the influence of external devices (shoes and orthoses) on the development of the longitudinal arch in children. The children, ages 11 months to 14 months at the time of enrollment, were divided into three study groups and one control group. At the end of the four-year study, neutral arches had developed regardless of the type of footwear worn, but had developed faster during the first 2 years with one type of arch support. Thereafter, arch development proceeded approximately equally regardless of the type of footwear worn.

Mosca VS: Calcaneal lengthening for valgus deformity of the hindfoot: Results in children who had severe, symptomatic flatfoot and skewfoot. *J Bone Joint Surg* 1995;77A:500–512.

A modification of the calcaneal lengthening osteotomy described by Evans corrected 31 severe, symptomatic valgus hindfoot deformities in 20 children with a variety of underlying medical conditions that were mostly neuromuscular. Only one foot deformity was a flexible flatfoot with a short Achilles tendon; however, the procedure was shown to effectively correct severe, intractably symptomatic valgus hindfoot deformity and eliminate the signs and symptoms associated with the deformity while avoiding arthrodesis.

Rao UB, Joseph B: The influence of footwear on the prevalence of flat foot: A survey of 2300 children. *J Bone Joint Surg* 1992;74B:525–527.

Screening in 6 schools in India occurred on one day in 1992 in order to obtain the footprints of 2,300 normal children ranging from 4 to 13 years of age. In the study, it was determined that if the width of the instep at the widest part was less than 1 cm (measured from the medial line of the footprint), the foot was considered to be a flatfoot. Approximately 30% of the children never wore shoes. In all age groups, flatfeet were more common in those children who wore shoes than in those who did not ($p < 0.001$).

Staheli LT, Chew DE, Corbett M: The longitudinal arch: A survey of eight hundred and eighty-two feet in normal children and adults. *J Bone Joint Surg* 1987;69A:426–428.

Footprints of 441 asymptomatic, normal subjects ranging from 1 year to 80 years of age were studied. The width of the footprint at the arch was divided by the width at the heel to determine the arch index. The values were plotted against the patients' ages on a chart. It was determined that there is a wide normal range of arch heights at all ages. Low arches are usual in infants, common in children, and within the normal range in adults. In the natural history of arch development, spontaneous elevation occurs during the first decade of life.

Theologis TN, Gordon C, Benson MK: Heel seats and shoe wear. *J Pediatr Orthop* 1994;14:760–762.

Helfet heel seats were used for 18 to 36 months in children with excessive heel valgus who ranged in age from 3 to 12 years. Shoe wear improved in 44 of 52 children. Six of the nine patients with pain reported improvement of their symptoms. Improvement in the height of the arch was not tested in this study. The authors acknowledged that previous studies had clearly shown that shoe inserts do not influence the natural history of arch development.

Vanderwilde R, Staheli LT, Chew DE, et al: Measurements on radiographs of the foot in normal infants and children. *J Bone Joint Surg* 1988;70A:407–415.

Weightbearing radiographs of 74 asymptomatic, normal subjects ranging in age from 6 to 127 months were studied. Means and standard deviations of 11 angles were determined. The range of normal values was wide for all angles at all ages. The angles reflected an increase in the height of the longitudinal arch with age.

Volpon JB: Footprint analysis during the growth period. *J Pediatr Orthop* 1994;14:83–85.

The length of the footprint and the medial longitudinal arch were evaluated in static footprints of 672 healthy white subjects ranging in age from newborn to 15 years. The author found that feet grew most rapidly up to 3 years of age, and then maintained an almost constant growth rate that was the same for both sexes until 12 years of age. At 12 years of age, girls' feet stopped growing, but boys' feet continued to grow. The author also found that flatfeet were common in infants. The arch developed spontaneously between 2 and 6 years of age in most children.

Wenger DR, Mauldin D, Speck G, et al: Corrective shoes and inserts as treatment for flexible flatfoot in infants and children. *J Bone Joint Surg* 1989;71A:800–810.

This was a prospective, controlled clinical and radiographic study on the influence of external devices (shoes and orthoses) on the development of the longitudinal arch in children. The children, enrolled between 1 and 6 years of age, were divided into three study groups and one control group. At the end of the three-year study, there was a significant improvement in the height of the arch in all groups, including the controls, and no significant difference between the controls and the treated groups.

Tarsal Coalition

Gonzalez P, Kumar SJ: Calcaneonavicular coalition treated by resection and interposition of the extensor digitorum brevis muscle. *J Bone Joint Surg* 1990;72A: 71–77.

Intermediate range follow-up of the results of this procedure demonstrated that 58 of 75 feet (77%) achieved good to excellent ratings. Three of the fair results improved to a good rating over time. The significance of the talar beak was not clear, as seven of 12 feet with this radiographic finding had good and excellent results following resection. The best results with this procedure are in patients with cartilaginous coalitions who undergo the operation before 16 years of age.

Grogan DP, Holt GR, Ogden JA: Talocalcaneal coalition in patients who have fibular hemimelia or proximal femoral focal deficiency: A comparison of the radiographic and pathological findings. *J Bone Joint Surg* 1994;76A:1363–1370.

Syme amputation specimens from 26 patients who had fibular hemimelia, proximal femoral focal deficieny (PFFD), or both conditions were analyzed anatomically. Talocalcaneal coalitions were found in 14 patients (54%)—one in nine patients who only had PFFD, six in eight patients who only had fibular hemimelia, and seven in nine patients who had both PFFD and fibular hemimelia. Only four talocalcaneal coalitions (15%) were identified on presurgical radiographs of these patients. Radiographic evaluation of 52 feet in 42 patients who had fibular hemimelia, PFFD, or both conditions revealed nine talocalcaneal coalitions (17%), a radiographic prevalence remarkably similar to that found in the anatomic study group. These 52 feet were not available for anatomic study. The prevalence of coalitions in these patients is underestimated by radiographs, particularly in young children.

Mosier KM, Asher M: Tarsal coalitions and peroneal spastic flat foot: A review. *J Bone Joint Surg* 1984; 66A:976–984.

This is an excellent review of all aspects of the subject, particularly pathomechanics. Conservative management should be used for all types of tarsal coalitions before resorting to surgical methods.

Moyes ST, Crawfurd EJ, Aichroth PM: The interposition of extensor digitorum brevis in the resection of calcaneonavicular bars. *J Pediatr Orthop* 1994;14:387–388.

Nine of ten feet that underwent resection of a symptomatic calcaneonavicular coalition with interposition of the extensor digitorum brevis became asymptomatic and mobile and showed no evidence of recurrence at a mean follow-up of 3.4 years. Three of seven feet in which the resection was not accompanied by extensor digitorum brevis interposition developed recurrence of the coalition in addition to pain and stiffness.

Munk PL, Vellet AD, Levin MF, et al: Current status of magnetic resonance imaging of the ankle and the hindfoot. *Can Assoc Radiol J* 1992;43:19–30.

Talocalcaneal tarsal coalitions are difficult to demonstrate by plain radiography. Conventional tomography, arthrography, and bone scanning are other imaging modalities that have been used to confirm that diagnosis. CT scanning has been shown to be superior to those other modalities for clearly identifying talocalcaneal coalitions. MRI also has the capability of demonstrating these coalitions three-dimensionally, non-invasively, without ionizing radiation, and can differentiate fibrous and cartilaginous coalitions.

Stuecker RD, Bennett JT: Tarsal coalition presenting as a pes cavo-varus deformity: Report of three cases and review of the literature. *Foot Ankle* 1993;14:540–544.

Three patients with tarsal coalitions and painful pes cavovarus are described. One of the patients had a calcaneonavicular coalition. Two of the patients had bilateral subtalar coalitions, of which only one was symptomatic in each patient. This is the first known report of an association between subtalar coalition and painful pes cavovarus. The calcaneonavicular coalition and one of the two symptomatic subtalar coalitions were treated by resection and muscle interposition. The other symptomatic subtalar coalition was treated by triple arthrodesis. Tarsal coalition should be considered in the differential diagnosis of progressive pes cavovarus along with neurologic etiologies.

Swiontkowski MF, Scranton PE, Hansen S: Tarsal coalitions: Long-term results of surgical treatment. *J Pediatr Orthop* 1983;3:287–292.

Thirteen talocalcaneal and 44 calcaneonavicular coalitions were treated by either resection, limited arthrodesis, or triple arthrodesis. The talar beak was carefully evaluated and believed to represent a talonavicular ligament traction spur related to increased stress at the talonavicular joint that was not necessarily associated with articular degeneration. Poor results were related to true degeneration of the talonavicular joint.

Takakura Y, Sugimoto K, Tanaka Y, et al: Symptomatic talocalcaneal coalition: Its clinical significance and treatment. *Clin Orthop* 1991;269:249–256.

A bony eminence was noted along the medial foot in the region of the sustentaculum tali in all 67 feet of 42 patients with talocalcaneal coalitions. A positive Tinel's sign over the eminence was found in 34% of the feet. A sensory disturbance on the sole of the foot consistent with a tarsal tunnel syndrome was seen in 25% of the feet. Conservative management in 31 feet resulted in 68% good and excellent results when evaluated at 5 years follow-up. Simple excision of the coalition in children and adolescents resulted in good and excellent results in 31 of 33 feet (94%) at 5.3-years average follow-up.

Wilde PH, Torode IP, Dickens DR, et al: Resection for symptomatic talocalcaneal coalition. *J Bone Joint Surg* 1994;76B:797–801.

Symptomatic talocalcaneal coalitions in 20 feet were treated by resection of the coalition. At short-term follow-up, excellent or good results were achieved in the ten feet in which the presurgical coronal CT had shown that the area of the coalition measured 50% or less of the area of the posterior facet of the calcaneus. These feet also demonstrated heel valgus of less than 16° and no radiographic signs of arthritis of the posterior talocalcaneal joint. Talar beaks were present in seven feet but did not impair the clinical result. Each of the ten feet that had a fair or poor result had a CT area of relative coalition greater than 50% and heel valgus greater than 16°.

26

Miscellaneous Foot Disorders

Bunions in Juveniles and Adolescents

A bunion is a mass, enlargement, or deformity at the first metatarsophalangeal joint. Hallux valgus is a deformity of the first metatarsophalangeal joint in which there is more than 20° of valgus angulation between the proximal phalanx and the first metatarsal. A varus angulation of the first metatarsocuneiform joint is usually present with hallux valgus. Associated deformities may include hallux rigidus, which is a limitation of dorsiflexion of the first metatarsophalangeal joint; pes plano valgus, often with a shortened Achilles tendon; metatarsus primus adductus; pronation of the large toe; subluxation of the first metatarsophalangeal joint; and hallux valgus interphalangeus.

The etiology of the bunion is multifactorial. Nearly 40 years ago, improperly fitting shoe wear was shown to be a contributing factor in the development of hallux valgus. An inheritance pattern, ligamentous laxity, pes planus, pronation of the hallux, and spasticity (cerebral palsy) have also been implicated as causative factors. The shape and alignment of the first metatarsophalangeal joint and the metatarsocuneiform joint may predispose the patient to the development of bunions and may complicate surgical management.

The incidence of bunions in adolescents is not known, partly because of its variable severity and the frequent lack of symptoms in those with mild deformities. When bunions occur, it is often in early adolescence. The onset often coincides with the wearing of stylish shoes that are too narrow. Progression of the deformity through adolescence, as well as recurrence following surgery, may be related to persistent ligamentous laxity and continued angular growth in the child's foot. Degenerative changes are rarely present in the adolescent. Although no sexual predilection has been documented, females undergo surgical correction more often than males. Deformities in adults in whom the onset of bunions occurred during adolescence are more difficult to correct surgically and are likely to have a higher recurrence rate.

The patient's complaints must be carefully assessed. The patient may be unable to find comfortable shoes, be displeased with the appearance of his or her feet, prefer to wear narrow or normal width shoes, or complain of pain. Pain in the metatarsal region (metatarsalgia) should be localized to the bunion, first metatarsophalangeal joint, or the metatarsal head. Other causes of pain, such as plantar fascia, hammertoes, first metatarsal stress fracture, ingrown toenail, accessory tarsal navicular, or sesamoiditis, should be ruled out first as the source of pain. The proper shoe fit can be assessed and demonstrated to the patient by tracing the patient's bare foot while weightbearing and matching the tracing to an outline of the patient's shoe.

The proper clinical evaluation of the condition includes assessment of not only the foot but of angular and rotational alignment, joint range of motion, and sensation of the entire lower extremity.

Proper radiographic assessment requires weightbearing anteroposterior (AP) and lateral views of both feet. The angles between the first and second metatarsals (normal range, 6° to 10°), first metatarsophalangeal joint (normal range, 10° to 20°), and cuneiform–first metatarsal joint should be measured. The shape, congruity, and orientation of these joints should be assessed. A bunion in the adolescent is present if the intermetatarsal angle between the first and second metatarsals exceeds 10° associated with hallux valgus greater than 20°.

Treatment of bunions in the adolescent can be difficult. Attempts to realign the great toe will not correct any underlying ligamentous laxity or generalized splayed foot. The orthopaedist, patient, and patient's parents must have a good understanding of the treatment options and the limitations of surgical correction. Surgery will not convert a wide, lax foot into a foot that will fit into a narrower, more attractive shoe. The painless wide foot should not be surgically changed into a stiff, painful foot in order to remove an unsightly bump. Surgical correction should be reserved for those patients with pain that regularly interferes with normal activities and who cannot find relief in shoe modification.

There are several shoe modifications that may lead to improved comfort and allow the patient to return to more normal activities, including sports. These modifications include wider shoes, bunion lasts, soft uppers, and metatarsal bars. Night splints have been reported to improve the alignment in 50% of patients surveyed. However, a recent study reported no benefit from orthotic use. In a survey of 6,000 children between the ages of 9 and 10 years of age, Kilmartin identified 122 children with unilateral or bilateral hallux valgus. Each child was then randomly assigned to one of two groups: observation only or treatment with foot orthoses. Radiographic follow-up of 93 children was obtained nearly 3 years later. The children treated with orthoses had a greater increase in the hallux valgus deformity than those children who were observed only.

Surgical correction should be postponed until skeletal maturity because of the high recurrence rates of bunions in young adolescent patients. Other surgical risks include physeal damage, shortening of the first metatarsal head, first metatarsophalangeal joint stiffness and pain, and the inability to return to sporting activities. Canale reviewed

30 adolescent patients treated with 51 Mitchell procedures to correct hallux valgus deformities. This study suggested that inadequate correction and/or fixation led to compromised results, as approximately 30% of the patients were rated fair to poor. Of 44 feet that underwent surgery for pain, 34% were still painful at the final follow-up.

Although the chevron, Mitchell, and other distal osteotomies have been performed in adolescents, the splaying of the first and second metatarsals (often more than 25°) is best managed by proximal first metatarsal osteotomy and distal soft-tissue realignment. A crescentic proximal metatarsal osteotomy may minimize shortening of the metatarsal. First metatarsophalangeal and medial cuneiform-metatarsal alignment and joint congruency must be carefully reviewed when planning osteotomies.

In a recent study, Peterson and Newman reported on their experience with 15 adolescent patients treated by double osteotomy of the first metatarsal. In all cases, indications for surgery included pain and difficulty wearing shoes. The authors reported that there was no loss of motion in the first metatarsophalangeal joint because the operation does not violate that joint.

Accessory Tarsal Navicular

An accessory tarsal navicular is a congenital enlargement of the medial tarsal navicular. Two types of accessory navicular have been described: type I is a small separate round or oval bone (possibly a sesamoid in the tibialis posterior) and type II is a large tuberosity at the medial aspect of the navicular that is either fused to the navicular or connected to it through a fibrocartilaginous plate (Fig. 1).

The incidence of accessory navicular has been reported to be as high as 10% to 14%. An association between the symptomatic accessory navicular and flexible flatfoot remains controversial. In 1929, Kidner, who believed that the posterior tibialis tendon abnormally inserted into the accessory navicular compromised its ability to support the arch, recommended that in addition to excision of the accessory navicular, the posterior tibialis tendon should be advanced and redirected to support the arch. Other researchers have not been able to document any improvement in the arch following Kidner's procedure when the procedure was compared with simple excision of the accessory bone. Macnicol concluded that advancement of the posterior tibialis tendon had no effect on the arch or the clinical outcome.

The majority of accessory naviculars are asymptomatic and are frequently bilateral. The most common finding upon presentation is intermittent tenderness directly over the accessory navicular prominence (with a time of onset between the ages of 8 and 14 years). A history of minor trauma is common. Careful examination can distinguish the painful accessory navicular from other painful areas along the medial aspect of the foot, such as painful sesamoids, stress fractures of the first metatarsal or tarsals, posterior tibial tendinitis, tarsal coalition, tarsal

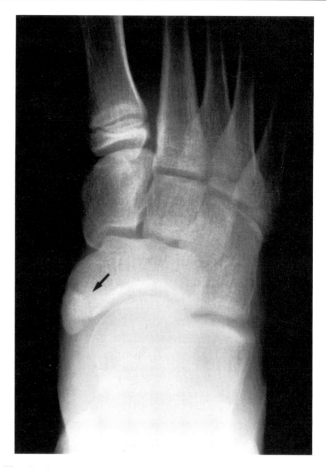

Fig. 1 Accessory tarsal navicular.

tunnel syndrome, plantar fasciitis, synovitis, arthritis, and tumors.

Standing AP and lateral and, occasionally, oblique radiographs of the foot will usually demonstrate the accessory naviculars and confirm the clinical diagnosis. In the very young child a mass may be palpable clinically but may not be seen on the radiograph because the navicular is not yet ossified.

Initial treatment of an accessory tarsal navicular consists of shoe adjustments that are made to avoid pressure on the tender prominence and reduction of sports activities. Many young athletes are unwilling to reduce their activities; therefore, use of arch supports to limit pronation onto the painful prominence of the accessory navicular may be useful. The patient may try using below-the-knee walking casts and temporary partial weightbearing with crutches to allow the symptoms to improve. One corticosteroid injection may be considered. Unfortunately, returning to sports activities too soon may result in recurrence of symptoms, particularly in the highly motivated athlete. At least 6 months of nonsurgical treatment should be provided before surgical intervention is considered.

When symptoms persist, surgical options can be considered. A simple excision of the accessory navicular is recommended. Advancement of the tibialis posterior has not been shown to improve the results. In a recent report of simple excisions on 75 feet, the results were excellent and good in 90%. Complete removal of the medial prominence was recommended because complaints persisted in six patients who had residual medial prominence. Surgical removal of an asymptomatic accessory navicular is unnecessary.

Congenital Vertical Talus

A vertical talus is a fixed congenital dorsolateral dislocation of the talonavicular joint. The term is descriptive of the radiographic appearance of the plantarflexed or vertical posture of the talus that results when the dorsally dislocated navicular presses downward on the talar neck. Clinically, the foot is deformed in a rocker bottom flatfoot or convex valgus alignment (also called congenital convex pes valgus) in which the heel is fixed in an equinovalgus position, the midfoot in valgus position, and the forefoot is dorsiflexed on the midfoot. The Achilles tendon, peroneal tendons, and anterior ankle tendons are contracted. The talar head is prominent in the medial aspect of the foot and can easily be felt.

This infrequent congenital deformity may be idiopathic or inherited. It is associated with arthrogryposis multiplex congenital syndrome, neurofibromatosis, and nail patella syndrome; chromosomal anomalies, trisomy 13–15 and 19; and neurologic conditions, such as myelomeningocele, tethered cord, lipoma of the cord, and sacral agenesis. Hip dysplasia and contralateral clubfeet have been identified in patients with this disorder. These syndromes and associated anomalies should be sought in all cases. The inability to correct (with or without surgery) causes of neuromuscular imbalance may result in recurrence of deformity.

It is likely that a neuromuscular imbalance leads to contracture of the posterior (gastrocnemius-soleus complex), lateral (peroneus longus and brevis), and anterior (tibialis, extensor digitorum longus, and extensor hallucis, and possibly the peroneus tertius) muscles. In utero, the talonavicular joint dislocates dorsolaterally, forcing the navicular to rest on the dorsolateral talar neck and subsequently plantarflexing the talus in the mortise. The os calcis is laterally rotated under the talus. The lateral column of the foot is deformed into valgus position with various amounts of bony deformity present.

The differential diagnosis includes calcaneovalgus foot, flexible flatfoot with midfoot sag and short Achilles tendon, the rigid flatfoot associated with tarsal coalition and peroneal spasticity, and the young ligamentous lax flatfoot. Only the true vertical talus deformity has the four fixed components: hindfoot equinovalgus, midfoot valgus, forefoot dorsiflexion, and dislocation of the talonavicular joint.

The diagnosis can be confirmed radiographically with three views: AP, dorsiflexed lateral, and plantarflexed lateral (Fig. 2). The AP view demonstrates the midfoot valgus and increased talocalcaneal angle. The dorsiflexed lateral view demonstrates the dislocation of the navicular on the talar neck, as well as the fixed equinus position of the hindfoot. The increased talocalcaneal angle confirms the hindfoot valgus. The plantarflexed lateral view demonstrates that the talonavicular dislocation is not reducible; a line drawn through the long axis of the talus and another drawn through the first metatarsal will not meet in front of the talar head. In the infant, only metatarsals, the talus, and the calcaneus are likely to be ossified. Drawing lines through these three bones on the radiograph will still confirm the diagnosis.

While this deformity may produce few problems in shoe wear or ambulation in the very young child, the older child will develop a painful callus over the weightbearing talar head, have difficulty with shoe fit, and have degenerative arthritis and pain at the dislocated talonavicular joint. Surgical options are limited in the older child.

Stretching exercises and serial casting may be partially successful when used to lengthen the contracted tendons, but they will not help reduce the talonavicular dislocation. Surgical correction must reduce the talonavicular dislocation, derotate the subtalar joint, and lengthen the contracted posterior, lateral, and dorsal muscles and subtalar (talocalcaneal and talonavicular) capsules and ligaments. Failure to release the soft tissues may lead to compression and subsequent osteonecrosis and growth disturbance of the talus and navicular. The Cincinnati incision allows sufficient exposure to accomplish a complete release. K-wire fixation will hold the reduction in place. Postoperative casting for 3 months is recommended. Residual or untreated deformity of the vertical talus in the older child may be salvaged by resection arthrodesis or talectomy, which may produce a plantigrade but short, wide, and stiff foot.

Sever's Disease

Sever's disease, an apophysitis of the skeletally immature calcaneus, may account for heel pain in the adolescent. The radiographic appearance is one of sclerosis and fragmentation of the calcaneal apophysis. This finding also has been observed commonly in normal asymptomatic individuals.

Typically, the presenting findings of calcaneal apophysitis include a history of chronic, intermittent pain related to sports, pain located along the calcaneal apophysis medially and usually plantarly, and a history of running in hard heels or on concrete surfaces. Swelling medially about the heel may be evident.

Standing AP and lateral, oblique, and Harris view radiographs should be obtained to rule out other abnormalities, such as a bone cyst or stress fracture.

Although calcaneal apophysitis is common, other conditions also may lead to foot pain. These include Achilles

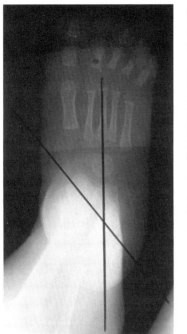 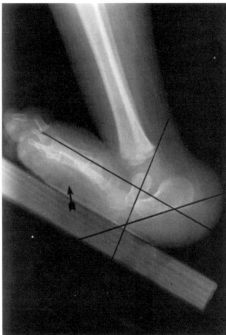 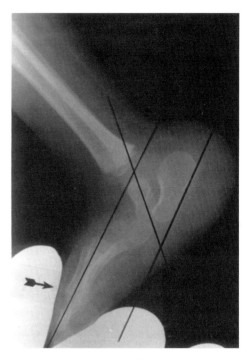

Fig. 2 Congenital vertical talus. **Left,** On the AP radiograph, the angle between the talus and calcaneus is increased. **Center,** On the dorsiflexion stressed lateral radiograph, the calcaneus remains in the equinus position. **Right,** On the plantarflexion stressed lateral radiograph, the forefoot remains dorsally dislocated on the talus (the talar line and first metatarsal line should be parallel upon each other).

tendinitis, stress fracture of the os calcis, plantar fasciitis, entrapment of the calcaneal or plantar nerves, medial facet talocalcaneal coalitions, accessory navicular, and, infrequently, cysts and tumors.

Treatment of calcaneal apophysitis should begin with a period of ice, rest, and limitation of activities. Footwear can be modified to include padding and, when appropriate, arch supports to limit pronation. Cast immobilization may be considered for symptom relief. Fortunately, the problem is limited to those who are skeletally immature. Surgical intervention is not indicated.

Freiberg's Infraction

Freiberg's infraction is an osteochondrosis of the second or, less commonly, third metatarsal head and is typically seen in healthy, often athletic, adolescent females aged 10 to 18 years. It can occur bilaterally. Typically, the patient develops vague pain, swelling, and loss of motion of the involved metatarsophalangeal joint following increased activity. Over time, the symptoms may be present with limited activities, such as walking.

The exact etiology of Freiberg's infraction is not known. Theories include acute trauma, repetitive trauma, and vas-

cular insufficiency. Surgical findings have included synovitis, inflammation, loose bodies of cartilage and bone, and osteophytes. Necrotic bone is often observed histologically. Clinically, the differential includes two other entities: metatarsalgia and stress fracture.

An AP radiograph of the forefoot may demonstrate varying degrees of involvement. In the earliest stages, the radiographs are usually normal although bone scan, especially pinhole collimation, may reveal abnormal vascularization. Osteopenia may be present. In more advanced stages of disease, a subchondral fracture may be evident with joint widening, sclerosis, and flattening of the metatarsal head. Collapse, fragmentation, osteophytes, revascularization, and healing may be evident with even further disease progression. Degenerative arthrosis may ensue.

Nonsurgical treatment appears to be most effective in the early stages of Freiberg's infraction. Treatment includes a reduction of activities, shoe modification using stiff rocker soles or metatarsal bars, cast immobilization, avoidance of weightbearing, and judicious use of corticosteroids. Return to regular sports activities should be gradual. It may be months or years before pain-free activity can be resumed.

Surgical intervention is rarely necessary. Potential surgical procedures include joint debridement, partial or complete metatarsal head excision, joint replacement, excision of the proximal portion of the proximal phalanx, shortening osteotomy of the metatarsal, replacement and pinning of large fragments, and metatarsal neck osteotomy to redirect the articular surface. Although most reports have claimed success with any of these treatments, study size has been small and studies have not been comparative. Joint debridement and partial metatarsal head resection are more likely to be successful in less involved cases.

Cavus Feet

A cavus foot is a deformed foot with an excessively high arch. Anatomically, the deformity can be caused by problems in the forefoot, such as plantarflexion of the first metatarsal, pronation of the forefoot, or clawing of the toes; midfoot, such as contracture of the plantarfascia or plantarflexion of the talonavicular or naviculocuneiform joints; and hindfoot, such as heel varus or calcaneus deformity. Additionally, fixed deformity in the forefoot can cause abnormal posture in the hindfoot during weightbearing. For example, the fixed plantarflexion of the first metatarsal will invert the heel in stance if the subtalar joint is flexible.

Neurologic etiologies of cavus feet include hereditary motor and sensory neuropathies, such as Charcot-Marie-Tooth, Dejerine-Sottas, and Refsum diseases; cord anomalies including spina bifida, tethered cord, and lipoma of the cord; and polio. Many of these conditions progress in their neuromuscular involvement and lead to progressive foot deformity. Spinal cord anomalies may often lead to unilateral involvement; neuropathies lead to symmetrical deformities.

The various causes of cavus or cavovarus feet mandate that the patient undergo a complete physical examination. The foot is evaluated in stance and in the nonweightbearing position, and the forefoot, midfoot, and hindfoot are then evaluated separately. Coleman's lateral block test is useful to differentiate rigid hindfoot varus from flexible hindfoot varus. This differentiation is important because it affects the extent of surgical treatment required to correct the deformity.

Standing AP and lateral radiographs demonstrate the deformity (Fig. 3). Hindfoot talocalcaneal and first metatarsal–talus angles are measured on the lateral projection. The first metatarsal–talus angle, which is normally 0°, will increase as a cavus deformity worsens.

Correct diagnosis of the patient's condition is extremely important in order to initiate appropriate treatment. For example, an individual whose foot deformity is a result of a tethered spinal cord must have the tethered cord released prior to correction of the foot. Many patients with cavus feet recreationally participate in sports in spite of cavovarus deformities. Shoe modifications can accommodate claw toes, forefoot pronation, metatarsalgia, high instep,

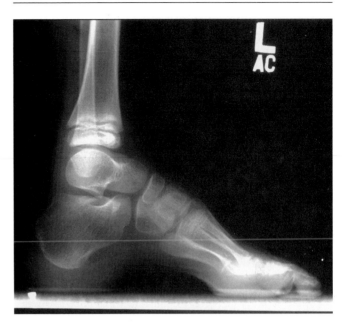

Fig. 3   The cavus foot has an exaggerated arch on the standing lateral radiograph.

and heel varus. Stretching exercises may be beneficial and molded ankle-foot orthoses may allow for recreational sports participation throughout the school years. Unfortunately, many of these patients will not return to sports after osteotomy or arthrodesis.

Soft-tissue releases, such as plantar fascia, intrinsic muscles, and peroneus longus, and tendon transfer of the posterior tibialis to the dorsum of the foot may improve the flexible foot. The transferred posterior tibialis may eventually be weakened by the disease process, limiting the benefit of the transfer.

Osteotomy and/or arthrodesis may be required to correct the rigid mature deformities. Commonly employed osteotomies include dorsal closing wedge osteotomy of the first or, infrequently, all the metatarsals; tarsometatarsal wedge osteotomies; and valgus, posterior, and/or lateral sliding osteotomies of the os calcis. Soft-tissue release prior to osteotomy and arthrodesis will reduce the amount of bony correction that is needed. Arthrodesis should only be used to correct severe deformity because loss of joint motion may transfer stresses to adjacent joints and lead to subsequent degenerative changes.

Persistent neuromuscular imbalance and/or progression of the disease process may lead to a recurrence of deformity despite properly performed surgery early in the course of the disease. An understanding that the disease and associated deformities are progressive and that the patient's needs will change with time may reduce the patient's disappointment with the long-term outcome.

Annotated Bibliography

Bunions in Juveniles and Adolescents

Canale PB, Aronsson DD, Lamont RL, et al: The Mitchell procedure for the treatment of adolescent hallux valgus: A long-term study. *J Bone Joint Surg* 1993;75A: 1610–1618.

Thirty patients who as adolescents had had a total of 51 Mitchell procedures to correct hallux valgus deformities were examined. The average age of the patients at the time of the operation was 15 years. Results were excellent in 19 feet, good in 16, fair in six, and poor in ten. A plantar callosity beneath the second metatarsal head in 17 feet suggested increased loadbearing by the second metatarsal.

Coughlin MJ, Mann RA: The pathophysiology of the juvenile bunion, in Griffin PP (ed): *Instructional Course Lectures XXXVI*. Park Ridge, IL, American Academy of Orthopaedic Surgeons, 1987, pp 123–136.

The authors thoroughly review the history and understanding of the pathophysiology of the bunion in juveniles.

Kilmartin TE, Wallace WA: The significance of pes planus in juvenile hallux valgus. *Foot Ankle* 1992;13:53–56.

This study compares the degree of pes planus in normal and hallux valgus feet. An unpaired *t*-test determined that there was no significant difference between the arch index of 32 11-year-old children with hallux valgus and 32 11-year-olds with no first metatarsophalangeal joint deformity ($p > 0.05$). The height of the arch is not relevant to the hallux valgus deformity. Arch supports designed to raise the height of the arch can play a palliative role in the management of the condition.

Kilmartin TE, Barrington RL, Wallace WA: A controlled prospective trial of a foot orthosis for juvenile hallux valgus. *J Bone Joint Surg* 1994;76B:210–214.

In a survey of 6,000 children between 9 and 10 years of age, 122 were found to have unilateral or bilateral hallux valgus. These children were randomly assigned to observation only or the use of a foot orthosis. About 3 years later, 93 children underwent radiography again. The metatarsophalangeal joint angle had increased in both groups but more so in the group treated with orthoses. During the study, hallux valgus developed in the unaffected feet of children with unilateral deformity, despite the use of the orthosis.

Mann RA: Decision-making in bunion surgery, in Greene WB (ed): *Instructional Course Lectures XXXIX*. Park Ridge, IL, American Academy of Orthopaedic Surgeons, 1990, pp 3–13.

This article is an excellent overview of the approach to bunion surgery on children and adolescents.

Peterson HA, Newman SR: Adolescent bunion deformity treated with double osteotomy and longitudinal pin fixation of the first ray. *J Pediatr Orthop* 1993;13:80–84.

Double osteotomy and longitudinal pin fixation of the first ray was performed on 15 feet. This procedure is technically easy, provides excellent correction and stability, and has a low rate of recurrence of deformity. The operation is indicated for severe deformities and should be applicable to adults.

Accessory Tarsal Navicular

Bennett GL, Weiner DS, Leighley B: Surgical treatment of symptomatic accessory tarsal navicular. *J Pediatr Orthop* 1990;10:445–449.

In a retrospective review of 75 feet with accessory tarsal naviculars treated by excision of the accessory tarsal navicular, the authors found 90% good and excellent results without altering the course of the tibialis posterior tendon.

Macnicol MF, Voutsinas S: Surgical treatment of the symptomatic accessory navicular. *J Bone Joint Surg* 1984;66B:218–226.

The authors compared 26 patients treated by the Kidner operation with 21 patients in which the accessory navicular ossicle was excised. The authors concluded that the excision was as effective as the Kidner technique, provided that the prominence was completely removed. Additionally, they believed that correction of the flatfoot was secondary to growth and maturation of the foot rather than to the Kidner operation.

Congenital Vertical Talus

Schrader LF, Gilbert RJ, Skinner SR, et al: Congenital vertical talus: Surgical correction by a one-stage medial approach. *Orthopedics* 1990;13:1233–1236.

The authors describe their experience with 14 feet with a single stage medial approach to the congenital vertical talus. In this procedure, they released the posterior ankle, posterior and medial subtalar joint, as well as the talotibial capsule anteriorly. The Achilles tendon is lengthened. Results were rated as excellent in one foot, good in 11 feet, and poor in two feet.

Wirth T, Schuler P, Griss P: Early surgical treatment for congenital vertical talus. *Arch Orthop Trauma Surg* 1994;113:248–253.

The authors review their experience with 13 feet with congenital vertical talus. Excellent results were reported in ten out of 13 children with a one-stage operation that reduced the talonavicular joint and corrected the hindfoot equinus while trying to avoid tendon lengthenings and transfers. Follow-up averaged 3.5 years.

Freiberg's Infraction

Katcherian DA: Treatment of Freiberg's disease. *Orthop Clin North Am* 1994;25:69–81.

This is a detailed review of Freiberg's infraction and its treatment stages.

Kinnard P, Lirette R: Freiberg's disease and dorsiflexion osteotomy. *J Bone Joint Surg* 1991;73B:864–865.

Intra-articular dorsal wedge osteotomy through the distal metaphysis with sufficient bone removal to bring the healthy plantar part of the metatarsal head into articulation with the phalanx was performed on 15 patients. Advanced disease was present in nine patients. The authors reported that all of the patients were able to return to sports, although three had mild discomfort after prolonged jogging. Although the authors observed about 2.5 mm of shortening, the technique appears to restore congruity of the joint.

Smith TW, Stanley D, Rowley DI: Treatment of Freiberg's disease: A new operative technique. *J Bone Joint Surg* 1991;73B:129–130.

The authors discuss metatarsal shaft shortening (4 mm) in 15 patients (16 feet) and the application of a "T" plate. The plate was removed after 12 months. Pain was relieved within 12 months (mean 5 to 7 months) in all but one patient. Swelling was improved in four patients and stiffness was observed in seven of the 16 feet postoperatively. In four feet the toe did not contact the ground in stance. Results were assessed as excellent in five patients; nine were pleased with the results.

Sproul J, Klaaren H, Mannarino F: Surgical treatment of Freiberg's infraction in athletes. *Am J Sport Med* 1993;21:381–384.

The authors reviewed 11 cases of Freiberg's infraction in athletes. All patients underwent debridement and all were reported to have had improvement in symptoms with 80% normal range of motion. Nine of ten patients returned to presurgical sports activities.

Cavus Feet

Alexander IJ, Johnson KA: Assessment and management of pes cavus in Charcot-Marie-Tooth disease. *Clin Orthop* 1989;246:273–281.

In this article, the authors thoroughly reviewed assessment and management of pes cavus in Charcot-Marie-Tooth disease.

Watanabe RS: Metatarsal osteotomy for the cavus foot. *Clin Orthop* 1990;252:217–230.

The authors reviewed their experience with 39 patients with pes cavus deformities treated by plantar fasciotomy and proximal dorsal closing wedge osteotomies of all five metatarsals. An appropriate lateral wedge was removed as needed to correct varus deformity of the mid- or forefoot. Good or excellent results were reported in 84% of patients.

Wukich DK, Bowen JR: A long-term study of triple arthrodesis for correction of pes cavovarus in Charcot-Marie-Tooth disease. *J Pediatr Orthop* 1989;9:433–437.

The authors review their long-term (12-year follow-up) experience with triple arthrodesis for cavovarus in Charcot-Marie-Tooth disease. Radiographic evidence of degenerative joint disease was observed.

IV
Trauma

Paul D. Sponseller, MD
Section Editor

27

Femur Fractures

Introduction

The treatment of femur fractures is changing. For some fractures, closed management is evolving toward interventional approaches to minimize sequelae. The orthopaedist must consider the potential short- and long-term problems related to each fracture. With the availability of viable treatment options, the risks and benefits of the individual treatment modalities are becoming more obvious. No longer is one method of management applicable for all of these injuries.

Hip Fractures

Hip fractures in children historically have accounted for less than 1% of all pediatric fractures. Unlike the adult with osteporosis, hip fractures in the pediatric age group are typically associated with high energy trauma unless there is an underlying pathologic process (eg, solitary bone cyst, fibrous dysplasia). Hip fractures in the skeletally immature population have sequelae in about 60% of the patients.

The proximal femur begins as a single physis separating into two separate centers of ossification—the capital epiphysis with its physis and the trochanteric apophysis. At birth, the blood supply to the femoral head is from metaphyseal vessels traversing the neck, which are derived from the medial and lateral circumflex arteries. As the subcapital physis develops, these metaphyseal vessels no longer significantly penetrate the femoral head. By the age of 4 years, the contribution of these vessels to the blood supply is negligible. At this time, the posterosuperior and posteroinferior retinacular systems derived from the medial circumflex artery provide the major blood supply to the femoral head. The physeal anatomy and the blood supply to the proximal femur explain the high incidence of problems following fractures of the hip in children.

The classification system of Delbet reported by Colonna in 1929 is still used. A type I fracture is a transepiphyseal separation with or without dislocation of the femoral head from the acetabulum. A type II injury is a transcervical fracture. A type III injury is a cervicotrochanteric fracture. The type IV fracture is at the intertrochanteric level (Fig. 1).

Type I fractures are the least common of these injuries and tend to occur in younger children compared to types II, III, and IV entities. Almost half of these transepiphyseal separations have dislocation of the capital femoral epiphysis. With dislocation of the femoral head, the rate

of osteonecrosis approaches 100%. As for all femoral neck fractures in children, the initial displacement seems to most directly affect the risk of osteonecrosis.

Treatment of type I injuries should consist of an attempt at closed reduction for partially displaced fractures using longitudinal traction, abduction, and internal rotation, followed by pin fixation. In patients younger than 2 years of age, the reduction may be relatively stable. Spica cast treatment alone can sometimes be used in this age group. If there is any doubt about stability, however, internal fixation should be used. If closed reduction is unsuccessful, open reduction will be necessary. For fractures with posterior dislocation of the capital epiphysis, the dislocation should be approached posteriorly. Conversely, if the dislocation is anterior, the anterior or anterolateral approaches

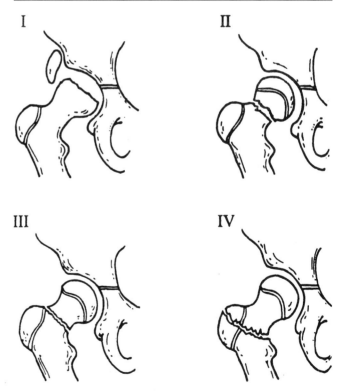

Fig. 1 The hip fracture classification system of Delbet for children. Type I is a transepiphyseal separation with or without dislocation of the head from the acetabulum. Type II is a transcervical fracture. Type III is a cervicotrochanteric fracture. Type IV is an intertrochanteric fracture. (Reproduced with permission from Hughes LO, Beaty JH: Fractures of the head and neck of the femur in children. *J Bone Joint Surg* 1994;76A:283–292.)

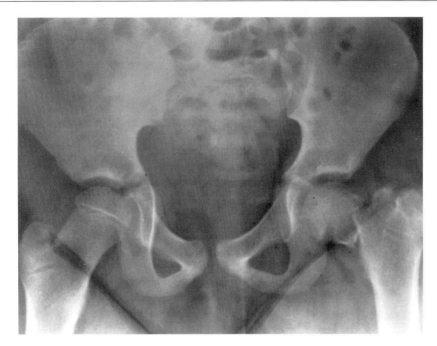 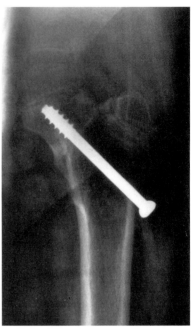

Fig. 2 **Left,** Radiograph showing a type III femoral neck fracture. **Right,** This fracture was manipulated with traction and abduction on the fracture table and a percutaneous 4-mm screw was placed. The patient was placed in a spica cast with the hip and knee in extension. There is residual medial translation of the proximal fragment that potentially could have led to varus angulation. This patient went on to uneventful healing.

should be used. CT can be helpful in visualizing the location of the femoral head dislocation.

In a type I fracture, internal fixation can be accomplished either with pins or screws that, by necessity, must cross the physis. In the young child, smooth pins across the physis should be used, followed by a spica cast. Some have advocated threaded pins or screws in children older than 9 years of age; however, chronologic age and skeletal maturity do not always correlate. The capital epiphysis contributes about 15% of the total length of the extremity. Obviously, premature physeal closure in the older patient nearing skeletal maturity is less significant than in the younger child. Both skeletal maturity and gender (females typically complete skeletal growth sooner than males) should be a consideration for smooth versus threaded fixation.

Proximal femoral epiphysiolysis can occur in the newborn. In this age group, the capital femoral epiphyseal separation typically follows a breech delivery with a clinical appearance of "pseudoparalysis" of the limb. The differential diagnosis includes infection and developmental dislocation of the hip. Aspiration of the hip and arthrogram are of benefit here. If recognized initially, skin traction should be used to restore alignment. If recognized after callus formation is visible radiographically, simple immobilization alone is used. Open surgical reduction is not advocated for these injuries. These epiphyseal separations in

the newborn tend to remodel if the physis does not close prematurely, so observation after healing is warranted.

Type II (transcervical) fractures are the most common of the neck fractures in children. Most are displaced. Osteonecrosis occurs in about 50%. Fractures that are displaced have a higher risk for osteonecrosis than nondisplaced injuries.

Type III (cervicotrochanteric) fractures are the second most common of the pediatric hip fractures. Osteonecrosis occurs in about 25% of these injuries. Again, displacement of the fracture increases the risk of this sequela.

Treatment of type II and type III fractures is aimed at achieving anatomic reduction either by closed or open means. If open reduction is needed, a capsulotomy should be done anteriorly because of the proximal femur's blood supply. If possible, the internal fixation should stop short of the physis; however, at times it is necessary to cross the physis to achieve stability. If the physis can be avoided, screw fixation here is desirable. Cannulated 4.0- to 4.5-mm screws can often be used in children, and the cannulated 6.5- to 7.0-mm screws for older children and teenagers. After reduction and internal fixation, a spica cast is generally used for those patients who have not yet reached adolescence. In these younger patients, the smaller diameter of the femoral neck limits the size and number of screws that can be placed (Fig. 2).

Nondisplaced type II and III fractures have been

treated with cast immobilization alone. Close follow-up is mandatory if this method is chosen because of the potential for loss of reduction, producing coxa vara. In general, internal fixation is recommended for most of these nondisplaced injuries, in order to decrease the risk of displacement and coxa vara.

Type IV (intertrochanteric) fractures have a lower incidence of sequelae than the femoral neck fractures. These can be treated with traction followed by a spica cast with the leg abducted. If reduction cannot be accomplished by closed means, open reduction and internal fixation should be used to prevent varus malunion. In children older than 8 years of age and in multitrauma patients, surgical intervention should be considered initially. Screw and side plate combinations are available in pediatric sizes, and the screw fixation should stop short of the physis, if possible.

Complications of Hip Fractures

Osteonecrosis remains the most serious of the complications following hip fractures in children. Both fracture types (type I and type II fractures) as well as age (older than 10 years) are associated with an increase in the risk of osteonecrosis. Evacuation or aspiration of the hematoma has been recommended by some; however, the type of treatment does not seem to affect the rate of osteonecrosis. This leaves the value of evacuation of the hematoma unproved. The factor most correlated with osteonecrosis in the literature is the initial displacement of the fracture.

Ratliff has described three patterns of osteonecrosis following hip fractures in children. Type I osteonecrosis involves the entire proximal fragment. This group is the most common and the most severe type and has the worst prognosis. Type I osteonecrosis is thought to be related to injury to all of the lateral epiphyseal vessels. Type II osteonecrosis, which involves only a portion of the femoral head, has been explained as being due to localized injury to the lateral epiphyseal vessels at the anterolateral femoral head. Type III osteonecrosis involves the femoral neck to the physis with the capital epiphysis spared. This pattern is thought to be related to injury of the metaphyseal vessels. Although rare, the long-term prognosis for type III may be better for some individuals compared to the group with necrosis of the entire femoral head.

Treatment of osteonecrosis following femoral neck fracture has been aimed at maintaining motion and containment because of a lack of treatment alternatives to improve the natural history of this process. Osteotomies to rotate either an uninvolved portion or a less-deformed area of the femoral head into the weightbearing region may improve congruity and symptoms for some patients. Whether vascularized bone grafting has a role for osteonecrosis following hip fracture in the skeletally immature remains to be seen.

The sequelae of these fractures also include coxa vara, premature physeal closure, and nonunion. Coxa vara can be due to malunion or premature physeal closure with relative trochanteric overgrowth. The overall prevalence of coxa vara has been about 20% in the literature. Internal fixation decreases the likelihood of varus from malunion, provided an anatomic reduction is obtained. If the hip has a neck shaft angle less than 110°, it is unlikely that this will correct with growth. Subtrochanteric valgus osteotomy is useful for those deformities that do not improve with observation.

Premature physeal closure occurs even without internal fixation crossing the physis, and closure is often related to osteonecrosis. A decrease in the number of patients with physeal closure that may have been related to the avoidance, when possible, of crossing the physis with pins or screws has been reported. Nonunion occurs in about 4% to 7% of patients. The risk of nonunion seems to be related to a failure to obtain or maintain an anatomic reduction. Valgus osteotomy is recommended for nonunion to create a compression force at the fracture site. Chondrolysis has also been reported, but the cases have been in conjunction with osteonecrosis.

Subtrochanteric Femur Fractures

Subtrochanteric femur fractures in the pediatric age group are those fractures that occur 1 to 2 cm distal to the lesser trochanter. In these fractures, the proximal fragment is markedly flexed, abducted, and externally rotated, and the distal fragment must be matched to this position if traction or spica cast immobilization is used. These fractures can be very difficult to manage by closed methods, so it is not uncommon to use one of the surgical treatments available. The guidelines and principles of treatment are the same as discussed for fractures of the diaphyseal femur.

Fractures of the Femoral Diaphysis

Fractures of the femoral diaphysis are common and can occur in children in distinctly different settings. The clinical situation can vary from an injury occurring on the playground to high-energy trauma, as in a motor vehicle accident. In children younger than 1 year of age, about 70% of femur fractures are related to abuse.

Good results from a variety of treatment options have been obtained in children. Treatment methods have included traction followed by spica cast, early spica cast application, external fixation, flexible intramedullary rods, interlocking nails, and compression plate fixation. All of these modalities have a role in fracture treatment in the skeletally immature patient. The choice of treatment depends on several factors. Age, mechanism of injury, open versus closed fracture, ipsilateral tibial fracture, neurovascular injury, head injury, multitrauma, pathologic fractures, and social environment are all a part of this decision process.

Traction followed by cast treatment has been a very traditional and reliable method of care. The patient is placed in traction for 2 to 4 weeks until early consolidation occurs, and then a cast is applied. The fracture fragments are allowed to overlap 1 to 1.5 cm because of femoral overgrowth. Good results from traction followed by cast application can be expected in children younger than 10 years of age.

In the small child weighing less than 30 lb, skin traction is used. Because of the potential for neurovascular compromise in Bryant's traction, variations on split-Russell traction have become quite popular. In the older child, 90-90 skeletal traction is an effective method. The hip and knee are flexed to 90°. The distal femur is the preferred pin site and allows direct pull without transmitting the traction forces across the knee. Pin placement in the proximal tibia creates a risk of injury to the tibial physis near the tubercle with growth disturbance. Knee subluxation and dislocation have been reported following proximal tibial pin traction in the skeletally immature patient.

Early spica cast treatment either on the day of injury or within the first couple of days has become quite popular for a number of reasons. First, it obviates the need for prolonged traction, so the hospital stay is minimized and the patient can go home. It has been shown to be a very effective mode of treatment, and early cast application provides significant economic savings when compared to inpatient hospital traction.

The concerns with early spica cast application have centered on the ability to maintain adequate alignment. The acceptable amount of angulation in a cast is less than 10° of varus or valgus, 10° of posterior bowing, and 20° of anterior bowing. The cast should have a flat lateral border on the thigh because there is a tendency for the fracture to angulate into varus. Shortening in the cast of 1 to 1.5 cm is desirable because of femoral overgrowth. In children 2 to 10 years of age, the overgrowth averages 1 cm. There can also be slight overgrowth of 0.2 to 0.5 cm of the tibia on the ipsilateral leg. The amount of shortening in a cast should not exceed 2 to 2.5 cm on follow-up radiographic examination.

Not all patients are suitable candidates for early spica cast treatment. Multitrauma patients have other injuries that may be difficult to care for in a cast. Spasticity of the extremities following a head injury complicates maintaining control of the fracture fragments. Some children 6 to 10 years of age are large enough that it is hard for the family to lift and care for them. The "floating knee" is another example of a clinical situation in which rigid fixation of at least one fracture simplifies the treatment and improves the result.

Some patients do develop excessive shortening in the cast. These patients then require removal from the cast with subsequent treatment by traction, an external fixator, or other means of surgical stabilization. In patients with fractures secondary to high-energy trauma, more soft-tissue and periosteal stripping occur, potentially allowing for greater shortening of the fracture fragments. Greater disruption of the soft-tissue envelope compromises stabil-

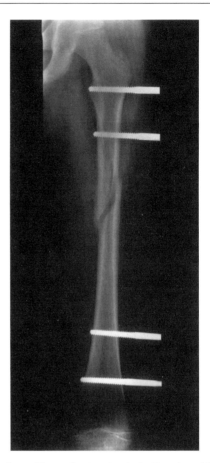

Fig. 3   Diaphyseal femur fracture treated with external fixation.

ity. This important concept illustrates the need for weekly radiographs during the first 3 weeks to monitor the patient for excessive angulation and shortening.

Although early spica cast application and traction can provide good results for many of these fractures, there is a role for surgical intervention. Patients between the ages of 10 and 12 years are, in general, best managed with surgical fixation, and most adolescent patients are treated surgically. In this older age group, traction and cast application are not as reliable. Children younger than 10 years of age may require surgical intervention in instances of multitrauma, head injury, open fractures, neurovascular injury, ipsilateral tibia fracture, and excessive shortening of the fracture fragments.

External fixation of femur fractures has been quite useful in children. It can be applied relatively easily with minimal blood loss, often requiring only two pins above and two pins below the fracture, unless there is concern that fracture healing may be prolonged because of severe comminution or unless there is a severe open injury (Fig. 3). In these cases, it may be advisable to use three pins on each side of the fracture. The fractures can be placed out to length or overlapped 1 to 1.5 cm, depending on the age of the patient and the surgeon's preference. Progressive weightbearing is encouraged after callus is visible. Depending on the school and family environment, some of these children can return to school. Patients are also allowed to shower.

As with any treatment, there are disadvantages to external fixation. Pin care is necessary and pin-tract inflammation and infection can occur in up to 10% of patients. The combination of the fracture and the pins in the lateral soft tissues of the thigh do tend to limit the knee range of motion (ROM). Some patients do exceptionally well having full ROM with the external fixator in place, while others will have significant limitation of motion. Once the frame is removed, the patients tend to regain their motion within 6 weeks. Occasionally, patients may need gentle manipulation when the external fixator is removed if there is very limited active ROM.

The average duration of external fixation is about 10 to 12 weeks. Excellent callus formation should be visible radiographically and it is recommended that the patient fully bear weight on the frame prior to removal. If possible, the stiffness of the frame should be decreased or the frame should be "dynamized" as fracture healing progresses. Because there is a small incidence of refracture after the external fixator is removed, if there is concern about the amount of callus visible, cast bracing should be considered.

Intramedullary rod fixation has been quite successful in the adult population and has been extended to adolescents and older children. Locked intramedullary fixation is most useful in those 12 years of age and older. Reamed intramedullary antegrade nails have been used in children younger than 10 years of age; however, there are potential complications. Theoretically, in the very young patient, reaming could create a trochanteric growth arrest with subsequent coxa valga. Fortunately, this does not seem to be a problem in children older than 10 years of age. Another potential complication is osteonecrosis of the femoral head, which has been reported in the adolescent age group. Reaming in the pyriformis fossa may injure the vessels at the base of the neck.

Elastic or flexible intramedullary nailing is gaining acceptance for the treatment of pediatric femur fractures given the concerns about osteonecrosis with reamed nailing in the older child. The use of Rush or Ender type of nails requires skill and planning. To achieve rotational stability, the canal can be stacked with multiple nails or a combination of "C" and "S" shaped nails can be used. Alternatively, two "C" shaped nails can be inserted from medial and lateral portals proximal to the distal physis. Retrograde and antegrade placement can be used. Cast immobilization may be necessary in some fractures if adequate stability cannot be achieved. This type of fixation is not as suitable for severely comminuted fractures and injuries with bone loss (Fig. 4).

Another option for the treatment of pediatric femur

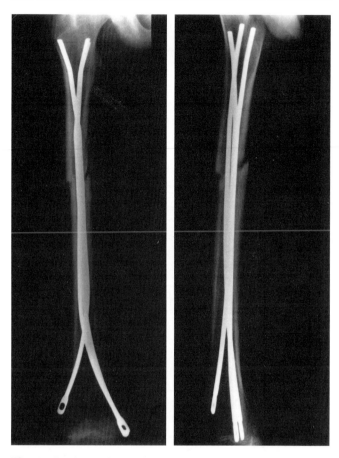

Fig. 4 Diaphyseal femur fracture treated by retrograde flexible intramedullary rods as seen on the anteroposterior **(left)** and lateral **(right)** radiographs. The entry site into the bone is above the physis.

fractures is compression plate fixation. The primary role is in the patient with polytrauma or head injury to assist in easing nursing care and rehabilitation. Broad 4.5-mm plates should be used. If there is any evidence of medial comminution at the fracture site, the patient should be cautioned that unprotected weightbearing may cause the plate to break. The plate can break even after the sixth postoperative week. There is also a risk of fracture through a screw hole after the plate is removed.

The published series of femur fractures treated surgically have shown that the leg length discrepancies have not been a problem for most patients. Most patients are within 0.5 to 1 cm of length equality; however, in each series there may be a small number of patients that do have a significant difference of 2.5 cm or greater. Unfortunately, there does not seem to be a means by which to predict which individuals will have significant overgrowth. A few patients have seemingly had an increase in their discrepancy as a result of overgrowth following the removal of an intramedullary nail.

When treating femur fractures in children, lower limb lengths should be followed after healing, regardless of the treatment used. Approximately 78% of the overgrowth occurs in the first 18 months, and by 42 months after fracture healing, 85% of all patients have reached their maximum discrepancy. From this it is clear that these patients need periodic follow-up to determine whether or not lower limb length discrepancy will be a clinical problem.

In summary, for diaphyseal fractures, early spica cast application in infants and children up to 6 years of age is reliable and should be the treatment of choice. If the patient is in a high-energy accident and requires several days of observation, skin traction (split-Russell) can be used until a cast is appropriate. Excessive femoral shortening in the cast (> 2 to 2.5 cm) can be corrected by conversion to traction or external fixation. Patients with other clinical issues, such as multitrauma, open fracture, head injury with spasticity, and "floating knee," may often be more easily managed with external fixation.

Children 6 to 10 years of age have more variability in treatment options. Early spica cast application can be used in this group as well. Again, excessive shortening can be managed by conversion to another treatment plan. The considerations of patient size and the family's ability to care for the child in a cast are important. These factors,

along with multitrauma, head injury, open fractures, and "floating knee," are reasons to consider other modalities of treatment. External fixation, flexible intramedullary rodding, and compression plating are excellent options. In general, in this age group reamed intramedullary nailing is not advocated because of the small pyriformis fossa and possible injury to the vessels at the base of the femoral neck with resultant osteonecrosis.

Adolescents 10 years of age and older are best managed with surgical stabilization, such as external fixation, flexible intramedullary rods, compression plating, and antegrade locked nailing systems. Currently, compression plating is not being advocated in the adolescent population when locked nailing is appropriate. Concerns regarding osteonecrosis and reamed nailing remain, especially in children 12 years of age and younger. With the reports of osteonecrosis, even in the young adolescent, care should be taken with the entry site in the region of the pyriformis fossa.

Supracondylar Femur Fractures

Supracondylar femur fractures, those that occur above the level of the gastrocnemius origin, typically produce hyper-

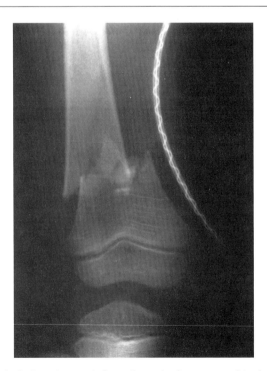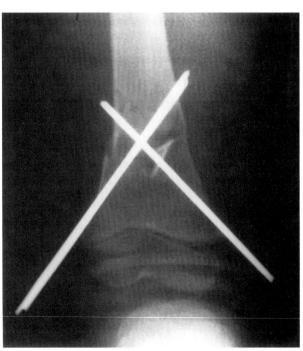

Fig. 5   Left, An anteroposterior radiograph of a supracondylar femur fracture. **Right,** This fracture was unstable and difficult to hold by closed methods. Cross pin fixation was performed and a cast was applied. Plate fixation could be used but would probably require a cast because of the small distal fragment available for screws above the physis. A disadvantage of external fixation here would be restriction of knee range of motion with half pins through the iliotibial band distally, as well as the potential for intra-articular sepsis from pin penetration of the joint capsule.

extension of the distal fragment with apex posterior angulation between the two fragments. To achieve adequate alignment with cast application or traction, the knee must be flexed to reduce the pull of the gastrocnemius. Achieving and maintaining alignment by closed methods can be difficult. The proximal fragment can be "buttonholed" through the quadriceps mechanism. The acceptable amount of angulation in a cast is again less than 10° of varus or valgus, 10° of posterior bowing, and 20° of anterior bowing.

If a satisfactory reduction cannot be maintained, the treatment options include cross pin fixation with cast application, or open reduction with a plating system such as a blade plate, screw plate combination, or compression plate. External fixation at this level is not as ideal. Loss of knee motion with half pins in the distal iliotibial band can exacerbate the development of adhesions in the quadriceps mechanism that can occur following these fractures. Joint sepsis secondary to inadvertent penetration of the capsule by the distal half pins is another drawback to external fixation at this level (Fig. 5).

Fractures of the Distal Femoral Physis

These fractures often result from a hyperextension force. Angular and growth disturbances, common sequelae of these injuries, occur in up to 30% of patients. With thicker periosteum, a greater force is required to produce these injuries in the child than the adolescent. This helps explain the occurrence of sports-related distal femoral physeal fracture separations in the adolescent.

Distal femoral physeal fractures related to a breech delivery can be managed with skin traction or cast immobilization. If a length discrepancy or angular deformity occurs, the tendency is for resolution in the majority, in this age group, but some patients do develop severe deformity.

In the child and adolescent, the Salter-Harris classification remains the most widely used. Nondisplaced injuries can be managed in a well-molded long leg cast or hip spica with the knee slightly flexed. Positioning the knee in extreme flexion to hold the fracture reduced should be avoided because of the risk of neurovascular compromise.

Salter-Harris types I and II displaced fractures require reduction (Fig. 6). To obtain reduction, manual longitudinal traction is followed by gentle correction of residual angulation and translation. Adequate sedation or anesthesia is required because forceful manipulations may further damage the physis. Percutaneous smooth pin fixation across the physis is often used to help maintain the reduction. If the metaphyseal spike is larger than 2.5 cm, pin or screw fixation across this fragment can be used, thus avoiding the physis. Because these forms of internal fixation are not rigid, a cast is necessary. Depending on the age of the patient and the fracture pattern, sufficient healing may be present to allow early ROM 4 to 6 weeks after injury.

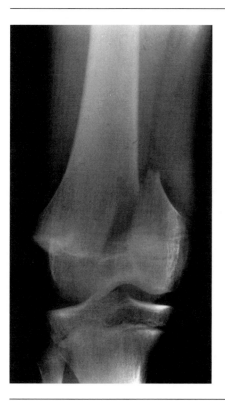 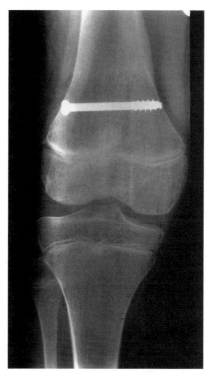

Fig. 6 **Left,** Salter-Harris type II distal femur fracture. **Right,** This fracture could not be reduced by closed manipulation. The lateral side remained displaced with a gap between the epiphysis and metaphysis. A lateral approach to the distal femur allowed removal of the intervening soft tissue and the fracture was anatomically reduced. Lateral exposure screw fixation to the large metaphyseal fragment was done and a cast applied. More than one screw could have been used. Screws can also be placed from the medial side.

When placing smooth pins from the epiphysis through the metaphysis, intra-articular pin positioning is of concern. The starting point of the pin should be proximal on the epiphysis in a plane slightly posterior to the midpoint of the femoral condyle. The pins should cross above the physis in the metaphysis and engage the opposite cortex.

Displaced types III and IV fractures require anatomic reduction (open if necessary) and fixation. Pins or screws can be used. The screw fixation can be placed between the two epiphyseal regions or between the metaphyseal spike and the metaphysis of the femur. Threaded fixation should avoid the physis. A cast may be needed and ROM is started within 4 to 6 weeks.

Complications of Distal Physeal Femur Fractures

Angular deformity and limb length discrepancy are major concerns following a distal physeal femur fracture. These fractures should be aligned without residual angulation, because angular correction during growth is not a dependable phenomenon in the child and adolescent with these fractures. Lower limb length discrepancies can be significant because of physeal bar formation. Growth arrest is not as closely linked to the Salter-Harris classification as it is related to the initial severity of the injury and the amount of displacement. Patients require close observation for development of a physeal bar and growth arrest. Radiographs at 6 months and 1 year after healing can alert the physician to early physeal problems. If there is no evidence of growth arrest or angular deformity after the first year, the patient can be followed annually with a clinical examination until skeletal maturity. Reconstructive procedures, such as bar resection, contralateral epiphysiodesis, lengthening, or angular correction by osteotomy will be necessary for some patients.

Annotated Bibliography

Hip Fractures

Canale ST: Fractures of the hip in children and adolescents. *Orthop Clin North Am* 1990;21:341–352.

The author discusses the types of fractures, the complications, and recommended treatment regimens and updates an earlier series of hip fractures in this age group. Comparison between the two series of hip fractures shows differences in results and complications, providing support for surgical management of these injuries.

Forlin E, Guille JT, Kumar SJ, et al: Transepiphyseal fractures of the neck of the femur in very young children. *J Pediatr Orthop* 1992;12:164–168.

This discusses the results of nonsurgical treatment of displaced femoral neck fractures in children 8 to 26 months of age. In the two patients with an open proximal femoral physis after healing, the varus femoral neck shaft angle corrected spontaneously. Two patients had closure of their physis and required a later valgus osteotomy. No patient developed osteonecrosis.

Forlin E, Guille JT, Kumar SJ, et al: Complications associated with fracture of the neck of the femur in children. *J Pediatr Orthop* 1992;12:503–509.

The authors reviewed 16 patients with displaced femoral neck fractures and complications. As expected, osteonecrosis, nonunion, and chondrolysis were associated with a poor outcome. Even with secondary osteotomy, the clinical course following complete femoral head necrosis remained poor.

Hughes LO, Beaty JH: Fractures of the head and neck of the femur in children. *J Bone Joint Surg* 1994;76A:283–292.

The authors of this article provide a review of the previously reported hip fracture series in the literature. Fracture types, complications, and treatment regimens are discussed. This is an excellent overview of these injuries, and specific treatment guidelines are included for each fracture type in the Delbet classification.

Femoral Shaft Fractures

Aronson J, Tursky EA: External fixation of femur fractures in children. *J Pediatr Orthop* 1992;12:157–163.

Forty-four femur fractures were treated by external fixation. External fixation was used both in multitrauma and in single extremity injury situations. Patients were encouraged to progressively bear weight. Complete consolidation and bridging of the fracture should be visible prior to fixator removal to avoid refracture. Time in the external fixator averaged 10 to 12 weeks.

Beaty JH, Austin SM, Warner WC, et al: Interlocking intramedullary nailing of femoral-shaft fractures in adolescents: Preliminary results and complications. *J Pediatr Orthop* 1994;14:178–183.

Thirty-one fractures were treated in 10- to 15-year-olds, all of which healed. One 11-year-old patient developed segmental osteonecrosis. The average femoral overgrowth was 0.51 cm; however, two patients with no other injuries had an increase in length of 2.5 and 3.2 cm. One of these two patients had an increase in the amount of femoral overgrowth after nail removal.

Heinrich SD, Drvaric D, Darr K, et al: Stabilization of pediatric diaphyseal femur fractures with flexible intramedullary nails (a technique paper). *J Orthop Trauma* 1992;6:452–459.

This discusses nail size as well as surgical technique in the placement of these devices. The surgical methods described are very helpful in achieving reliable nail insertion and results.

Heinrich SD, Drvaric DM, Darr K, et al: The operative stabilization of pediatric diaphyseal femur fractures with flexible intramedullary nails: A prospective analysis. *J Pediatr Orthop* 1994;14:501–507.

The authors of this series examine the results of 73 fractures treated with flexible nailing. In the 50 fractures with more than 12 months follow-up, 88% had normal varus/valgus alignment and 94% had a normal anterior-posterior alignment. The rotational profile was symmetric in 94% of this greater than 12-month follow-up group. Four patients in the study required reoperation—one for refracture following hardware removal, one for valgus angulation, and two for fracture collapse and rod migration. The authors clearly state their indications for surgical management.

Irani RN, Nicholson JT, Chung SM: Long-term results in the treatment of femoral-shaft fractures in young children by immediate spica immobilization. *J Bone Joint Surg* 1976;58A:945–951.

The authors report satisfactory results with early spica cast application. At the time this article was written, this was a departure from the standard treatment of initial traction that was followed by conversion to a spica cast several weeks later. The amount of angulation accepted in this series would be regarded as excessive by most orthopaedists today.

Mileski RA, Garvin KL, Crosby LA: Avascular necrosis of the femoral head in an adolescent following intramedullary nailing of the femur: A case report. *J Bone Joint Surg* 1994;76A:1706–1708.

This is a case report of a 14-year-old with osteonecrosis of the ipsilateral femoral head following femoral shaft fracture and intramedullary rodding. The concerns are discussed regarding osteonecrosis with antegrade reamed nailing in the adolescent and pediatric age groups.

Newton PO, Mubarak SJ: Financial aspects of femoral shaft fracture treatment in children and adolescents. *J Pediatr Orthop* 1994;14:508–512.

The article compares the costs of early spica cast application, traction (both inpatient and home traction), and intramedullary rodding for the treatment of femur fractures. Early spica cast treatment had the lowest patient charges while inpatient skeletal traction and intramedullary rodding were the most expensive.

Shapiro F: Fractures of the femoral shaft in children: The overgrowth phenomenon. *Acta Orthop Scand* 1981;52:649–655.

The author examines the amount of femoral overgrowth in patients younger than 13 years of age and provides useful guidelines on the amount of overgrowth and the time span over which this phenomenon occurs. The amount of overgrowth averages 9.2 mm, and 78% of the overgrowth occurs in the first 18 months. However, overgrowth can continue over several years. At 18 months, only 12% of patients had completed their femoral overgrowth.

Ward WT, Levy J, Kaye A: Compression plating for child and adolescent femur fractures. *J Pediatr Orthop* 1992;12:626–632.

Twenty-four patients had compression plating with broad 4.5-mm AO dynamic compression plate. Plating was most commonly done in patients with either multitrauma or head injury. Periosteal bone healing was common, and primary bone healing, as would be expected with AO technique, was seen in only six of 24 fractures. Medial cortical comminution can lead to plate failure. The discussion in this article is cogent and addresses the advantages and disadvantages of plate fixation.

Fractures of the Distal Femoral Physis

Beaty JH, Kumar A: Fractures about the knee in children. *J Bone Joint Surg* 1994;76A:1870–1880.

The authors discuss fractures about the knee—both distal femoral and proximal tibial. Clear treatment guidelines are provided for the distal femoral physeal fracture separations.

Lombardo SJ, Harvey JP Jr: Fractures of the distal femoral epiphyses: Factors influencing prognosis. A review of thirty-four cases. *J Bone Joint Surg* 1977;59A:742–751.

This series documents the sequelae of distal physeal injuries of the femur. Thirty-six percent of these patients had a limb length discrepancy of 2 cm or more. The development of late deformity seems to be related to the amount of initial displacement rather than the Salter-Harris classification.

Riseborough EJ, Barrett IR, Shapiro F: Growth disturbances following distal femoral physeal fracture-separations. *J Bone Joint Surg* 1983;65A:885–893.

Again, the high rate of complications following these injuries is documented. The juvenile age group was likely to have a worse outcome than the adolescent group. This was thought to be in part due to the higher energy trauma associated with the physeal fracture separation in the younger age group. When central growth arrest occurs, limb length discrepancy can be expected. The authors provide in the discussion an overview of the pathophysiology that could lead to growth arrest regardless of the Salter-Harris classification.

28

Injuries of the Humerus and Elbow

Injuries of the humerus in children primarily involve the proximal and distal ends of the bone. The fracture types, immobilization times, and associated neurologic injuries are different from injuries in adults. This chapter will discuss pediatric humeral and elbow injuries beginning with proximal injuries and ending with distal injuries, dealing with those lesions most likely to pose problems.

Fractures of the Humerus

Fractures of the Proximal Humerus

Fractures of the proximal humerus usually result from a torsional force that is applied to the outstretched arm. This type of injury is first seen at birth, at which time a neonate may sustain a Salter I fracture of the humerus caused by abduction–external rotation forces in delivery. The infant fails to move the extremity, giving the impression of an Erb's palsy, but tenderness reveals the actual location of the injury. Radiographs may show what appears to be a shoulder dislocation, but ultrasonography reveals the true cartilaginous nature of the injury. Immobilization of the arm to the infant's side with an elastic bandage for 2 weeks is sufficient treatment. Rarely, shortening or a varus deformity of the humerus may develop in the long term.

A Salter II fracture of the proximal humerus occurs most commonly in adolescents. This type of fracture results from a hyperextension mechanism to the shoulder either in abduction or adduction. Several classifications have been proposed, but they are not useful in treatment decisions. Both physeal growth arrest and neurovascular injury are rare with this type of injury. Fracture reduction need not be anatomic because of the adolescent's exceptional growth and remodeling potential. Usually, the fracture alignment improves (when the patient is sitting or standing) once muscle spasm has subsided. A consensus is emerging that the only indication for formal reduction is in the patient who has reached skeletal maturity with an angulation greater than 25° in the coronal or sagittal plane. The rest may be treated with sling and swathe. In situations in which active treatment is needed, closed or open reduction with percutaneous pin fixation is well tolerated.

Metaphyseal fractures of the proximal humerus occur by the same mechanism. Significant associated deltoid injury may be present with metaphyseal fractures. Internal fixation may not be needed if satisfactory position of the fracture fragments is attained in a sling. Because shaft fractures are not common in children, underlying abnor-malities such as unicameral cysts or fibrous dysplasia must be ruled out. Treatment with a functional humeral brace and sling yield excellent long-term results.

Supracondylar Fractures of the Humerus

Historically, the highest rate of associated complications and the poorest results of all pediatric fractures have occurred with supracondylar fractures of the humerus. Problems must and can be minimized by using an orderly approach to assessment and treatment.

Approximately 2% of supracondylar fractures result from flexion type injuries (eg, landing on the point of the elbow). The vast majority of these fractures result from hyperextension injuries, which are the childhood equivalent of elbow dislocations in individuals older than 10 years of age.

Wilkins has classified the supracondylar fracture caused by hyperextension injuries into three types of fractures. Type I are undisplaced, type II are displaced but hinged on an intact posterior cortex, and type III are complete and displaced. The prevalence of associated neurologic injury in type III fractures ranges from 7% to 15%. Median nerve injuries are somewhat more common than radial nerve injuries in the majority of series, and ulnar injuries are least common, although the percentages are close. It is extremely important to check and record the function of the radial, median (including anterior interosseous branch), and ulnar nerves separately, even if the child is young or uncooperative. If necessary, these nerves can be tested by stimulus withdrawal. It is in the surgeon's best interest to detect all existing neurologic injuries before reduction in an effort to eliminate concern that injury may have been caused by treatment.

Correct assessment of vascularity can be very difficult. It should include temperature of the extremity, capillary refill, pulses, pain on passive stretch, and active muscle function. None of these parameters is definitive either by its presence or its absence; all parameters should be evaluated together. Pulse oximetry has not been adequately correlated with muscle perfusion and, therefore, does not by itself provide sufficient information. If vascular impairment is suspected, treatment must not be delayed by taking the time to obtain an arteriogram. There are several reasons for not delaying treatment. First, the site of compromise is already known; it is at the level of the fracture. Second, the blood flow may often be restored simply by reducing the fracture. Finally, the arteriogram may be done intraoperatively using fluoroscopy, which is already needed to assess fracture reduction.

The patient should be under general anesthesia during

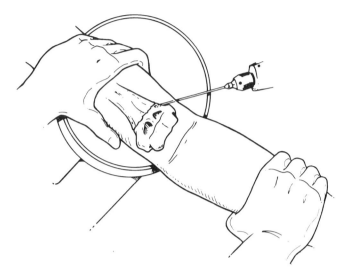

Fig. 1 Method of closed reduction and percutaneous pin fixation of a supracondylar fracture of the humerus. Traction is applied in a distal direction and 30° anteriorly to provide a reduction force. This will allow visualization of the carrying angle and fluoroscopic visualization of pin placement.

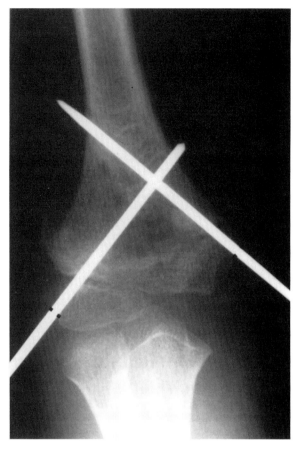

Fig. 2 Placement of medial and lateral pins in a supracondylar fracture of the humerus. The medial pin enters the prominence of the medial epicondyle at an angle of about 45°; the lateral pin enters more distally at an angle of 30°.

fracture reduction, especially those who have sustained significantly angulated type II fractures or type III fractures.

An unacceptable varus/valgus component may be present in type II fractures. It is important to examine the elbow in extension to assess whether the varus/valgus component exists. Any deformity in excess of 10° of varus/valgus or 20° of extension should be reduced. Reduction can be accomplished by correcting the deformity in all planes, as in a greenstick fracture, and ensuring that the fragment does not "spring back" into a displaced position. If the fragment becomes displaced, it should be pinned.

Some displaced supracondylar fractures (type III) may be successfully treated by closed manipulation and cast immobilization or by traction. The best results, however, are achieved by anatomic reduction and pin fixation, procedures that should be taught as the standard of care. If neurovascular status is intact, reduction can be electively scheduled within 24 hours of the injury; however, it is not wise to wait longer than 24 hours.

Closed Reduction and Pin Fixation   A general anesthetic is used during closed reduction and pin fixation of supracondylar fractures. To minimize soft-tissue swelling, formal closed reduction is not attempted until the extremity has been sterilely prepared. The patient is moved while supine to the side of the operating table, and the fluoroscopy unit is kept close to the patient's body, perpendicular to the extremity and out of the way. The large (receiving) end of the unit is draped and used as a platform for the procedure (Fig. 1). Reduction is achieved by correcting the translation of the fracture edges. The patient's upper arm

is stabilized using one hand while anterior and distal traction is applied with the other hand. Stabilization can be accomplished with elbow flexion of 30°, so that the view of the distal fragment is not obscured by the forearm. The quality of reduction in both the anteroposterior (AP) and lateral planes can be determined on the AP view. If the fracture gap is obliterated, the fragment widths match, and Baumann's angle is restored, it may be presumed that the lateral projection is also satisfactory. A relatively stable fracture can then be fixed using two pins, either two lateral pins or a medial and a lateral pin. Use of medial and lateral pins has been shown to be the most biomechanically sound. Lateral crossed pins must be avoided because of their extremely low torsional resistance.

When using a medial or lateral pin, a skilled assistant should maintain axial traction (in slight flexion) as the lateral pin is inserted first. It is important to insert the pin distal enough to obtain purchase in the distal fragment. The pin should enter at the level of the ossific nucleus of the lateral condyle, not at the metaphysis (Fig. 2). The point of insertion should be slightly anterior to the mid-

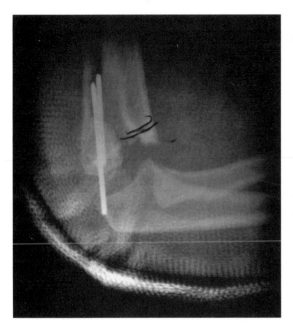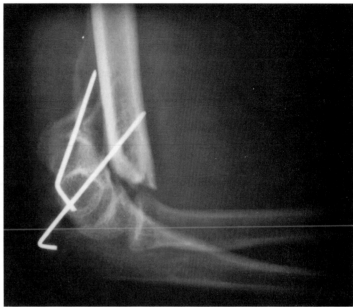

Fig. 3 Common pitfalls of percutaneous pin fixation. **Left,** Pins exit at fracture site and intraoperative lateral film is not scrutinized. **Right,** Displacement follows.

line, because of the anterior inclination of the distal humerus. The angle of the lateral pin in the frontal plane should be about 30° to the long axis of the humerus. The pin should engage both cortices and be large enough to resist bending (usually .062 in or .075 in). When the lateral pin has been inserted, a good lateral view can be obtained by externally rotating the flexed elbow. The medial pin may then be inserted using caution because of the nearby location of the ulnar nerve. If the elbow is swollen, pressure over the medial epicondyle may be applied to compress the edema and highlight this landmark. Beginning the procedure on the anterior edge of the epicondyle helps the surgeon stay clear of the ulnar nerve. Making a small incision through the skin, clearing a tract with a hemostat, and using a hollow pin-guide also promote safe pinning. The angle of the medial pin should be about 45° to the axis of the humerus to allow for the flare of the epicondyle. The elbow should be kept in less than 90° flexion during pinning to permit the ulnar nerve to remain posterior to the epicondyle. Both cortices should be engaged. If swelling prevents confident pin placement medially, the second pin may be placed laterally, parallel to and apart from the first pin. Portions of the pins should protrude from the skin, as the pulse is checked and an intraoperative permanent radiograph is obtained to document satisfactory pin placement. The most common errors in this type of pin fixation are pin entry close to or through the fracture line, failure to engage the proximal fragment as seen on the lateral film (Fig. 3), and pins crossing at the fracture site. The normal Baumann's angle is 72° ± 4° (Fig. 4).

Open Reduction If a satisfactory closed reduction cannot be achieved after two or three attempts, the surgeon should proceed to an open reduction. An open reduction will not cause permanent stiffness, as has been commonly thought. The surgical approach should be on the side of the greatest fracture gap, which is usually the lateral side. Obstructions to reduction, such as brachialis muscle, artery, or nerve, should be sought and relieved. Pin fixation is then performed as previously described.

After surgery, the elbow should be immobilized in a comfortable amount of elbow flexion, generally 80° to 90°. The antecubital fossa should not be compressed by the cast or padding. Any impaired tissue perfusion should be noted by absent Doppler pulse or impaired temperature, capillary refill, and muscle function. Nerve function should be rechecked when the patient awakens from anesthesia. After a splint has been worn full-time for 4 weeks, the pins are removed. The splint is then reapplied and removed twice daily for supervised range of motion exercises for an additional 2 weeks. These time guidelines may be prolonged in the case of an open fracture, which heals more slowly.

If satisfactory perfusion is not restored by fracture reduction, the vascular surgeon may decide to perform an intraoperative arteriogram or direct exploration of the artery. An anterior Henry approach is preferred. If the artery appears to be in spasm or impaled on bone, disengagement and bathing with lidocaine may restore blood flow. An intimal tear is addressed by arteriotomy and a gross tear is addressed by repair. Although it is known that

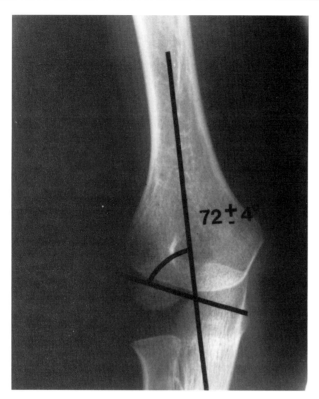

Fig. 4   The normal Baumann's angle is 72° ± 4° and does not vary significantly with age or sex.

the brachial artery flow across the elbow may be replaced by collateral flow in children, in this age of skilled vascular surgery, it is common practice to restore brachial artery flow if interruption is diagnosed. The fracture should first be pinned to stabilize the elbow and protect the vascular repair. Forearm compartment pressures should be measured after reperfusion, and fasciotomies performed if the pressures are elevated or if there has been a long ischemic period.

If a neurologic deficit is recognized preoperatively, observation only of the deficit is recommended. Approximately 75% of neurologic deficits will resolve spontaneously. If no improvement is seen within 3 to 5 months, an electromyogram (EMG) should be obtained. If no signs of reinnervation are present, the EMG should be followed by exploration and neurolysis of the involved nerve. This procedure has been shown to be effective in most cases, provided that the nerve is intact. By contrast, if a neurologic deficit occurs as a result of reduction and pinning, the nerve should be explored to ensure that it is not trapped within the fracture site or by the pin.

Associated forearm fractures occur with 5% of supracondylar fractures. These forearm fractures can be treated by closed reduction as long as the supracondylar fracture is stable.

In a large series of supracondylar fractures, the outcome was good to excellent in 75% of the patients. If cubitus varus occurs, it is usually caused by malreduction, although less frequently it may develop secondary to osteonecrosis of the trochlea. Varus or valgus malreduction does not cause much functional impairment, although it may be cosmetically significant if the deformity is greater than 10° to 15°, especially if it is accompanied by hyperextension. Varus deformity may also increase the risk of a lateral condyle fracture occurring later. If the varus deformity is excessive and the patient wishes it, a corrective supracondylar osteotomy may be performed. Correction of any rotational component is not necessary; only the coronal plane and, occasionally, the sagittal plane deformities need to be corrected. Disappointing results following corrective osteotomy in some series may be caused by inadequate fixation of both medial and lateral columns. Full correction or slight overcorrection, stabilization of medial and lateral columns by predrilled pins or an intact hinge, and lateral epiphysiodesis in the presence of medial growth arrest lead to a predictably good result.

Intercondylar Fractures of the Distal Humerus

Intercondylar fractures of the distal humerus occur in an older age group than the typical supracondylar fracture, but still may be seen in children as young as 8 years of age. They result from a direct fall on the elbow. The usual criterion for closed reduction of intra-articular fractures, displacement of less than 2 mm, must be observed or open reduction must be performed, no matter what the patient's age.

Physeal Fractures of the Distal Humerus

Physeal fractures of the distal humerus occur in the very young child but may be seen in children up to 6 years of age. Although physeal fractures may occur in the process of a difficult childbirth, if they occur in the infant or toddler, child abuse must be considered. Clinically and radiographically, a physeal fracture resembles an elbow dislocation. In the child whose capitellum has not yet ossified, there may be no clue that the distal humerus is displaced. The key to the correct diagnosis is to remember that elbow dislocations are extremely rare in children younger than 6 years of age. The distal humeral physeal fracture may be a Salter I or II injury. In a Salter II injury, the metaphyseal fragment is most often lateral and may radiographically resemble a lateral condyle fracture. The distinction may be made, however, by the more circumferential swelling seen in the Salter II injury, and presence of medial as well as lateral tenderness. In addition, in a Salter II injury the radius and ulna are translated as a unit with the entire distal humeral fragment; in a lateral condyle fracture the ulna does not shift. If the diagnosis is in question, a magnetic resonance imaging (MRI) scan, ultrasonography, or an arthrogram may confirm the correct diagnosis. If an MRI is obtained, the elbow should be splinted in extension.

Treatment of the newborn with a physeal fracture should include simple immobilization of the elbow in flexion to allow the thick periosteal hinge to guide reduction. In the older child with significant displacement, the fracture is treated like a supracondylar fracture with percutaneous pin fixation. Because the medial epicondyle is not ossified at this young age, fixation with two lateral pins has been recommended. These physeal fractures are more stable than supracondylar fractures because they occur through the broad metaphyseal surface. Usually, immobilization for 3 to 4 weeks is all that is necessary. Osteonecrosis of the trochlea has been reported, presumably due to interruption of the lateral trochlear transphyseal vessels.

Lateral Condyle Fractures

Lateral condyle fractures are commonly associated with problems that occur later. This is, in part, because the rather innocuous initial appearance of the injury may lead to undertreatment. Two principles are important regarding lateral condyle fractures. First, lateral condyle fractures are one of the few pediatric fractures in which nonunion is not rare, particularly when displacement of the intra-articular lateral condyle fracture is greater than 2 mm. Second, a cast is rarely able to obtain or maintain reduction of a displaced fracture, because there is little external means of applying a reduction force. Remembering these two principles should help in selecting the proper treatment method.

In lateral condyle fractures, the cleavage plane is usually oblique, which may not be fully appreciated on the AP or lateral radiographs. Oblique films are helpful if an occult lateral condyle fracture is suspected. Neurovascular injuries are not commonly associated with this fracture.

If the fracture is displaced less than 2 mm in any plane, close observation may be justified. Radiographs must be checked at 5 and 10 days in order to detect any displacement of the fragment. A fiberglass splint or cast will allow better radiographic visualization of the fracture than plaster. Recently, however, there has been a strong trend toward percutaneous pin fixation of all lateral condyle fractures, including those that are minimally displaced. Choice of treatment options should be a matter of individual discretion. If the surgeon senses that compliance with follow-up instructions may be poor, then pin fixation should be chosen so that detection of fragment displacement is not delayed until a time when reduction becomes impossible.

If the initial radiograph shows a displacement of 2 mm or more between the fracture fragments, reduction and pin fixation is necessary. If the fracture has an intact medial hinge and occurred less than 48 hours earlier, a closed reduction and percutaneous pinning may be attempted. An arthrogram is obtained to prove that the articular hinge is intact. If an anatomic position cannot be achieved with closed reduction, the surgeon should proceed to an open reduction.

Pin Fixation of Lateral Condyle Fractures An arthrogram of the lateral condyle may be performed if joint surface congruity is in doubt. Reduction of a minimally displaced fracture is achieved by percutaneous pressure on the fragment, perpendicular to the plane of the fracture, which is oriented posterolaterally. At least one pin may need to traverse the capitellar cartilage; however, two widely spaced or divergent pins should be used in order to prevent redisplacement. Each pin should engage two cortices. If an anatomic reduction cannot be obtained by closed means, open reduction through a lateral Kocher incision is necessary. Dissection should be limited to the region around the fracture, not distal or posterior to the fracture, because the blood supply to the lateral crista of the trochlea enters from the posterior side. The metaphysis should not be extensively exposed subperiosteally. If visualization of the joint is necessary, it should be anterior. The entry sites for the pins should be posterolateral, not directly lateral. The surgeon should not hesitate to traverse some of the capitellar cartilage or even some of the epiphysis with the pin (Fig. 5). Usually, this is necessary because the metaphyseal fragment is small and not adequate for purchase. Growth will not be altered by the temporary presence of a smooth pin across the epiphysis. It is important to restore the normal tilt to the distal humerus. The pins may back out if the far cortex is not engaged. Elbow range of motion exercises may be started at 4 to 6 weeks and the pins may be removed at 6 weeks.

Complications

If a fracture is treated with only a cast and union is not achieved within 8 weeks, bone graft in situ across the metaphyseal fragment should be undertaken. Internal fixation may be used. Care should be taken to avoid excessive dissection. The bone graft should be packed gently into the fracture cleft and a bone peg inserted into the humeral metaphysis (Fig. 6).

Nonunion presenting late (after 12 weeks) may create a dilemma. If the nonunion remains in good position and is pain-free, it may be left untreated to avoid loss of elbow motion that grafting may cause. Some lateral condyle fractures are prone to develop progressive cubitus valgus with tardy ulnar nerve palsy, a progression that usually takes many years to develop. If this progressive shift into valgus is seen, the ulnar nerve should be transposed and the fracture should be bone grafted in situ. The fracture should not be reduced to anatomic position, in order to avoid stiffness or osteonecrosis. If a tardy ulnar palsy is present, anterior transposition of the ulnar nerve should be performed. In patients with cubitus valgus, the indications for varus osteotomy are instability with loading or cosmetic concerns. Osteotomy will not help a nerve palsy or improve elbow range of motion.

In some cases, cubitus varus may occur. Statistically, cubitus varus is more common than cubitus valgus and problems resulting from cubitus varus are less severe than those

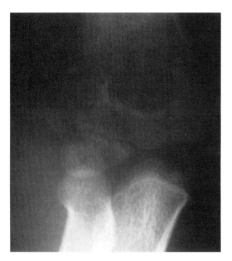 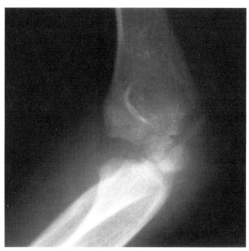 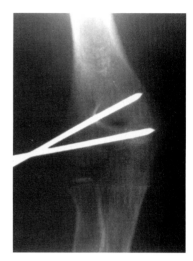

Fig. 5 **Left,** Displaced lateral condyle fracture. **Center,** Oblique view shows fracture plane best. **Right,** Proper pin placement for lateral condyle fracture after reduction.

from cubitus valgus. Cubitus varus results either from mal-reduction of the fracture or from overgrowth of the condyle secondary to hyperemia (Fig. 7). Additionally, cubitus varus may result from osteonecrosis of the lateral portion of the trochlea. Later development of a "fish-tail" or inverted-V appearance of the distal humerus may develop because of undergrowth of this avascular segment. This change may cause slight restriction to joint range of motion, but no major impairment or symptoms.

Medial Epicondyle Fractures

Medial epicondyle fractures occur most commonly in children between 9 and 14 years of age. These fractures result from valgus stresses to the elbow. A medial epicondyle fracture may sometimes occur with elbow dislocation and, if so, the epicondylar fragment may become entrapped within the joint. Fractures with significant soft-tissue disruption will be more difficult to rehabilitate. Properly differentiating the ossification center of the medial epicondyle from that of the trochlea is the key to making the correct diagnosis.

Epicondylar displacement is well tolerated by the patient unless significant repetitive forceful loading is anticipated in the future. Documentation in long-term follow-up studies has shown that the presence of a displaced fragment does not cause significant discomfort. The studies also show that a chronic fibrous union will most likely function satisfactorily, but may cause aching of the elbow during athletic activities. The limited indications for open reduction include an entrapped medial epicondyle fragment within the joint that fails to be extracted with closed manipulation or a patient with a displaced medial epicon-

dylar fragment in a dominant arm in which significant valgus loading may be expected (eg, tennis or baseball). An entrapped medial epicondyle may be successfully freed from the joint by applying tension through the flexor-pronator mass with the forearm supinated and the wrist and fingers extended.

Traumatic ulnar neuritis or palsy may occur acutely but will resolve spontaneously in most instances. Long-term studies of medial epicondylar fractures treated conservatively have shown good results as long as the fragment is not in the joint. After nonsurgical treatment, slightly more than half of epicondyles form a pseudarthrosis, but this pseudarthrosis does not appear to be correlated with increased symptoms.

During fixation, the patient is placed prone, with the arm on a hand table, or supine with the arm abducted and externally rotated, to allow access to the posteromedial side and a tourniquet is applied. A curvilinear Kocher-J incision is made posteromedially, the fracture fragments and nerve are identified, and the fracture edges cleared. If the fragment is incarcerated in the joint, the flexor-pronator mass is followed until it leads to the bone fragment. After reduction, the fragment is provisionally fixed in place with a threaded pin, then definitively stabilized with an appropriate size compression screw. Care must be taken with the screw to avoid excessive compression or the medial epicondyle may be crushed under the pressure of the screw head. Countersinking the screw head or using a washer may prevent damage to the medial epicondyle. An anterior transposition of the ulnar nerve is not necessary. Range of motion exercises are started at 4 to 6 weeks after surgery and the screw is removed only if it is significantly prominent. Permanent complications are rare, other than

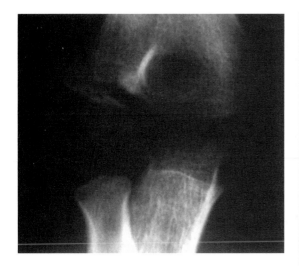

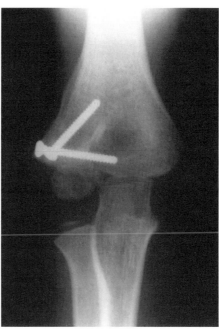

Fig. 6 **Left,** Lateral condyle fracture that was initially displaced 2 mm. Delayed union followed. **Right,** The fracture was treated by bone graft in situ across the metaphyseal portion, with subsequent union.

the occasional prominence, varus, or mild restriction of extension. The same problems may occur with nonsurgical treatment, although there is less restriction of extension.

If an elbow dislocation is encountered with a medial epicondyle fracture, the dislocation is reduced first. If the medial epicondyle remains entrapped (or significantly displaced in the dominant arm of an athlete), open reduction of the fragment is performed through a medial approach (Fig. 8).

Elbow Dislocations

Elbow dislocations occur most commonly in children older than 6 years of age and virtually never occur before age 6. Usually, the mechanism of injury is hyperextension of the elbow with abduction. The associated fractures that commonly occur with elbow dislocations are radial head fractures, medial epicondylar and lateral condylar fractures, and coronoid avulsion fractures. It is important to detect radial neck fractures before reduction to prevent displacement.

Neurologic injury occurs in 10% of elbow dislocations and is usually associated with entrapment of the ulnar nerve by the medial epicondyle. The majority of nerve injuries will resolve spontaneously. Radial nerve abnormalities are rare, but median nerve damage may result if the nerve kinks inside the joint, courses behind the medial epicondyle, or is entrapped in an epicondylar fracture. Arterial injuries with elbow dislocation are very rare, and most

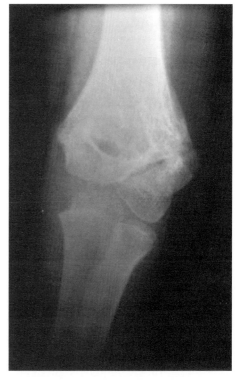

Fig. 7 Cubitus varus caused by incomplete reduction following lateral condyle fracture.

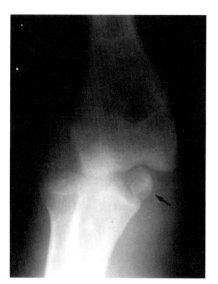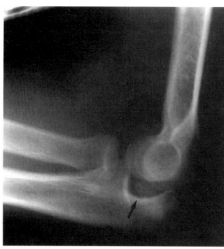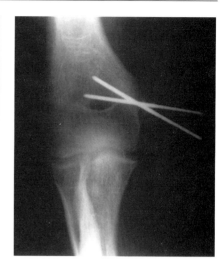

Fig. 8 **Left** and **center,** Medial epicondyle fracture-dislocation. **Right,** Open reduction was required to extract the epicondyle, so pin fixation was performed.

reported cases occurred with an open injury. Decreased range of motion follows most elbow dislocations but usually is not severe.

After an uncomplicated elbow dislocation has been reduced, circulation and muscle function must be monitored, either in the hospital or by close observation at home. The decision whether to hospitalize the patient depends on the amount of soft-tissue injury that is present and the parents' understanding of the problem. Elbow range of motion exercises should be begun within 2 weeks of treatment.

Recurrent elbow dislocations and posterolateral instability are recently described conditions. Virtually all patients with recurrent elbow dislocations had the initial episode occur in childhood. The pathology primarily is an attenuation of the posterolateral capsular structures. If repair is necessary, it is performed by reattaching the lateral capsule to the epicondyle.

Late unreduced elbow dislocations are seen mainly in patients who have sustained polytrauma or head injury, or who have not sought medical attention for their elbow dislocation. If treatment is delayed for longer than 1 week, closed reduction should be avoided and an open reduction performed. Open reduction may be performed successfully as late as 2 years after the dislocation. Early controlled joint range of motion exercises should be begun and medications to prevent heterotopic ossification should be prescribed. Patients with very late recognized dislocations who have a reasonable range of motion in the dislocated position (an arc greater than 60°) should be observed, due to the likelihood of satisfactory function.

An isolated radial head dislocation may be caused by trauma. It is important to differentiate a traumatic dislocation from a congenital dislocation. A congenital dislocation has a more rounded appearance to the radial head, incongruity with the capitellum, relative overgrowth of the radius, and hypoplasia of the capitellum. Because there is little likelihood of a successful outcome, congenital dislocations should not be reduced. However, if detected early, closed reduction of a traumatic dislocation is often successful. Correction of any subtle ulnar plastic or greenstick deformity must be achieved at the same time. In late cases—up to 2 years after injury—consideration may be given to reducing and stabilizing the radial head using an annular ligament reconstruction, such as the procedure described by Bell Tawse. In this method, a strip of triceps fascia is harvested, left attached distally, then woven around the radial neck and through a tunnel in the ulna.

Fractures of the Radius and Ulna

Fractures of the Radial Head and Neck

The articular surface of the radial head forms an angle of approximately 10° valgus, with respect to the long axis of the radius. This mild angulation is seen well on an AP radiograph, and slightly less well on a lateral radiograph. Maintaining this angle and avoiding significant translation of the radial head are critical to restoring full range of forearm rotation following a radial neck fracture.

The neck of the radius may be fractured by one of three injury mechanisms: valgus force to the extended forearm; shearing force during elbow dislocation or reduction; or fracture dislocations such as Monteggia variants.

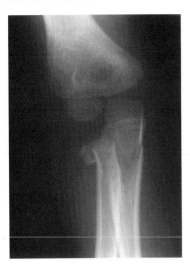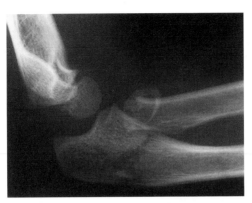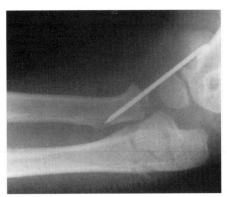

Fig. 9 **Left** and **center,** Radial neck fracture. The coexisting fracture of the olecranon is a clue to the valgus mechanism. **Right,** Closed manipulation of the radial head fracture was followed by intraosseous pin fixation.

When a radial neck fracture results from a valgus force injury, often there is an associated fracture of the olecranon or an avulsion of the medial epicondyle (Fig. 9). The radial head fragment may be impacted into the metaphysis, making manipulative reduction difficult. Translation may be minimal in these valgus force injuries. Radial neck fractures associated with dislocation usually are not impacted and have a greater amount of translation. In these dislocation injuries, there have been several reports of the radial head being "flipped" 180°, resulting in the fracture surface of the radial neck articulating with the capitellum (Fig. 10).

Early motion is recommended treatment of radial neck fractures in which angulation is less than 30° and translation less than 5 mm. Such minimal malposition is less likely to decrease elbow range of motion than are additional adhesions following reduction and immobilization. Fractures with angulation between 30° and 60° warrant closed reduction, but do not justify open reduction. Only in those fractures with angulation greater than 60° or translation over 5 mm is the added soft-tissue reaction from an open reduction justified, should closed reduction attempts fail.

There are several methods of attempting closed reduction of radial neck fractures. Manipulation of the fracture with the elbow in extension has been described. The elbow is rotated until the maximum deviation of the fracture can be palpated or visualized with fluoroscopy, then a varus stress is applied to open the lateral side, and digital pressure is applied over the angulated fragment. Manipulation with the elbow in flexion has also been described. A thumb is placed anteriorly over the displaced radial head, and with pronation the fragment may be forced into place.

Both of these techniques are difficult when the radial head fragment is severely impacted.

The most common technique for reduction of severely angulated radial neck fractures uses a percutaneous Steinmann pin to lever the fragment back into place. This is done in the operating room using fluoroscopy. The forearm is rotated until maximum fracture profile is seen, then a Kirschner wire (K-wire) is introduced percutaneously into the radial head. To avoid irritation of the posterior interosseous nerve, the K-wire is introduced posteriorly near the ulna. The wire is used, in combination with some axial traction on the arm, to push the radial head back into place.

If closed or percutaneous methods fail to reduce the severely angulated fracture, open reduction through a lateral approach may be necessary. Minimum stripping, dissection, or devascularization should be done no matter how the reduction is obtained. If the reduction is stable through a reasonable range of rotation, no fixation is needed. If the reduction is not stable, fixation is necessary and is best done by an intraosseous technique. A percutaneous K-wire is passed from the proximal-lateral corner of the proximal radius, across the fracture site, to engage the distal cortex. Use of a transcapitellar pin is less desirable because of the significant risk of intra-articular pin breakage. Sequelae of this fracture include premature growth arrest of the radial neck, overgrowth of the radial head, synostosis of the radius to the ulna, and elbow stiffness.

Monteggia Fractures

A Monteggia fracture consists of a radial head dislocation in conjunction with an ulnar fracture. The radial head dis-

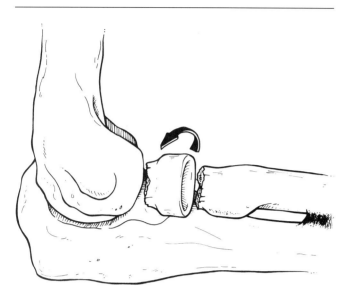

Fig. 10 Radial neck fractures that occur with elbow dislocation may displace with reduction and become completely rotated.

locates in the direction of the apical ulnar angulation. A type I Monteggia fracture, an ulnar fracture with anterior dislocation of the radial head, is the most common, occurring in 70% of patients with Monteggia fracures. A type II fracture is an ulnar fracture with posterior dislocation that occurs in 5% of patients and a type III is an ulnar fracture with lateral dislocation that occurs in 25% of patients. A type IV is a fracture of both the ulna and radius with a dislocation of the radius, and is rare. "Monteggia-equivalent lesions" are isolated radial head dislocations without ulnar fracture, or ulnar shaft fractures with radial neck fracture.

Most Monteggia fractures in children may be treated by closed reduction. The strong ulnar periosteum usually allows a satisfactory ulnar reduction that in turn allows the radial head to be reduced. If the ulnar fracture is relatively oblique, comminuted, or otherwise hard to control, however, primary stabilization may be needed. To reduce the radial head dislocation in type I injuries, the elbow should be flexed and fully supinated. In type II injuries, the elbow should be extended and the forearm placed in 45° pronation. Type III injuries are treated with the elbow flexed to 90° with supination. Type IV injuries are usually treated with the elbow in flexion. Closed reduction of the radial head can usually be obtained as late as 2 weeks after the fracture. If the radial head cannot be reduced, it may be because of imperfect reduction of the ulna, an infolded annular ligament, or buttonholing of the radial head through the joint capsule. Unsatisfactory closed reductions should be treated first by internal fixation of the ulna

and followed by open reduction of the radial head, if necessary. Late cases with radial head dislocation may be treated up to 2 years after the injury and still achieve satisfactory, though limited, range of motion. Ulnar angulation must be corrected and can be stabilized with an intramedullary rod. In the preferred annular ligament reconstruction, described by Bell Tawse, a long lateral incision is used, and a strip of triceps fascia based distally on its ulnar insertion is harvested and routed around the radial neck back upon itself.

Complications of Monteggia fractures include restriction of motion, recurring dislocations, and nerve palsy. The radial or posterior interosseous nerve is the most commonly injured nerve, occurring mainly in type III injuries. Spontaneous neural recovery can be expected.

Olecranon Fractures

Fractures of the olecranon are quite rare and may be apophyseal or metaphyseal. The average patient age is 9 years and one third of these patients have additional elbow fractures. Most apophyseal fractures of the olecranon are caused by hyperflexion injuries and most metaphyseal fractures occur with flexion, extension, or shear injuries. A "sleeve" fracture is an apophyseal avulsion that occurs when the elbow is flexed. Stable fractures are those with no displacement or those with minimal separation but no movement upon flexion and extension. Stable fractures may be treated by immobilization only. Some displaced flexion-type fractures reduce in extension and, because it is well tolerated, may be treated by immobilization in extension. Unstable fractures should be treated with open reduction and internal fixation.

Elbow Capsular Contracture

Although children rarely lose significant range of motion following elbow fractures, there are exceptions. The useful arc of elbow flexion–extension needed for activities of daily living is from 30° to 130°. If elbow flexion is limited to 90°, significant impairment may result. Initial treatment should include static and dynamic splinting followed by open surgical release of capsular contracture if improvement is not seen. This procedure is performed through a lateral incision, incising the entire anterior or posterior capsule, as needed, and removing any obstacles that prevent motion. In one series of nine children, a mean improvement of 50° was noted after open surgical release of capsular contracture.

The successful treatment of pediatric elbow fractures depends on an understanding of the patterns of ossification and fractures, and knowing who is at risk for nonunion and who is at risk for stiffness. If the principles presented in this chapter are followed, satisfactory results will be achieved most of the time.

Annotated Bibliography

Fractures of the Humerus

Cramer KE, Green NE, Devito DP: Incidence of anterior interosseous nerve palsy in supracondylar humerus fractures in children. *J Pediatr Orthop* 1993;13:502–505.

In 101 supracondylar fractures, there were 15 patients with nerve palsy; 12 had involvement of the anterior interosseous nerve alone. In two patients with median nerve palsy and absent pulses, the median nerve was entrapped in the fracture. Complete resolution of the nerve palsy was found in 14 of the 15 patients.

Culp RW, Osterman AL, Davidson RS, et al: Neural injuries associated with supracondylar fractures of the humerus in children. *J Bone Joint Surg* 1990;72A:1211–1215.

In 101 supracondylar fractures, 18 nerve injuries in 13 patients were seen. Only nine of the injured nerves recovered spontaneously by 5 months; the rest displayed no improvements on EMG. Of the remaining nine nerves, neurolysis was successful in eight that were found entrapped in scar or callus. The remaining nerve was found to be lacerated, and nerve grafting was unsuccessful. The authors recommend observation with EMG at 3 to 5 months, with neurolysis if no improvement is seen by 5 months.

Ellefsen BK, Frierson MA, Raney EM, et al: Humerus varus: A complication of neonatal infantile, and childhood injury and infection. *J Pediatr Orthop* 1994;14:479–486.

In this article, 16 cases of humerus varus are described, some as sequelae of childhood and infantile fractures.

Flynn JC: Nonunion of slightly displaced fractures of the lateral humeral condyle in children: An update. *J Pediatr Orthop* 1989;9:691–696.

Causes and treatment of 23 nonunions are reviewed. In one quarter of the cases, the patient did not seek medical attention or the diagnosis of fracture was missed. Undertreatment of a displaced fracture occurred in more than one half of the cases. Treatment of 14 of the nonunions was by "peg" bone graft with limited dissection. All nonunions healed, and only three patients experienced growth disturbances.

Josefsson PO, Danielsson LG: Epicondylar elbow fracture in children: 35-year follow-up of 56 unreduced cases. *Acta Orthop Scand* 1986;57:313–315.

Fifty-one consecutive fractures of the medial epicondyle treated nonsurgically were examined at a minimum of 20 years follow-up. A pseudarthrosis was present after healing in 60%. Only 25% of patients had residual symptoms, none of which were limiting. There was no significant difference in elbow pain whether or not the epicondyle had healed. Minor ulnar nerve symptoms were slightly more common in the group with pseudarthrosis.

Masada K, Kawai H, Kawabata H, et al: Osteosynthesis for old, established non-union of the lateral condyle of the humerus. *J Bone Joint Surg* 1990;72A:32–40.

Nonunions more than 5 years old were studied in 30 patients. The authors concluded that the goals of treatment should be separated into treatment of pain, deformity, or prevention of ulnar palsy. Osteosynthesis was effective in relieving pain, but produced a significant postsurgical decrease in motion.

Mintzer CM, Waters PM, Brown DJ, et al: Percutaneous pinning in the treatment of displaced lateral condyle fractures. *J Pediatr Orthop* 1994;14:462–465.

Closed reduction and percutaneous pinning was successful in 12 patients who had lateral condyle fractures with displacement greater than 2 mm, but with intact articular cartilage as documented by arthrogram. Excellent range of motion and function resulted.

Pirone AM, Graham HK, Krajbich JI: Management of displaced extension-type supracondylar fractures of the humerus in children. *J Bone Joint Surg* 1988;70A:641–650.

This classic review of 230 displaced extension-type supracondylar fractures treated by four different methods shows that best results (78% excellent) were achieved by percutaneous pin fixation and worst results (51% excellent) were in patients treated by closed reduction and cast.

Rockwood CA Jr, Wilkins KE, King RE (eds): *Fractures in Children,* ed 3. Philadelphia, PA, JB Lippincott, 1991, vol 3.

This definitive reference provides excellent information on history, anatomy, treatment, and complications of fractures in children.

Voss FR, Kasser JR, Trepman E, et al: Uniplanar supracondylar humeral osteotomy with preset Kirschner wires for posttraumatic cubitus varus. *J Pediatr Orthop* 1994;14:471–478.

In this series of 36 patients, 97% of posttraumatic cubitus varus deformities were corrected and maintained to within 5° of the contralateral side. Preservation of a medial hinge and the use of two preset, widely-spaced pins is helpful.

Williamson DM, Coates CJ, Miller RK, et al: Normal characteristics of the Baumann (humerocapitellar) angle: An aid in assessment of supracondylar fractures. *J Pediatr Orthop* 1992;12:636–639.

In this study of 114 children between ages 2 and 13 years, the normal Baumann angle was 72° ± 4°. It did not vary significantly with age or sex.

Zionts, LE, McKellop HA, Hathaway R: Torsional strength of pin configurations used to fix supracondylar fractures of the humerus in children. *J Bone Joint Surg* 1994;76A:253–256.

In resistance to rotational torque, medial and lateral pins were most stable, followed by three lateral, then two parallel lateral pins. Two crossed lateral pins produced 80% less stability.

Elbow Dislocations

Fowles JV, Slimane N, Kassab, MT: Elbow dislocation with avulsion of the medial humeral epicondyle. *J Bone Joint Surg* 1990;72B:102–104.

Retrospective comparison of surgical and nonsurgical management of medial epicondylar fractures followed for at least 18 months showed an increased incidence of flexion contractures in the group receiving surgical treatment.

Fractures of the Radius and Ulna

Bernstein SM, McKeever P, Bernstein L: Percutaneous reduction of displaced radial neck fractures in children. *J Pediatr Orthop* 1993;13:85–88.

This technique often eliminates the need to open significantly displaced fractures that cannot be treated with closed reduction.

Graves SC, Canale ST: Fractures of the olecranon in children: Long-term follow-up. *J Pediatr Orthop* 1993;13:239–241.

In this review of 44 fractures, with follow-up occurring a mean of 29 months after injury, results were generally good; only one fourth of displaced fractures had minor loss of motion.

Elbow Capsular Contracture

Mih AD, Wolf FG: Surgical release of elbow-capsular contracture in pediatric patients. *J Pediatr Orthop* 1994;14:458–461.

A mean 50° improvement in flexion-extension arc in nine children ages 5 to 17 years was found, with traumatic or nontraumatic contractures.

29

Forearm and Wrist Fractures

Forearm fractures are the most common long bone fractures in children, accounting for 45% of all childhood fractures and 62% of upper extremity fractures. Approximately 75% to 84% of these forearm fractures occur in the distal third; 15% to 18%, in the middle third; and less than 5%, in the proximal third. Much less commonly, children will suffer injuries to the distal radioulnar joint, carpal bones, or intercarpal ligaments. The most common carpal bone fracture is of the scaphoid, and yet it accounts for only 0.45% of all upper extremity fractures in children.

Fractures of the Diaphyseal Radius and Ulna

Diaphyseal fractures are classified as: plastic deformation; buckle or torus; greenstick or incomplete; and complete. Approximately 50% of diaphyseal fractures are greenstick and most often occur in children younger than 8 years of age. Greenstick fractures most commonly have apex volar malalignment and supination rotational deformity. Complete fractures are more common in the preadolescent and adolescent age groups and tend to be unstable.

The forearm rotates an average of 150° to 180° with the mechanical axis of rotation extending from the proximal radius to the distal ulna. Rotational malalignment of a forearm fracture leads directly to loss of this rotation in a ratio of at least 1:1. In middle third diaphyseal malrotated fractures, this loss of rotation may have a ratio as high as 2:1.

Frontal or sagittal angulation will also limit forearm rotation. Angular deformity greater than 20° significantly decreases pronation and supination. Fortunately, remodeling of angular deformity occurs in children but is dependent on the age of the patient, proximity of the fracture to the physis, amount of deformity, and direction of the angular deformity. Remodeling of angular deformity of the radius may be as rapid as 10° per year. A new index, axis deviation, may better assess remodeling potential and outcome than the amount of angulation alone. Axis deviation is the deviation of the fracture apex from a straight line between the articular surfaces and is calculated from reference tables. The clinical outcome of forearm rotation does not always correlate with the degree of malunion, however. Criteria for acceptable reduction of diaphyseal fractures have not been definitively established and clearly depend on the age of the patient and location of the fracture.

By definition, torus or buckle fractures are stable; cortical failure occurs only in compression and not in tension. Immobilization in a short arm cast for 3 to 4 weeks provides pain relief and prevents further injury. If both cor-tices are fractured, there is a risk that malangulation will occur gradually, and a well-molded long arm cast should be used. Greenstick fractures generally are stable after a closed reduction and can be treated in a long arm cast with appropriate three-point fixation, interosseous mold, and straight ulnar border. Because most of these fractures have apex volar malangulation and supination malrotation, reduction should first correct the malrotation by pronating the forearm, followed by correction of the apex volar angulation using three-point molding.

Displaced complete diaphyseal fractures are difficult to reduce closed and are frequently unstable. Closed reduction requires aligning the distal fragment with the proximal fragment by correcting the malrotation, angulation, and translation sequentially. If both bones are displaced, it is often best to reduce the ulna first. Open reduction is indicated for: (1) irreducible fractures; (2) unstable fractures, especially in the adolescent; (3) displaced segmental fractures; (4) fractures associated with unstable Monteggia, Galeazzi, or supracondylar fractures; and (5) refracture.

Fractures of the Distal Radius and Ulna

Metaphyseal Fractures

Seventy-five percent to 84% of pediatric forearm fractures involve the distal radius. Most of these radial fractures are metaphyseal and are associated with metaphyseal fractures of the ulna. Although closed reduction and long arm cast immobilization is indicated for fractures with greater than 10° of malalignment, several recent studies indicate a high incidence of loss of reduction with closed treatment of these fractures. Poor casting techniques, isolated radius fractures, associated displaced ulna fractures or plastic deformation, and initial malangulation greater than 30° have all been implicated as predicators. The need for repeat closed reduction has been cited to be as high as 34%. Percutaneous pin fixation may decrease the need to re-reduce the difficult distal radius fractures. Remodeling of malunited fractures in the flexion/extension plane will occur and, to a lesser extent, will also occur in the radial deviation/ulnar deviation plane. Rotational malunion will not remodel, however. Currently, what represents an acceptable alignment after reduction is controversial but clearly depends on the age of the patient, fracture location, and other injuries.

Percutaneous pinning may be indicated for fractures associated with neurovascular compromise, significant soft-

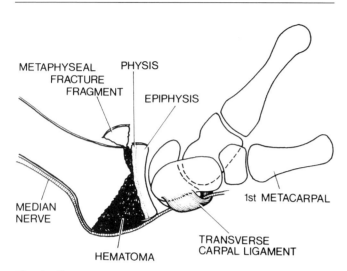

Fig. 1 The potential compression of the median nerve from tenting of the nerve over the metaphyseal fragment, local hematoma, and the dorsally displaced physis and transverse carpal ligament. (Reproduced with permission from Waters PM, Kolettis GJ, Schwend R: Acute median neuropathy following physeal fractures of the distal radius. *J Pediatr Orthop* 1994;14:173–177.)

tissue swelling, initial angulation greater than 30°, displacement more than 50% of the diameter of the radius, or concomitant fractures of the elbow. A smooth K-wire is inserted obliquely from distal to proximal, starting in the radial metaphysis just proximal to the physis. Care must be taken to avoid the radial sensory nerve with insertion. This may be done with a 5- to 10-mm incision and clearing pin track. A second, crossing K-wire can be inserted from between the third and fourth dorsal extensor compartments while avoiding the extensor pollicus longus tendon at the level of Lister's tubercle.

Physeal Fractures

Most distal radial physeal fractures are Salter-Harris type II injuries that occur in the adolescent. Displacement is typically dorsal with apex volar angulation. Atraumatic closed reduction and long arm cast immobilization is indicated for fractures with greater than 10° of malangulation. The most significant concerns with these fractures are future growth arrest and acute neurovascular compromise. The incidence of associated nerve injuries was 8% in a recent prospective study (Fig. 1). Another retrospective series reported that patients with signs or symptoms of median nerve injury at the time of presentation would be

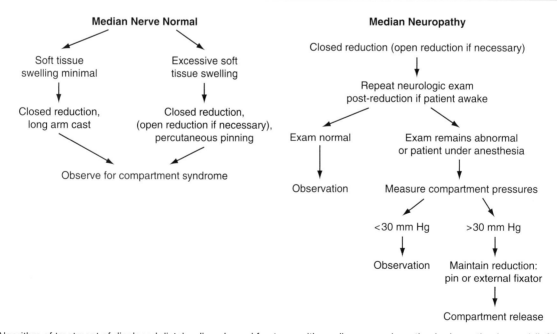

Fig. 2 Algorithm of treatment of displaced distal radius physeal fractures with median nerve dysesthesias/paresthesias and (**left**) normal median nerve or (**right**) median neuropathy. (Reproduced with permission from Waters PM, Kolettis GJ, Schwend R: Acute median neuropathy following physeal fractures of the distal radius. *J Pediatr Orthop* 1994;14:173–177.)

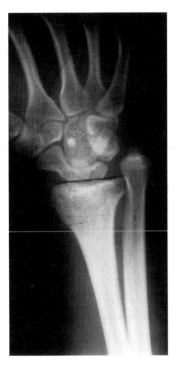 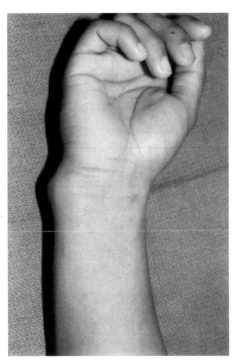 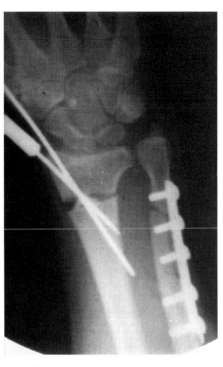

Fig. 3   Left, Radiograph shows distal radial physeal arrest after repetitive closed reductions of a Salter-Harris type II fracture. **Center,** Clinical photograph. **Right,** Because of signs and symptoms of ulnar-carpal impaction syndrome and limited forearm rotation, the patient underwent a corrective ulnar shortening and opening wedge radial osteotomy as shown. The ulnar bone from the Z-shortening was used as radial bone graft.

managed best by percutaneous pin fixation rather than cast immobilization in order to lessen the risk of forearm compartment syndrome, acute carpal tunnel syndrome, or median neuropathy (Fig. 2). A single oblique smooth K-wire inserted from the radial styloid distally and directed to the ulnar aspect of the radial metaphysis proximally provides sufficient fixation. As with metaphyseal fractures, care must be taken to avoid the radial sensory nerve during pin insertion. If left percutaneous, the K-wire can be readily removed in the office after 4 weeks.

Growth arrest is related to two factors: the amount of initial trauma affecting the physis and iatrogenic injury with late reduction. Patients with redisplacement or late presentation should not undergo repeat reduction after 7 days from fracture in order to avoid iatrogenic physeal arrest. Late open reduction should be avoided for the same reason (Fig. 3). Because these fractures displace in the plane of motion of the wrist joint and are juxtaphyseal, there is tremendous potential for remodeling of a malunion in the younger adolescent (Fig. 4). If the malunion does not remodel with growth, a dorsal opening wedge osteotomy with bone graft and internal fixation may be needed for the skeletally mature patient with greater than 10° apex dorsal malangulation. Finally, patients with dis-

placed physeal fractures should be examined 1 to 2 years after fracture to rule out growth disturbance.

Salter-Harris types III and IV fractures are rare but require anatomic reduction to restore articular and physeal congruity. Open reduction is indicated for those fractures that fail closed reduction. Wrist arthroscopy can be used in adolescents to aid and assess closed reductions and percutaneous fixation (Fig. 5).

Galeazzi Fractures

Galeazzi fractures are rare in children. More common is a Galeazzi equivalent, with an ulnar physeal fracture associated with a distal radius metaphyseal or physeal fracture. Anatomic reductions of both the radius and ulna fractures are required to restore normal function. In children, reduction can often be achieved closed. Inability to achieve a closed reduction of the ulna physeal fracture may result from extensor tendon or periosteal interposition and, if so, then requires an open reduction. Late instability is rare following this fracture, but premature ulnar physeal arrest and ulnar shortening has been reported in more than 55% of patients with distal ulnar physeal fractures (Fig. 6).

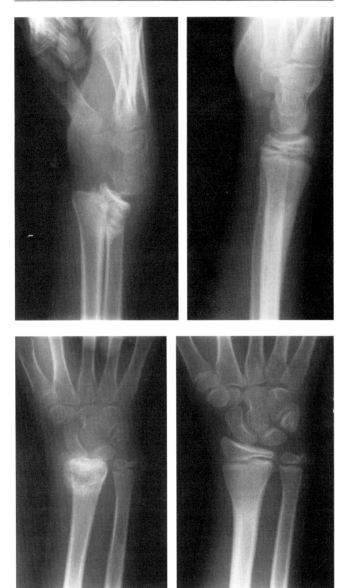

Fig. 4 **Top left** and **bottom left,** Radiographs of an 11-year-old boy who presented late with a significantly displaced Salter-Harris type II distal radial physeal fracture. It was decided to monitor his remodeling with growth. **Top right** and **bottom right,** Subsequent radiographs 1 year after fracture show anatomic alignment of the radius with open physes.

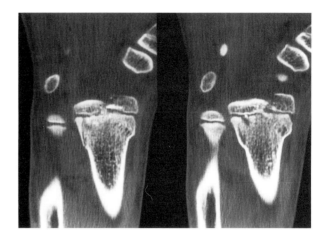

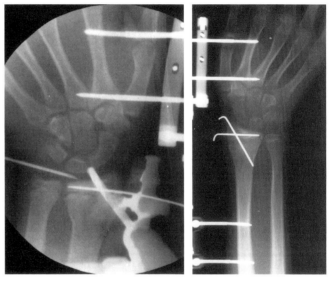

Fig. 5 **Top,** Computed tomogram of a displaced, combined Salter-Harris types IV and II fractures of the distal radius in a 15-year-old boy. **Bottom left,** Intraoperative fluoroscopic radiograph showing the reduction with the external fixator, utilization of the wrist arthroscope to visualize the reduction of the articular surface and assist in percutaneous pinning of the physis. **Bottom right,** Follow-up healed radiographs at the time of pin and external fixator removal.

Less common are true Galeazzi injuries, with ligamentous disruptions of the distal radioulnar joint and triangular fibrocartilage. Classically, the most common instability pattern, both acutely and chronically, has been described in adults as dorsal dislocation. This instability pattern is more rare in children than adults. Although rarer acutely, volar dislocation of the ulna in supination appears to be the more common late instability pattern. Soft-tissue reconstruction with a portion of the retinaculum of the fifth and sixth dorsal extensor compartments and a distally based slip of the extensor carpi ulnaris tendon can stabilize the joint. Any malunion leading to instability should be corrected with osteotomy.

Carpal Injuries

Triangular Fibrocartilage Complex Tears
The presence of an ulnar styloid nonunion in an adolescent with persistent ulnar-sided wrist pain after a radius and ulna fracture often represents ulnocarpal impaction

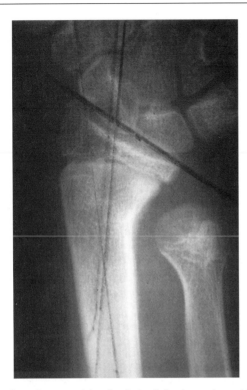

Fig. 6 Growth arrest of the distal ulna following a physeal fracture with subsequent deformity of the radius.

and a peripheral triangular fibrocartilage complex (TFCC) tear. In patients who fail nonsurgical therapy, excision of the nonunion and repair of the TFCC tear is helpful.

Diagnostic wrist arthroscopy has led to an appreciation that unresolved ulnar-sided wrist pain may indicate an unrecognized TFCC tear. Wrist arthrograms and magnetic resonance imaging have both been shown to have an unacceptably high rate of false-negative results when compared with wrist arthroscopy in prospective studies comparing multiple imaging techniques. The development of the 2.5- to 3.0-mm diameter arthroscopes and small instruments has offered easy access to the radiocarpal, midcarpal, and radioulnar joints. Isolated tears of the TFCC are now being diagnosed with increasing frequency in adolescents. There are presently insufficient long-term clinical data to comment on the efficacy of open versus arthroscopic repairs.

Scaphoid Fractures

Most scaphoid fractures in the skeletally immature patient are fractures or avulsions of the distal pole. These fractures heal readily with thumb spica cast immobilization for 4 to 8 weeks with essentially no risk of nonunion or osteonecrosis. Scaphoid waist fractures, however, carry the same risks of nonunion and osteonecrosis in the child as they do in an adult. Scaphoid waist fractures should be assessed with tomograms for fracture displacement. If nondisplaced, thumb spica cast immobilization is indi-

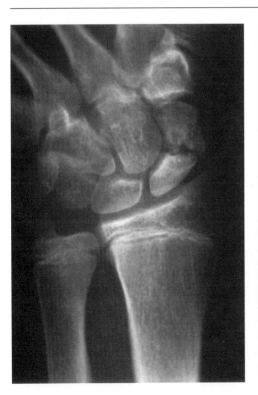 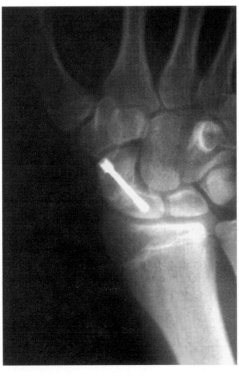

Fig. 7 **Left,** Scaphoid nonunion in a skeletally immature patient. **Right,** Treatment with iliac crest bone graft and Herbert screw fixation was successful.

cated for 3 to 6 months until healing. The issue of long arm or short arm thumb spica cast immobilization is unresolved. An established nonunion in a child should be treated with open reduction, bone grafting, and potentially internal fixation. Herbert screws have been used in children both with acute displaced waist fractures and established nonunions (Fig. 7). The issue of whether a bipartite scaphoid, even if bilateral, is congenital or post-traumatic is unresolved; however, if a bipartite scaphoid is symptomatic, it should be treated as a nonunion with open reduction and bone grafting.

Annotated Bibliography

Radius and Ulna Diaphyseal Fractures

Price CT, Scott DS, Kurzner ME, et al: Malunited forearm fractures in children. *J Pediatr Orthop* 1990; 10:705–712.

The authors present a retrospective series of 39 patients treated initially with closed reduction for a forearm fracture and followed for longer than 2 years (average follow-up, 5.75 years). All patients had fracture malunion as defined by more than 10° angulation, displacement of more than 50%, malrotation, or encroachment on the interosseous membrane. Good to excellent results were reported in 92%. Only 8% of these patients had a fair clinical result by their criteria.

Younger AS, Tredwell SJ, Mackenzie WG, et al: Accurate prediction of outcome after pediatric forearm fracture. *J Pediatr Orthop* 1994;14:200–206.

The authors introduce a new index, axis deviation, and correlate it with clinical outcome in terms of forearm rotation after fracture. They propose that an axis deviation of less than 5° be the goal for acceptable reduction and clinical union. The reference matrices in Figure 5 of their text are necessary for clinical application.

Distal Radius Metaphyseal Fractures

Gibbons CL, Woods DA, Pailthorpe C, et al: The management of isolated distal radius fractures in children. *J Pediatr Orthop* 1994;14:207–210.

The authors present a prospective series of 23 patients with displaced isolated distal radius fractures. Ten cases were treated with percutaneous pinning and 13 cases were treated with long arm cast immobilization. Ninety-one percent of the cast group had loss of reduction (averaging 24.6°) that required repeat reduction. None of the pinning group had loss of reduction or complications.

Holmes JR, Louis DS: Entrapment of pronator quadratus in pediatric distal-radius fractures: Recognition and treatment. *J Pediatr Orthop* 1994;14:498–500.

Three cases of irreducible distal radius fractures are described, all of which were approximately 3 cm proximal to the distal radial physis and had failed attempts at closed reduction. At open reduction all three had interposed pronator quadratus muscle that blocked the closed reduction. After extraction of the muscle, all had uneventful open reduction.

Mani GV, Hui PW, Cheng JC: Translation of the radius as a predictor of outcome in distal radial fractures of children. *J Bone Joint Surg* 1993;75B:808–811.

The authors present a retrospective analysis of 94 distal radius fractures in children treated with primary closed reduction and cast immobilization. Loss of reduction was 29%. Initial translation of the radius more than half the diameter of the radius had a 60% rate of loss of reduction compared with an 8% rate if the initial translation was less than half the diameter of the radius. The authors recommend primary percutaneous pinning of severely displaced fractures and open reduction for irreducible fractures (12% of their study group).

Proctor MT, Moore DJ, Paterson JM: Redisplacement after manipulation of distal radial fractures in children. *J Bone Joint Surg* 1993;75B:453–454.

In this review of 68 fractures of the distal radius in children treated with primary reduction and cast immobilization, loss of reduction occurred in 34%. Initial complete displacement and failure to achieve a perfect reduction were associated with loss of reduction. The authors advocate percutaneous pinning for those children at risk for loss of reduction by these criteria.

Radius Physeal Fractures

Waters PM, Kolettis GJ, Schwend R: Acute median neuropathy following physeal fractures of the distal radius. *J Pediatr Orthop* 1994;14:173–177.

Case series describing eight cases of median neuropathy associated with displaced Salter-Harris type II fractures of the distal radius. The authors outline the etiology of median nerve injury, including direct contusion, tenting of the nerve over a displaced fracture, and the development of an acute compartment syndrome. The authors outline an algorithm for treatment that includes percutaneous pinning of those fractures most at risk for compartment syndrome.

Galeazzi Fractures

Golz RJ, Grogan DP, Greene TL, et al: Distal ulnar physeal injury. *J Pediatr Orthop* 1991;11:318–326.

The authors review 18 patients who had distal ulnar physeal injuries with associated radial metaphyseal or physeal fractures. Ulnar styloid fractures were excluded. Physeal fractures by Salter-Harris classification were: I (8 fractures), II (1), III (6), and IV (1); two fractures were not classified. Premature physeal closure of the ulna occurred in 55% of patients. Seven of those ten patients had angular deformity in the radius and ulnar translocation of the carpus.

Letts M, Rowhani N: Galeazzi-equivalent injuries of the wrist in children. *J Pediatr Othop* 1993;13:561–566.

The results of ten cases of Galeazzi fracture (distal radius fracture with dislocation of the distal ulna) and Galeazzi-equivalent fractures (distal radius fractures with ulnar physeal separation) are described and a classification system is proposed. Closed reduction of both the radius fracture and ulnar dislocation is usually successful in children. Open reduction is indicated for an irreducible ulna and often heralds interposed extensor tendons or periosteum. Long-term problems were persistent instability of the distal radioulnar joint in Galeazzi injuries and ulnar growth arrest in the Galeazzi-equivalent fractures.

Carpal Injuries

Doman AN, Marcus NW: Congenital bipartite scaphoid. *J Hand Surg* 1990;15A:869–873.

The authors present a single case report of bilateral bipartate scaphoid. This is a thorough review of the literature surrounding the controversy of the congenital versus traumatic etiology of the bipartate scaphoid.

Mintzer CM, Waters PM, Simmons BP: Nonunion of the scaphoid in children treated by Herbert screw fixation and bone grafting: A report of five cases. *J Bone Joint Surg* 1995;77B:98–100.

The authors present a case series of five skeletally immature patients with scaphoid nonunions treated with open reduction, bone grafting, and Herbert screw fixation. Average age at fracture was 12.7 years, with average follow-up 3.3 years. All healed radiographically without a carpal instability pattern. All had excellent clinical results.

30

Knee Injuries and Tibial Fractures

Knee Injuries

Ligament Injuries

Ligament injuries of the knee are less common in children than in adults. Much more common are physeal fractures, particularly of the distal femur. The ligaments of the knee arise from the epiphyses of the distal femur, proximal tibia, and proximal fibula with the exception of the superficial portion of the medial collateral ligament (MCL), which inserts into the tibial metaphysis. As a result, stress concentration occurs within the region of the physes when bending or twisting forces are exerted across the knee. Because ligament injuries about the knee are uncommon in children, treatment recommendations are often based on anecdotal evidence or on series involving a small number of patients. However, once the physes begin to close, the treatment recommendations become similar to those given for adults.

The physical examination aids in differentiating physeal injury from collateral ligament injury. Swelling and tenderness are more circumferential and are located at the level of the physis in cases of physeal fracture. MCL injury usually produces swelling with tenderness localized to the region of the ligament. Clinical instability to valgus stress may be secondary to either a physeal or MCL injury. Radiographic stress views may be useful in differentiating these injuries, although stable nondisplaced physeal fractures may not open when stressed. A short period of immobilization may be useful in differentiating distal femoral physeal injury from MCL disruption. Within 3 weeks, periosteal new bone and/or physeal widening may be present radiographically following injury to the distal femoral physis. Rarely, a collateral ligament injury and a physeal fracture may occur together.

Classifying MCL injuries by severity aids in treatment planning. Grade I MCL injuries are stable and may be treated symptomatically. Grade II injuries have mild instability and grade III injuries have severe instability to valgus stress. Both respond well to nonsurgical treatment. In adolescents, a brief period of immobilization followed by 3 to 6 weeks of unlimited motion in a hinged knee brace with rehabilitation allows for a return to preinjury activities within a reasonable period of time. If an MCL injury occurs in conjunction with an anterior cruciate ligament (ACL) injury, the ACL becomes the primary concern and its presence dictates the treatment.

Intrasubstance tears of the ACL are uncommon in children younger than 14 years of age. More frequently, a tibial spine avulsion fracture occurs. The incidence of ACL tears increases as maturity is approached. Most often these injuries are the result of a deceleration, external rotation, valgus stress injury to the knee. The patient may feel or hear a pop at the time of injury with the sensation that the knee subluxated. Continued participation in the activities at the time of injury usually is not possible. A hemarthrosis develops quickly and clinical swelling is present within hours. The Lachman test is the most sensitive examination to detect acute ACL insufficiency. The anterior drawer and pivot shift tests are difficult to perform in acute injuries because of muscle guarding secondary to pain. The joint line should be carefully palpated for tenderness, which, if present, may indicate an associated meniscal injury. This occurs in more than 40% of children and adolescents with ACL tears. Injuries to the collateral ligaments and physes must also be ruled out. The presence of an avulsion fracture of the tibial eminence should be evaluated radiographically. Magnetic resonance imaging (MRI) or diagnostic arthroscopy may be useful in the documentation of ligament or meniscal injury, but need not be performed in unequivocal cases. Unfortunately, children and adolescents generally have poor results with nonsurgical treatment of ACL injuries; however, the presence of open physes limits surgical options. Primary ligament repair and extra-articular reconstruction that avoids injury to the physes have both resulted in poor outcomes because of persistent instability. Intra-articular ligament reconstruction using tibial and femoral tunnels drilled through open physes may be used successfully in adolescents nearing skeletal maturity with limited risk for abnormal growth; however, in younger patients the risk of physeal injury with growth arrest precludes the use of tunnels through open physes. Therefore, primary treatment of the younger patient should consist of physical therapy, bracing, and activity limitation. Surgical reconstruction is postponed until skeletal maturity. If nonsurgical treatment fails and instability is experienced with activities of daily living, reconstruction may be performed using the semitendinosus and gracilis tendons without bone tunnels. The tendons are detached proximally at their musculotendinous junctions and left attached distally. The grafts are then passed over a groove on the anterior aspect of the tibial epiphysis and then are pulled to the over-the-top position of the distal femur, avoiding injury to the physes. Experience with this technique is limited.

Posterior cruciate ligament (PCL) injuries are rare in children and adolescents. Because of this rarity the natural history of the PCL-deficient knee in the skeletally immature patient is unknown. PCL injuries occur either secondary to forced posterior displacement of the tibia on the femur with the knee flexed 90° or secondary to knee hyper-

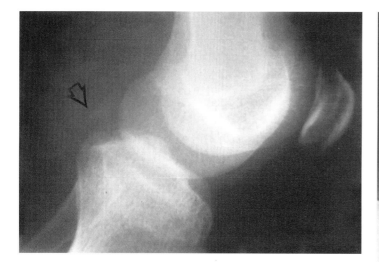
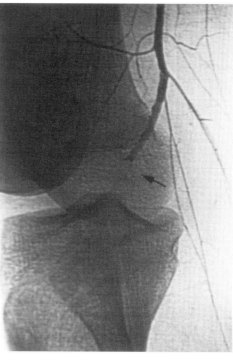

Fig. 1   Left, Lateral radiograph of the knee demonstrates an avulsion fracture of the PCL from its tibial insertion (open arrow) in an adolescent male. The injury occurred while playing basketball. Distal pulses were absent on physical examination. **Right,** Arteriogram demonstrates occlusion of the popliteal artery (arrow).

extension. PCL injuries may also be present following a spontaneously reduced knee dislocation. Therefore, a careful neurovascular examination is necessary in all patients who have an acute PCL injury (Fig. 1).

Following an acute injury, knee motion will be painful and weightbearing may be difficult. A knee effusion may not be present as the PCL is extrasynovial. Tenderness may be isolated to the posterior aspect of the knee and proximal calf. Joint line tenderness may indicate meniscal pathology. Posterior sag of the proximal tibia and the posterior drawer test may not be obvious in acute injuries; however, the quadriceps active drawer test is useful in detecting acute PCL injuries. The test is performed with the patient supine on the examination table with the knee flexed 70° and the foot flat on the table. The patient then contracts the quadriceps muscle. The tibial plateau will move anteriorly in the presence of PCL insufficiency. Accompanying collateral ligament injuries must also be ruled out. Stress radiographs of the knee may be necessary to distinguish between physeal fracture and ligament disruption. Radiographs must also be carefully evaluated for avulsion fractures from either the femur or tibia. MRI or diagnostic arthroscopy is useful in equivocal cases of ligament or meniscal injury. With regard to treatment of PCL injuries, isolated intrasubstance tears in the skeletally immature patient should be treated nonsurgically.

Displaced avulsion fractures from the tibia or femur are best treated with open reduction and internal fixation. Intraepiphyseal sutures for internal fixation may be used for either the femur or tibia. An intraepiphyseal cannulated screw with a soft-tissue washer (without violation of the proximal tibial physis) provides stable fixation for tibial avulsion injuries. Acute combined PCL and collateral ligament instability should be treated with primary repair of all injured ligaments. Some postoperative posterior instability should be expected. Children with chronic symptomatic PCL insufficiency should avoid ligament reconstruction until skeletal maturity to avoid injury to the physes.

Meniscal Injuries

The menisci aid in joint stabilization, load transmission between the femoral condyles and tibial plateau, and articular nourishment. Once thought expendable in children, the removal of menisci in children and adolescents is now known to lead to early degenerative changes.

The clinical diagnosis of meniscal injury is more difficult in children than in adults. There is a tendency for overdiagnosis of meniscal injury in children and adolescents because the symptoms of pain, giving way, and locking are frequently present in this age group without meniscal injuries. The differential diagnosis in children should include patellar instability, osteochondritis dissecans, loose body, inflammatory arthritis, and hip disease. Plain radiography remains the initial knee imaging modality. MRI is the most useful noninvasive study for establishing the presence of a meniscal injury; however, it should be used as an adjunct to the history, physical examination, and other studies.

With regard to treatment of meniscal injuries in children, the increased vascularity and cellularity of the menisci in children, particularly those younger than 10 years of age, suggests greater healing potential than adults. Meniscal tears should be repaired when possible, including tears in the less vascular white-white zone in young children. Adolescents should be treated the same as adults. Irreparable tears should be treated by partial meniscectomy. Total meniscectomy should be avoided. Meniscal tears in the presence of ACL disruption should be repaired when possible, although the presence of open physes may preclude simultaneous intra-articular ligament reconstruction. Ligament reconstruction should be delayed until skeletal maturity.

A discoid lateral meniscus must be considered in children and adolescents with symptoms of locking, giving way, and loss of knee motion. Lateral joint line tenderness may be present and the lateral meniscus may become prominent at the joint line with knee flexion. There are three types of discoid meniscus: complete, incomplete, and Wrisberg. The complete type has increased thickness and lacks any degree of the C-shape of normal menisci. The incomplete type has some degree of a semilunar shape but has increased thickness and occupies a larger area of the lateral compartment than normal. Both the complete and incomplete types have normal peripheral attachments. A tear is a frequent cause for symptoms. The Wrisberg type lacks posterior peripheral attachments and is unstable, although the Wrisberg ligament is intact. Plain radiography may show increased height of the lateral compartment with squaring of the lateral femoral condyle in the presence of a discoid meniscus, regardless of the type. MRI will show the abnormal meniscus.

Symptomatic complete and incomplete discoid menisci may be treated arthroscopically with partial resection of the meniscus. Attempts must be made to preserve a stable peripheral rim for load bearing. The Wrisberg type is the most difficult to treat. Consideration must be given for surgical repair with stabilization of the posterior peripheral attachments. Asymptomatic discoid menisci should not be resected.

Patella Fractures and Dislocations

Fractures of the patella are unusual in children because of the large cartilage-to-bone ratio and the patella's increased mobility. The patellar sleeve fracture is unique to children and adolescents. It occurs mainly through the unossified cartilage with only a small piece of bone attached and may be difficult to diagnose (Fig. 2). Although this is most often seen at the inferior pole of the patella, it may occur proximally and medially. Patellar tenderness following in-

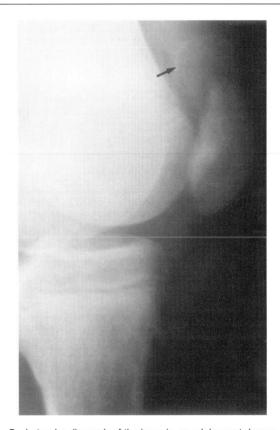

Fig. 2 Lateral radiograph of the knee in an adolescent demonstrates an avulsion fracture of the proximal pole of the patella.

jury should raise suspicion of a sleeve fracture. If the fracture is displaced and the retinaculum is torn, a palpable defect may be present or the child may be unable to actively extend the knee. Widely displaced fragments treated nonsurgically will result in an elongated patella with extensor lag, and therefore, the treatment of pediatric patella fractures does not differ significantly from that of the adult. Nondisplaced fractures should be treated with immobilization. Displaced fractures should be treated with open reduction and internal fixation, using a technique such as the tension band wire technique.

A fracture may occur at the bone-cartilage junction of a bipartite patella. Tenderness in the region of the bipartite patella may be the only finding. Immobilization is adequate treatment in nondisplaced fractures.

Acute patella dislocations may be secondary to a direct injury to the knee or may be indirect as occurs with a twisting injury. Most of these dislocations spontaneously reduce, and the patient may simply give a history of the "knee going-out" while being unaware that the patella dislocated. An effusion may not be present in patients with indirect injuries and generalized laxity. Furthermore, the torn joint capsule with traumatic injuries may allow joint fluid to extravasate into surrounding tissues, preventing accumulation of fluid within the knee. Tenderness along the medial border of the patella or the adductor tubercle may be present. Plain radiographs should be obtained to evaluate for osteochondral fractures. If present, these lesions should be examined arthroscopically. Small fragments should be removed. Larger fragments may be internally fixed with suture material, pins, or Herbert screws. ACL and MCL injuries can occur concomitantly with patella dislocation and must be ruled out.

Initial patella dislocations should be treated with a brief period of immobilization followed by a quadriceps rehabilitation program. Approximately 15% to 20% of pediatric patients will experience recurrent patella dislocations. Patients with predisposing factors, such as femoral condyle hypoplasia, an increased quadriceps angle, or atrophy of the vastus medialis, experience the highest recurrence rates. Generally, the frequency of subsequent dislocations decreases with advancing age into the third decade. The theoretical risk of degenerative joint disease secondary to articular damage following multiple dislocations in children and adolescents has not been substantiated clinically. Therefore, the primary indications for patella realignment surgery in patients experiencing recurrent patella dislocation should be for symptomatic relief and lifestyle considerations. Surgery should be considered only if a nonsurgical treatment program (consisting of physical therapy, activity modification, and patella bracing) has been unsuccessful.

Prior to the consideration of surgical intervention, the presence of tight lateral restraints, medial patellofemoral laxity, and an increased quadriceps angle must be assessed. The passive patella tilt test assesses tightness of the lateral restraints. The lateral edge of the patella is elevated from the lateral condyle with the knee extended. A 0° or negative patella tilt angle is indicative of excessive lateral tightness. The passive patella glide test determines the amount of medial patellofemoral laxity. The patella is pushed laterally with the knee in extension. Lateral subluxation of the patella of greater than 50% is indicative of insufficient medial restraints. A quadriceps angle of greater than 10° in boys and 15° in girls indicates an increased lateral vector of force for the patella. The active quadriceps angle is determined by having the patient contract the quadriceps muscles with the knee extended. The patella normally moves straight superior or lateral to superior in a 1:1 ratio. Abnormal lateral pull will result in more lateral than superior movement. A lateral release alone decreases the pull of the lateral retinaculum and may be considered in the patient with recurrent patella dislocation and tight lateral restraints. Insufficient medial restraints are treated with medial reefing and vastus medialis advancement, and distal realignment procedures are performed to correct an abnormal quadriceps angle.

Tibial tubercle transfer is to be avoided in skeletally immature individuals because of the risk of physeal damage and growth arrest. Semitendinosus tenodesis (Galeazzi procedure) or the Roux-Goldthwait procedure may be used in the skeletally immature patient requiring a distal realignment procedure. Frequently, in the child with recurrent patellar dislocations, the lateral release, medial reefing, and distal realignment must all be combined. The outcome of surgical intervention is less predictable in patients with connective tissue laxity such as may occur with Ehlers-Danlos syndrome or Down syndrome.

Tibial Fractures

Tibial Eminence Fractures

Most ACL equivalent injuries in children occur as avulsion fractures of the anterior tibial eminence. Prior to closure of the tibial physis, the ACL is actually more resistant to traction forces than is the intercondylar eminence. Avulsion from the femoral insertion is rare. Associated injuries to the collateral ligaments and menisci are common. An acute hemarthrosis will be present and anterior laxity may be evident. Concerning treatment, nondisplaced fractures are managed with immobilization. Elevated or displaced fractures should be reduced. Those that show some elevation without displacement of the entire fragment may be reduced by extending the knee and immobilized with the knee in extension. If this technique fails to achieve a reduction, it may be due to interposition of the meniscus within the fracture. Surgical removal of the meniscus from the fracture (with meniscal repair, if necessary) should be performed in such situations. Completely displaced fracture fragments are best reduced anatomically (either arthroscopically or open) and fixed internally. Internal fixation may be obtained with suture placed through the ACL near its tibial insertion and tied over an anterior bridge of epiphyseal bone or with intraepiphyseal screw fixation. Screws should not cross the physis except in adolescents nearing skeletal maturity. Regardless of treatment, most of these patients will demonstrate objective evidence of ACL laxity, although few will have subjective complaints of instability.

Tibial Tuberosity Fractures

Fractures of the tibial tuberosity are uncommon avulsion injuries. Most are sports-related and occur in older adolescents. Type I fractures represent an avulsion of a small fragment of the tuberosity. Type II fractures involve the entire anterior tuberosity with extension proximally to the level of the horizontal portion of the proximal tibial physis. Type III injuries involve the entire tuberosity with extension proximally into the articular surface, a Salter-Harris type III fracture. Patients present with pain, swelling, and tenderness over the tuberosity. Patella alta may be present. Surgical treatment of type I fractures is needed if patella alta (compared to the normal uninjured side) and a significant bony prominence are present. Displaced types II and III fractures are treated with open reduction and internal fixation. A cancellous interfragmen-

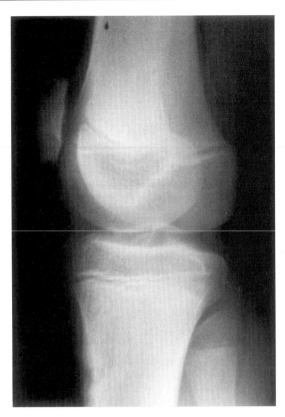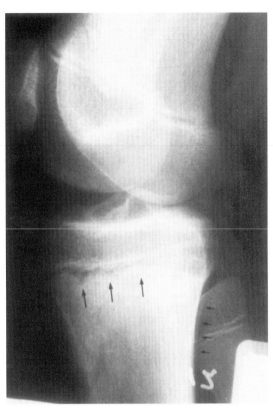

Fig. 3   **Left,** Normal lateral radiograph of the knee in a 15-year-old boy complaining of knee pain following an automobile accident. Tenderness was present circumferentially at the level of the physis. **Right,** Radiograph obtained 3 weeks later shows physeal widening (large arrows) and periosteal new bone (small arrows) indicative of a physeal injury.

tary screw may be placed through the tuberosity into the metaphysis. Because this injury occurs in patients near skeletal maturity, growth arrest with secondary genu recurvatum is rare.

Proximal Tibial Epiphyseal Fractures

Fractures of the proximal tibial epiphysis are uncommon. Most often these injuries are secondary to hyperextension of the knee. Rarely, hyperflexion is the cause. Most fractures are Salter-Harris type II injuries and tend to occur in older children and adolescents.

Patients present with pain, swelling, and tenderness at the level of the physis distal to the joint line. Recurvatum will be present distal to the tuberosity in angulated extension fractures. Popliteal artery injuries may occur with this fracture, so careful neurovascular evaluation is essential. Clinical evidence of arterial compromise at any point during treatment warrants an arteriogram. Angulated and displaced fractures will be obvious on radiographs. However, the radiographic diagnosis of a nondisplaced fracture may not be possible initially. Therefore, if a fracture is sus-

pected clinically, even though the radiographs appear normal, a short course of immobilization is warranted. Radiographs obtained 3 weeks later will demonstrate periosteal new bone and physeal widening if a fracture has occurred (Fig. 3).

Most Salter-Harris type I and II fractures may be treated with closed reduction and immobilization. Hyperextension injuries may be reduced by flexing the knee. The knee is casted in a position of flexion initially. After 3 weeks the knee is gradually extended. Total immobilization should not exceed 6 weeks. Displaced fractures may be treated with closed reduction and percutaneous pinning with the knee immobilized in extension. Salter-Harris type III and IV fractures may be treated with closed reduction and K-wire or cannulated screw fixation. If closed reduction is not possible, open reduction and internal fixation should be performed. Threaded internal fixation devices should not cross the physis. Physeal arrest with secondary angular deformity and limb-length discrepancy are the most common complications following this injury. Angular deformity occurs in 30% and limb-length discrepancy in 20% of the patients. Children sustaining proximal tibial physeal injuries should be followed for at least one year to determine whether these complications occur.

Proximal Tibial Metaphyseal Fractures

These injuries are more common than proximal tibial physeal fractures but less common than diaphyseal fractures. Most result from a valgus stress to the tibia. They tend to occur in younger children and are usually nondisplaced. Some may have an intact lateral hinge of intact cortex with valgus angulation of the tibia. Although these fractures may appear innocuous initially, they can lead to a late progressive valgus deformity. If a valgus deformity is noted acutely, the fracture should be reduced and immobilized. Soft-tissue interposition may prevent a successful closed reduction, thus necessitating open reduction. Parents should be advised of the possibility of a late valgus deformity because this occurs in nearly 50% of children with proximal tibial metaphyseal fractures. It is more common in greenstick and complete fractures and unusual in buckle fractures. The presence or absence of a fibula fracture does not appear to influence the development of a late valgus deformity of the tibia. The valgus deformity is most likely secondary to asymmetric growth of the proximal tibial physis. Surgical treatment for a late valgus deformity should be postponed for at least 2 to 3 years following the injury as the deformity will spontaneously correct in many patients. A valgus deformity greater than 20° may be too large for spontaneous correction to occur. If an osteotomy is needed at a later time, slight overcorrection is desired because there is a tendency for recurrence of the valgus deformity. Rigid fixation is advised. Bracing has not been shown to facilitate remodeling of late valgus deformity.

Fractures of the Tibial and Fibular Diaphyses

In comparison to adults, closed fractures of the tibia and fibula in children have fewer complications, heal faster, and have less morbidity. As long as significant shortening, angulation, and rotation are prevented, long-term sequelae are unusual. Infants may sustain nondisplaced oblique fractures of the distal tibia—the "toddlers fracture," as the result of an innocuous injury such as tripping over a toy or falling from a short height. These heal quickly and can be treated with only a short leg weight-bearing cast. More significant trauma is necessary to fracture the tibia in older children. Displaced or angulated tibia and fibula fractures should be reduced and immobilized in an above-the-knee cast until healed. Because remodeling is not predictable, angulation of more than 5° should not be accepted initially in adolescents. Angulation as much as 10° may be acceptable in younger children. Valgus angulation and apex posterior angulation are the least likely to remodel. Rotational malalignment should not be accepted because this does not remodel. Following a fracture, the tibia grows longer than the uninvolved side, an average of 5 mm in children 2 to 10 years of age. For this reason, shortening of more than 1 to 1.5 cm is unac-

Table 1. Classification of open tibia fractures

Type I	An open fracture with a clean wound less than 1 cm long
Type II	An open fracture with a wound more than 1 cm long without extensive soft-tissue damage, flaps, or avulsions
Type III	Either an open segmental fracture, an open fracture with extensive soft-tissue damage, a traumatic amputation, an open fracture caused by a farm injury, or an open fracture with accompanying vascular injury requiring repair

ceptable. With regard to surgical management, unstable tibia fractures may be treated with external fixation until radiographic evidence of healing is present. The presence of open physes precludes the use of rigid intramedullary rod fixation, although flexible intramedullary rods may be used in transverse fractures provided the physes are not violated during rod insertion. In cases of ipsilateral femur and tibia fractures, at least one and perhaps both of these long bones should undergo rigid fixation.

Although open fractures of the tibia in children are associated with osteomyelitis and delayed union, nonunion and late amputation are uncommon. Children are capable of healing serious soft-tissue injuries, recovering from osteomyelitis, and achieving a solid union (though delayed) when treated with current modalities. The classification of injury severity as described by Gustilo and Anderson is useful in predicting complications and selecting the appropriate antibiotics for children with open tibia fractures (Table 1).

With prompt treatment of the open tibia fracture, complications can be minimized. Antibiotics should be started in the emergency department, tetanus prophylaxis administered, and the wound covered with a sterile dressing. A broad-spectrum cephalosporin is used for type I and II open fractures with an aminoglycoside added for type III open fractures. Penicillin is included for lawn mower injuries and injuries sustained in a farm environment. Following resuscitation in the emergency department, the fracture is irrigated and debrided in the operating room. Fracture stabilization may be achieved with cast immobilization for most type I and II open fractures. External fixation is used for type III open fractures and those with unstable fracture patterns. Soft-tissue and arterial injuries are managed according to the principles outlined for adults. Free muscle flaps may be successfully used in children. For vascular injuries, the small caliber of childrens' vessels does not preclude successful repair or grafting. The indications for primary amputation are not clearly defined in children. However, the mangled extremity severity score (MESS) described for adults appears to be applicable for children and adolescents. An open tibia fracture in the presence of an avascular lower extremity with disruption of the posterior tibial nerve and an insensate foot is probably best treated with primary amputation.

Annotated Bibliography

Ligament Injuries

Engebretsen L, Svenningsen S, Benum P: Poor results of anterior cruciate ligament repair in adolescence. *Acta Orthop Scand* 1988;59:684–686.

Eight adolescents were followed 3 to 8 years after primary repair of a midsubstance tear of the ACL. Only three of the patients had good function, while five had unstable knees. The authors conclude that primary suture of the ACL should not be used in children and adolescents.

Graf BK, Lange RH, Fujisaki CK, et al: Anterior cruciate ligament tears in skeletally immature patients: Meniscal pathology at presentation and after attempted conservative treatment. *Arthroscopy* 1992;8:229–233.

Of 12 patients (average age, 14.5 years) treated for arthroscopically documented acute midsubstance ACL tears; eight were treated nonsurgically (brace and return to sports) and four had surgical reconstruction (two intra-articular, two extra-articular). Six patients also had eight meniscal tears, none of which were repaired. All eight nonsurgically treated had giving way and seven of eight had further meniscal damage. In both patients with extra-articular reconstructions, the knee became unstable and had new meniscal injury. The authors did not address the concept that lack of activity modification despite brace use, especially in the face of untreated meniscal injury, can be expected to produce continued ligamentous and meniscal damage.

McCarroll JR, Shelbourne KD, Porter DA, et al: Patellar tendon graft reconstruction for midsubstance anterior cruciate ligament rupture in junior high school athletes: An algorithm for management. *Am J Sports Med* 1994;22:478–484.

Sixty children nearing skeletal maturity were treated with patellar tendon graft reconstruction with tibial and femoral tunnels drilled through open physes for ACL insufficiency. Postoperatively, 55 of the children returned to their original sport. No incidence of abnormal growth related to the intra-articular reconstructive surgery was noted. Patients were considered candidates for intra-articular surgery if they had radiographs demonstrating closing physes, had undergone an adolescent growth spurt, were within 2.5 to 5 cm of the height of siblings and parents, and were a Tanner stage 4 or 5. The authors reported poor results with nonsurgical treatment as well as with extra-articular reconstruction for this population of patients.

Parker AW, Drez D Jr, Cooper JL: Anterior cruciate ligament injuries in patients with open physes. *Am J Sports Med* 1994;22:44–47.

This is a small series of five patients with ACL disruption and open physes treated surgically. The reconstruction used the hamstring tendons placed through a groove on the front of the tibia and a groove over the lateral femoral condyle in the over-the-top position. The distal femoral and proximal tibial physes were not violated. The patients were followed for a minimum of 25 months. Four of the five had returned to their preinjury level of sports participation. None had a positive pivot shift. There were no growth plate injuries. This surgical technique may provide a valuable alternative to the other methods of intra-

articular knee stabilization without significant risk of injury to the physes.

Stanitski CL: Anterior cruciate ligament injury in the skeletally immature patient: Diagnosis and treatment. *J Amer Acad Orthop Surg* 1995;3:146–158.

This is a comprehensive review of ACL injury in skeletally immature patients with emphasis on accuracy of diagnosis and establishment of maturity state by physiologic (Tanner stages) and radiographic (bone age) criteria. Lesions were classified as acute (less than 3 weeks), subacute (3 to 12 weeks), and chronic (more than 12 weeks). Reconstruction can be by intra-articular physeal sparing, partial transphyseal, or complete transphyseal techniques, depending on physeal maturity status. Extra-articular reconstructions alone have not been successful. Nonsurgical management emphasizes rehabilitation and activity modification to eliminate sports with high demand deceleration/rotation stresses.

Stanitski CL, Harvell JC, Fu F: Observations on acute knee hemarthrosis in children and adolescents. *J Pediatr Orthop* 1993;13:506–510.

Seventy patients with acute, traumatic hemarthrosis of the knee were arthroscoped. Forty-seven percent of preadolescents (aged 7 to 12 years) had meniscal tears and 47% had ACL tears. Forty-five percent of adolescents (aged 13 to 18 years) had meniscal tears and 65% had ACL tears. Hemarthrosis of the knee may indicate significant intra-articular injury in both children and adolescents.

Meniscal Injuries

Wroble RR, Henderson RC, Campion ER, et al: Meniscectomy in children and adolescents: A long-term follow-up study. *Clin Orthop* 1992;279:180–189.

Thirty-nine patients who underwent total meniscectomy in childhood were evaluated an average of 21 years postoperatively. Only four of the patients had ACL insufficiency noted at the time of meniscectomy. At follow-up, 71% reported pain; 68%, stiffness; 54%, swelling; and 41%, giving way. Ninety percent had abnormal radiographs with abnormalities most often in the meniscectomized compartment. Follow-up longer than 26 years, substantial instability, and male gender predisposed to poorer results. Few differences existed between medial and lateral meniscectomies. Total meniscectomy should be avoided in children.

Patella Fractures and Dislocations

Grogan DP, Carey TP, Leffers D, et al: Avulsion fractures of the patella. *J Pediatr Orthop* 1990;10:721–730.

Forty-seven skeletally immature patients with marginal fractures of the patella were studied. Avulsion fractures involved the superior, inferior, and medial margins of the patella. Separation occurred through the subchondral bone along the margins of progressive chondro-osseous transformation. The small size of the osseous fragment may not represent the true size of the more peripheral, radiolucent cartilaginous component. Minimally displaced fractures with an intact quadriceps mechanism may be treated nonsurgically.

Maguire JK, Canale ST: Fractures of the patella in children and adolescents. *J Pediatr Orthop* 1993;13: 567–571.

Twenty-four patients with patella fractures were followed for greater than 2 years. One third of the fractures were associated with ipsilateral fractures of the tibia or femur. These associated injuries frequently dictated the treatment. Ten fractures were treated closed; four, with open reduction/internal fixation; one, partial patellectomy; five, total patellectomy; and four, traction/ spica casting. Most patients had a good result. Displaced, comminuted fractures in patients with ipsilateral fractures of the tibia or femur had the worst results.

Tibial Fractures

Buckley SL, Smith G, Sponseller PD, et al: Open fractures of the tibia in children. *J Bone Joint Surg* 1990;72A:1462– 1469.

Forty-two open fractures of the tibia were retrospectively studied. All fractures were treated with either external fixation or cast immobilization. The average time to fracture union was 5 months. The time to fracture healing was related to the severity of the soft-tissue injury, the pattern of the fracture, the amount of segmental bone loss, the occurrence of infection, and the use of external fixation. Twenty percent of the patients with severe injuries treated with external fixation developed a centimeter or greater of overgrowth of the tibia. All infections were successfully treated, all fractures united, and there were no late amputations.

Janarv PM, Westblad P, Johansson C, et al: Long-term follow-up of anterior tibial spine fractures in children. *J Pediatr Orthop* 1995;15:63–68.

Sixty-one patients with tibial eminence fractures were evaluated at an average follow-up of 16 years. Treatment varied. Most with type III injuries had an open reduction and internal fixation. Five had type I injuries; 22, type II; and 19, type III. Eighty-seven percent had excellent or good results. Pathologic sagittal plane laxity occurred in 38% but was not related to poor subjective function. Arthroscopic evaluation of type II and III lesions is recommended to rule out associated meniscal and/or articular damage. The following recommendations were made. Type I should be treated with closed reduction and casting; type II, with arthroscopically controlled reduction and casting; and type III, with arthroscopic reduction and fixation. ACL slackness was not eliminated by growth. Only type III fractures had correlation between laxity and functional score. This study encompasses a broad time frame with many surgeons and treatment protocols.

Kreder HJ, Armstrong P: The significance of perioperative cultures in open pediatric lower-extremity fractures. *Clin Orthop* 1994;302:206–212.

The value of perioperative cultures in 86 open pediatric lower extremity fractures was assessed. Fifteen percent of the fractures became infected. In the infected wounds, the infecting organism was found on positive predebridement cultures 29% of the time, and on 60% of postdebridement cultures.

McLennan JG: Lessons learned after second-look arthroscopy in type III fractures of the tibial spine. *J Pediatr Orthop* 1995;15:59–62.

Ten knees with type III fractures had arthroscopy for other conditions 6 years after treatment at an average age of 17 years. Four patients had closed reduction (group 1), three had arthroscopic reduction and casting (group 2), and three had arthroscopic reduction and fixation (group 3). All had objective measurement and grading by objective and functional tests. The patients' primary complaints were anterior knee pain and not instability. Patellar malacic changes were primarily seen in group 1. Offset of more than 3 mm was seen in groups 1 and 2, suggesting loss of reduction and malunion. Sagittal laxity was greatest in group 1 and least in group 3. Functional tests were best in group 3.

Salter RB, Best TN: Pathogenesis of progressive valgus deformity following fractures of the proximal metaphyseal region of the tibia in young children, in Eilert RE (ed): *Instructional Course Lectures XLI.* Rosemont, IL, American Academy of Orthopaedic Surgeons, 1992, pp 409–411.

Twenty-one children with proximal tibial metaphysis fractures were reviewed. Sixty-two percent developed a significant valgus deformity (more than 10° greater than the valgus configuration of the opposite lower limb). The valgus deformity was the result of: (1) excessive valgus malunion; (2) transient acceleration of proximal tibial epiphyseal growth on the medial side; and (3) tethering effect of the fibula in the presence of overgrowth of the fractured tibia. Correction of any excessive valgus alignment of the fracture at the time of initial fracture treatment and immobilization in a long leg cast in extension is recommended by the authors. In deformities that do not resolve spontaneously, surgical treatment to avoid recurrence of the deformity includes shortening of the tibia approximately 0.5 cm in excess of the radiographically measured tibial overgrowth; osteotomy of the fibula; overcorrection of the tibial valgus deformity by a few degrees; and internal fixation of the osteotomy site with staples.

Shelton WR, Canale ST: Fractures of the tibia through the proximal tibial epiphyseal cartilage. *J Bone Joint Surg* 1979;61A:167–173.

Thirty-nine fractures of the proximal tibial physis were reviewed. Salter-Harris type I and II fractures were generally treated with closed reduction and immobilization, and displaced type III and IV fractures were treated with open reduction and internal fixation. Two patients had disruption of the popliteal artery, which were primarily repaired. Additionally, one patient experienced anterior compartment syndrome and another a peroneal nerve palsy. Twenty-eight fractures were followed to skeletal maturity. Four had unsatisfactory results because of limb length discrepancy, angular deformity, or osteoarthritis.

Willis RB, Blokker C, Stoll TM, et al: Long-term follow-up of anterior tibial eminence fractures. *J Pediatr Orthop* 1993;13:361–364.

Fifty patients were evaluated a minimum of 2 years following treatment for an anterior tibial eminence fracture. Clinical signs of anterior instability were noted in 64% of the patients. Twenty percent had a positive pivot shift. Only one patient had subjective giving way and was treated with an ACL reconstruction. The fracture classification of Meyers and McKeever (types I, II, and III) was predictive of subsequent clinical instability. The method of management (open versus closed) had no bearing on eventual outcome.

Zionts LE, MacEwen GD: Spontaneous improvement of post-traumatic tibia valga. *J Bone Joint Surg* 1986;68A: 680–687.

Seven children with posttraumatic tibia valga were reviewed. The valgus deformity appeared to progress during the period of fracture-healing as well as after union of the fracture for as long as 17 months. Clinical correction then occurred spontaneously in six of seven patients. The authors recommend a conservative approach to the management of both the acute fracture and the subsequent valgus deformity.

31

Traumatic Ankle and Foot Problems

Introduction

Ankle and foot problems in children are extremely common. Because there are ever-increasing opportunities for children to be injured as a result of accidents in recreational and motor vehicles, the number and variety of childhood injuries is very large. A more widespread awareness of these injuries unique to children and advanced diagnostic techniques will facilitate their management and treatment.

Distal Tibia and Ankle Fractures

Distal Tibial Metaphyseal Fractures

Distal tibial metaphyseal fractures in children are common and happen largely as a result of a direct blow to the lower leg area or a twisting injury of the ankle. Two types of injuries can occur. One is a complete fracture, in which the bone fails in tension. The other is a buckle fracture, in which the spongy metaphyseal bone fails in compression. In small children, failure to bear weight on the involved extremity may cause one to suspect a fracture of the distal tibial metaphysis. The diagnosis is suggested by tenderness in the distal tibial metaphyseal area. Plain radiographs will generally confirm the diagnosis. The buckle fracture is most common in toddlers, but may also occur in older

children. If angulation is greater than 15°, a buckle fracture should be reduced under anesthesia to enable a forceful disimpaction.

Distal Tibial Physeal Injuries

With common injury mechanisms in children, the distal tibial and fibular physes are more likely to fail than are the ligaments. These physes are susceptible to crush, shear, and distraction injuries. Such injuries result from twists, falls, and direct blows.

The diagnosis of physeal injury is suggested by a history of trauma, localized pain, deformity, and tenderness. Plain films will make the diagnosis in the majority of cases, although oblique views may be helpful if the fracture is nondisplaced. Although the mechanistic classification system is useful for many of these ankle injuries, the Salter-Harris classification will be both descriptive and prognostic for the vast majority of fractures around the ankle.

Distal Tibial Physeal Separation

Salter-Harris types I and II fractures have a very good prognosis for healing. Growth arrest is rare, although it has been described. Treatment of such injuries consists of closed reduction and cast immobilization. Analgesics, relaxing agents, and flexion of the knee will help relieve muscle tension in the calf and facilitate reduction. It is important to correct any external rotation deformity. This

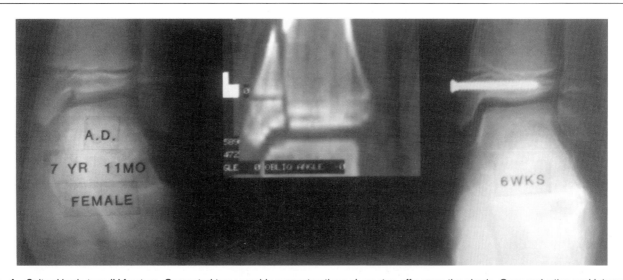

Fig. 1 Salter-Harris type IV fracture. Computed tomographic reconstructions show step-off across the physis. Open reduction and internal fixation was required to align growth plate and joint surface.

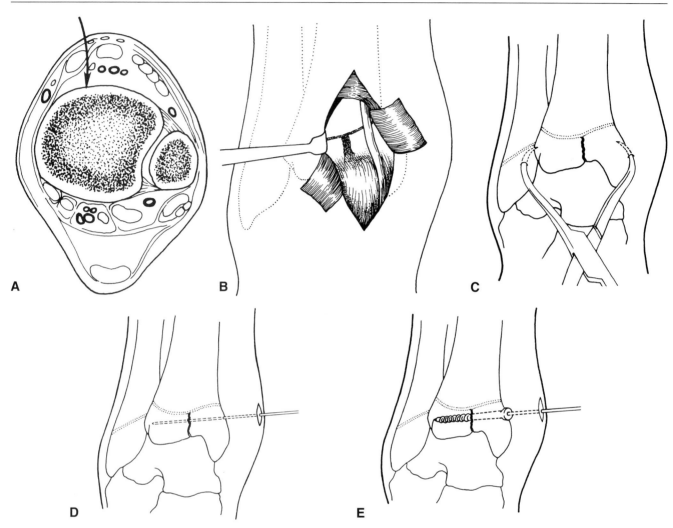

Fig. 2 **A,** Anterior approach to ankle joint is between the tibialis anterior tendon and the neurovascular bundle. **B,** The joint capsule is opened and sagittal fracture is easily seen. **C,** Direct reduction is accomplished. **D,** A guide wire is placed percutaneously from medial side under C-arm control. **E,** A cannulated screw is placed, which avoids joint surface and physis. (Reproduced with permission from Lintecum N, Blasier D: Direct reduction with indirect fixation of distal tibial physeal fractures: A report of a technique. *J Pediatr Orthop* 1996;16:107–112.)

deformity is common and is difficult to discern on plain films. Correctly assessing rotation requires an examination of the foot alignment with the knee flexed. An associated displaced fibular fracture will generally reduce closed. Because of rotational instability, an above-the-knee cast is required to prevent redisplacement. Healing usually occurs in 4 to 5 weeks.

Intra-articular Fractures

The majority of intra-articular fractures are types III and IV fractures as described by Salter and Harris. Many involve the medial malleolus; however, few of the fractures will completely displace because of the restraint of the tough, fibrous periosteum enveloping the distal tibia and fibula. If plain films clearly demonstrate less than 2 mm of

gap in the intra-articular surface, these fractures may be immobilized in a cast and followed closely. If displacement increases, surgical treatment is required. If the fracture displacement is more than 2 mm or cannot be determined, computed tomography (CT) will delineate the nature and extent of the intra-articular fracture. Specific indications for open reduction and internal fixation include: (1) a gap in the joint surface that is greater than 2 mm; (2) a step-off of the joint surface that is greater than 1 mm; (3) any misalignment of physis if significant growth (more than 1 year) is remaining; and (4) open fracture. Anatomic reduction and fixation are required to decrease the risk of growth arrest and intra-articular incongruity (Fig. 1).

An anterior approach will give good visualization of the intra-articular surface and allow manipulation of the fracture fragments to achieve anatomic reduction. Percutaneous screw fixation from medial or lateral may be useful in conjunction with an anterior approach (Fig. 2). Absorbable pins, which make hardware removal unnecessary, have been used for these fractures.

Transitional Fractures

Transitional fractures of the ankle occur during the period of transition from the fully open distal tibial physis of the child to the closed epiphysis of the adult. For this reason, these fractures typically occur in the adolescent. The transitional fractures include the juvenile Tillaux and the triplane fractures. These fractures occur when the ankle is forced into external rotation. In adolescence, the distal tibial physeal closure starts peripherally at the anteromedial aspect of the medial malleolus and extends posteriorly and laterally. The anterolateral quadrant of physis is the last to close, making the anterolateral physis most susceptible to separation. It is avulsed by the pull of the anterior tibiofibular ligament as the foot is twisted into external rotation. When this fragment alone is pulled away, the result is called a juvenile Tillaux fracture.

Triplane fractures also occur in external rotation. The fracture lines extend into the metaphysis, involve the physis, and may cross into the epiphysis. There are variable fracture patterns, which may consist of two, three, or four parts. Two general types have been described by von Laer. In the type I triplane fracture, the metaphyseal fracture line extends down to the physis but does not extend across it. In the type II triplane fracture, the metaphyseal fracture line extends across the physis into the epiphysis and joint. Type II fractures often require surgery. Triplane fractures may also occur in younger individuals with fully open growth plates. In this situation, the anteromedial portion of the immature physis is stabilized by a projection or hump in the physis, which tends to resist shear. The external rotation mechanism results in the same fracture.

The diagnosis of the transitional fracture is suspected by examination and confirmed with plain radiographs. Oblique films may be helpful in showing the Tillaux fracture. Triplane fractures are confirmed by the presence of a fracture through the epiphysis on the anteroposterior radiograph and a vertical metaphyseal fracture on the lateral view. Although triplane fractures are best visualized using CT, not all triplane fractures require CT examination. CT is indicated if: (1) the diagnosis is unclear; (2) the extent of displacement is unclear; or (3) surgery is contemplated but the planned exposure will not show the alignment of the physis or joint surface (Fig. 3).

Treatment for transitional fractures may be surgical or nonsurgical, depending on the amount of displacement. Closed reduction and cast immobilization are appropriate for fractures that can be reduced to within 2 mm of intra-articular separation. In late adolescence, when there is little growth remaining, harmful sequelae of physeal growth arrest are not significant. In younger children,

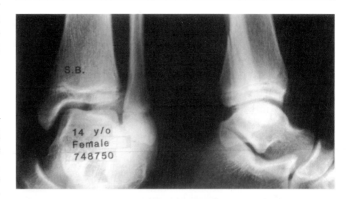
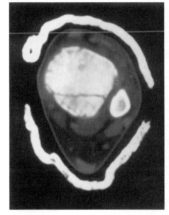
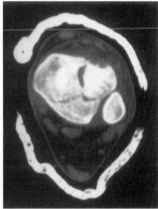
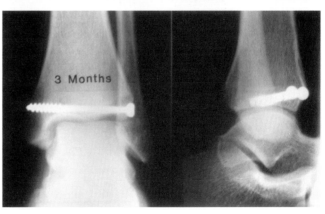

Fig. 3 **Top,** Triplane fracture. Anteroposterior view shows sagittal fracture line through epiphysis. Lateral view shows vertical metaphyseal fracture. **Center,** Computed tomographic cuts show a metaphyseal fracture, which is a coronal and displaced intra-articular fracture. **Bottom,** Open reduction and internal fixation was performed with anatomic reduction and fixation. (Reproduced with permission from Lintecum N, Blasier D: Direct reduction with indirect fixation of distal tibial physeal fractures: A report of a technique. *J Pediatr Orthop* 1996;16:107–112.)

however, compression screw fixation for displaced fractures may be helpful to restore joint congruity and physeal alignment. For fractures in the sagittal plane, anterior open reduction with indirect medial or lateral fixation will provide good exposure to the fracture site and allow for interfragment compression.

Foot

Talus

The child's talus is relatively resistant to fracture. A large proportion is cartilaginous and is more resilient to compression injury than is bone in the adult. Furthermore, children tend to have a much lower body mass, so that during a fall from a height there is less likelihood for a crush injury to the talus.

When they do occur, talus fractures in children result from forced ankle dorsiflexion. The diagnosis may be delayed because the fracture is usually nondisplaced and may not be visible on initial films. It may take 10 to 14 days for the fracture line to become easily distinguishable on plain films.

The treatment for a nondisplaced talus fracture in children is immobilization until healed. If the fracture is displaced more than 2 mm, anatomic open reduction and internal fixation should be considered. Osteonecrosis of the body of the talus may be seen, even if the fracture is nondisplaced. If this occurs, nonweightbearing is encouraged until revascularization is seen. Flattening of the talus and ankle stiffness are to be expected as sequelae of osteonecrosis, regardless of treatment.

Subtalar Dislocation

Subtalar dislocations are very unusual in children and are likely to be overlooked. These result from high-energy trauma, such as motor vehicle accidents or falls from heights. The diagnosis is suspected when there is significant pain, swelling, and deformity as seen on examination. The foot is most frequently displaced medially. The subtalar dislocation, although usually visible on plain films, is often not recognized because there is a tendency to focus on concomitant fractures. If the dislocation is recognized and diagnosed acutely, closed reduction is usually successful and stable. Open reduction is indicated if the dislocation is old (3 weeks or more) or if there is interposed soft tissue precluding closed reduction. After open reduction, pin fixation across the joint is recommended to maintain the reduction. Casting in a neutral position is appropriate. Healing is secure at approximately 3 to 6 weeks.

Calcaneus

Calcaneal injuries in children fare better than in adults for several reasons. Because a large portion of the calcaneus is cartilaginous, this bone is much more resilient in the child than in the adult. Furthermore, remodeling is possible in children with further growth. Associated injuries, which are common in adult calcaneal fractures, are much less frequent in children. Calcaneal fractures result from high-energy injuries, such as a fall from height or a motor vehicle accident. The diagnosis can be made on plain films

but, as with talus fractures, nondisplaced fractures may not be seen initially. A bone scan is helpful if the radiographs are normal and clinical suspicion is high.

Generally, in the absence of intra-articular displacement, nonsurgical measures lead to a satisfactory outcome. Open reduction and internal fixation may be needed if a large fragment is avulsed or the joint is disrupted. As a rule, these injuries will only be seen in older teenagers whose bony architecture and body habitus resemble those of an adult.

Midfoot Injuries

A bony mortise formed by the first and second cuneiforms contains the base of the second metatarsal. The first cuneiform-second metatarsal ligament is important in holding the second metatarsal base in the mortise. If this ligament is torn, lateral subluxation of the second and lesser metatarsals occurs with resultant joint incongruity, and late joint degeneration and pain are likely.

Lisfranc's joint injuries tend to result from forced plantarflexion, with or without rotation. The diagnosis is suspected with a history of a severe flexion force applied to the midfoot. Radiographic evaluation is key to making the proper diagnosis. There may be separation of the first and second metatarsals, loss of the second metatarsal base from the mortise, lateral translation of the lesser metatarsals, or a nutcracker compression fracture of the cuboid (Fig. 4). Furthermore, there may be a fracture or medial separation at the base of the first metatarsal, the so-called divarication injury.

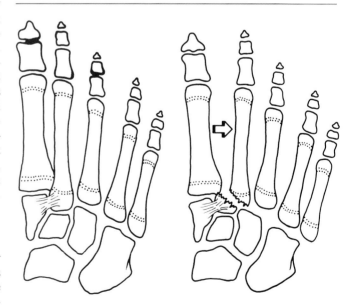

Fig. 4   Left, Normally, the base of the second metatarsal is held in the mortise formed by the cuneiforms, by the first cuneiform and metatarsal ligament. **Right,** With Lisfranc's injury, the lesser metatarsals may escape laterally. The cuboid may fail in compression laterally.

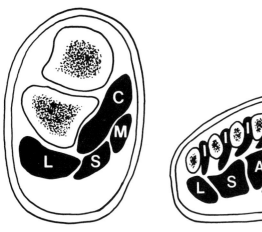

Fig. 5   Left, Axial cross-section of hindfoot at the level of the talar neck. **Right,** Axial cross-section of forefoot at the level of the mid-metatarsals. I, interosseous (four compartments); M, medial compartment; A, adductor compartment; S, superficial compartment; L, lateral compartment; C, calcaneal compartment.

A fracture unique to young children is the bunk bed fracture, an injury that occurs when a child falls from a height. The resulting flexion force wedges the first cuneiform-first metatarsal epiphysis into the first interspace.

Treatment of midfoot injuries is based on the severity and nature of the injury. If the tarsal-metatarsal joint is strained but there is no separation or dislocation of the metatarsal bases, immobilization is sufficient. If there is any lateral displacement of the metatarsal bases, closed reduction and pinning are indicated. Open reduction and pinning is indicated if anatomic reduction cannot be obtained closed.

Soft-Tissue Injuries

Peroneal Tendon Subluxation

The peroneal tendons pass posterior to the distal fibula in a fibular groove and are restrained there by the superior peroneal retinaculum. The tendons can bowstring laterally and anteriorly to this groove as a result of a hyperdorsiflexion injury of the ankle. The patient may present either with an acute injury to the peroneal retinaculum or as a result of a remote injury with chronic and recurrent subluxation of the tendons.

Radiographs are rarely helpful, but may show an avulsion of a ridge of bone with the retinaculum. The treatment of the acute condition is immobilization with the ankle in neutral or plantarflexion to allow the retinaculum to heal. In the chronic case with recurrent dislocation, repair or reconstruction of the retinaculum is suggested. The retinaculum can be directly imbricated; or, if retinacular tissues are not sufficient, strips of strong autogenous soft tissue, such as fascia lata or the Achilles tendon, may be used to reconstruct the retinaculum and secure it to bone.

Compartment Syndrome

Compartment syndrome results from severe crushing injuries or high-energy fractures of the foot. Anatomic studies have demonstrated nine compartments in the foot (Fig. 5). The diagnosis is based on clinical suspicion. There is tense swelling and pain that is out of proportion to that expected for the bony injury. Pallor, pulselessness, and paresthesia are not useful signs. Compartment pressure measurements will confirm the diagnosis. It is recommended that a compartment be released if the compartment pressure exceeds 30 mm Hg. Combinations of medial and dorsal approaches can be used, depending on the site of maximum swelling. Delayed skin closure or grafting will frequently be necessary.

Annotated Bibliography

Distal Tibia and Ankle Fractures

Böstman O, Mäkelä EA, Södergård J, et al: Absorbable polyglycolide pins in internal fixation of fractures in children. *J Pediatr Orthop* 1993;13:242–245.

Seventy-one children underwent internal fixation of fractures with absorbable pins. Fourteen of these fractures involved the ankle. Polyglycolide pins 1.5 or 2.0 mm in diameter were found to be satisfactory for fixation of fractures subject to low stress and did not cause growth disturbance when placed across the physis.

Caterini R, Farsetti P, Ippolito E: Long-term follow-up of physeal injury to the ankle. *Foot Ankle* 1991;11:372–383.

Sixty-eight children with physeal fractures of the distal tibia and fibula were followed for an average of 27 years. All but six had been treated conservatively. Sixty of 68 had a satisfactory result. The type of Salter-Harris lesion, the amount of initial displacement, and the quality of reduction were the main factors that affected the end result.

Hensinger RN, Beaty JH (eds): *Operative Management of Lower Extremity Fractures in Children.* Park Ridge, IL, American Academy of Orthopaedic Surgeons, 1992.

The section on ankle fractures in this monograph provides specific indications and techniques for surgical treatment of ankle fractures in children. Epiphyseal separation (Salter-Harris types I and II) fractures that are unstable after reduction can be stabilized with K-wires that pass from epiphysis to metaphysis. Multiple passes of the wire may damage the growth plate. Intra-articular fractures displaced more than 2 mm need to be accurately replaced and fixed. Pins or screws may be used. In younger children, an effort should be made to avoid traversing the physis by inserting wires parallel to it. In children with little growth remaining, fixation devices may cross the physis without the expectation of growth derangement.

Wilkins KE: Changing patterns in the management of fractures in children. *Clin Orthop* 1991;264:136–155.

Advances in imaging techniques have facilitated the diagnosis and treatment of childhood fractures. At the ankle, CT is useful in determining the number and displacement of fragments. Fluoroscopy-guided reduction and percutaneous fixation of selected fractures minimize the requirement for splintage and rehabilitation.

Transitional Fractures

Clement DA, Worlock PH: Triplane fracture of the distal tibia: A variant in cases with an open growth plate. *J Bone Joint Surg* 1987;69B:412–415.

Fifteen triplane fractures were reviewed. Although classically the triplane fracture is described to occur after fusion of the anteromedial portion of the growth plate, eight of these fractures were seen in the presence of a completely open growth plate. It was postulated that a hump or projection in the medial growth plate stabilizes the anteromedial portion of the epiphysis similar to the partial fusion seen in older children. This explains the occurrence of triplane fractures seen in the presence of an open growth plate.

Peterson HA: Physeal fractures: Part 2. Two previously unclassified types. *J Pediatr Orthop* 1994;14:431–438.

Two physeal fractures not previously classified are described. The first type, which occurs quite frequently, is a fracture completely across the metaphysis with an extension to the physis, but not along the physis. The second type, which is not common, is a fracture in which a portion of the physis is missing. This fracture generally results from a penetrating injury and develops premature physeal closure.

Schlesinger I, Wedge JH: Percutaneous reduction and fixation of displaced juvenile Tillaux fractures: A new surgical technique. *J Pediatr Orthop* 1993;13:389–391.

The intra-articular juvenile Tillaux fracture requires accurate reduction and fixation to restore the articular surface. The authors of this article describe percutaneous reduction of the fracture under fluoroscopic control with a Steinmann pin followed by K-wire fixation as an alternative to open reduction and internal fixation.

von Laer L: Classification, diagnosis, and treatment of transitional fractures of the distal part of the tibia. *J Bone Joint Surg* 1985;67A:687–698.

Three types of transitional fractures of the distal tibia were identified: a biplane lesion, which is restricted to the epiphysis; and two types of triplane fractures. In type I, the metaphyseal fracture ends in the physis; in type II, the fracture crosses the physis and enters the epiphysis and ankle joint. Intra-articular fractures with more than a 2-mm gap require open reduction.

Foot

Dimentberg R, Rosman M: Peritalar dislocations in children. *J Pediatr Orthop* 1993;13:89–93.

Peritalar dislocations are rare in children. This is a report of five cases of medial subtalar dislocation that occurred as a result of severe trauma. Closed reduction was successful unless delay in diagnosis or interposed tendon necessitated open reduction. The

presence of associated more-obvious injury tended to obscure the diagnosis of subtalar dislocation.

Johnson GF: Pediatric Lisfranc injury: "Bunk bed" fracture. *Am J Radiol* 1981;137:1041–1044.

The bunk bed fracture occurs after a fall from a height, with resulting flexion force at the first cuneiform-first metatarsal joint. This wedges the base of the first metatarsal into the first web space, causing a corner fracture of the metaphysis of the base of the first metatarsal which is angulated into varus, and lateral shift of the second metatarsal.

Schmidt TL, Weiner DS: Calcaneal fractures in children: An evaluation of the nature of the injury in 56 children. *Clin Orthop* 1982;171:150–155.

Sixty-two fractures of the calcaneus in 59 children were reviewed. Most occurred in falls from height or from motor vehicle accidents. Thirty-seven fractures were extra-articular and 22 were intra-articular. After age 15, the adult patterns of fracture were common. Twenty-seven percent of the fractures were initially unrecognized. Associated injuries were twice as likely to occur in children. It was estimated that two thirds of all children's calcaneal fractures could be expected to heal without functional sequelae.

Wiley JJ: Tarso-metatarsal joint injuries in children. *J Pediatr Orthop* 1981;1:255–260.

This is a review of 18 cases of tarsometatarsal joint injuries in children. The injuries were more common than usually thought and were often misdiagnosed. The injuries occurred as a result of an acute, forced plantarflexion of the forefoot often combined with rotation. Closed reduction was successful in seven. Four unstable reductions were secured with pins. No patient required open reduction. Short-term results were good in spite of extensive tarsometatarsal disruptions.

Soft-Tissue Injuries

Brage ME, Hansen ST Jr: Traumatic subluxation/ dislocation of the peroneal tendons. *Foot Ankle* 1992;13: 423–431.

The peroneal tendons are restrained in a bony groove behind the lateral malleolus by the superior peroneal retinaculum. Rupture or avulsion of the retinaculum allows the tendons to subluxate anteriorly. Immobilization or repair of the retinaculum is appropriate in the acute case. In cases of recurrent subluxation, tendon rerouting, groove-deepening, tenoplasty, or osteoperiosteal flaps will yield 95% satisfactory results.

Manoli A II, Fakhouri AJ, Weber TG: Concurrent compartment syndromes of the foot and leg. *Foot Ankle* 1993;14:339–342.

The coexistence of compartment syndrome of the foot and leg suggests that communications between compartments of the foot and leg may be important. Increased compartment pressure in the foot or leg remote from an obvious fracture should be suspected and treated appropriately.

Manoli A II, Weber TG: Fasciotomy of the foot: An anatomical study with special reference to release of the calcaneal compartment. *Foot Ankle* 1990;10:267–275.

Anatomic studies of the foot reveal nine fascial compartments: medial, lateral, adductor, four interosseous, superficial plantar, and calcaneal. The calcaneal compartment is newly described. It contains the quadratus plantae muscle, which, if damaged, may contract and cause clawing of the toes. Surgical release of all nine compartments requires a three-incision technique.

32

Spine Trauma

Transport of Small Injured Children

Infants and children up to the age of 5 years who are suspected of having cervical injuries must be transported in a different manner than adults. Suspicion of cervical spine injury in the child should be high if there is loss of consciousness and/or lacerations to the head, face, or chest. In the field, small children with these findings should have a neurologic examination documented by paramedical personnel before they are moved. In transport, the child's position should not be changed, and the child's position should be moved as a unit. Flexion of the neck in the small child and infant is contraindicated in transport because the most common level of injury in the small child involves the occiput–C1–C2 complex. If the odontoid process is intact but the atlantoaxial ligaments have been disrupted, spinal cord compression may occur if the child's head and neck are held in a flexed position. Compared to the adult, the small child has a disproportionately large head in relation to the torso. Therefore, if a small child is transported positioned on a flat spine board, the neck will be flexed. To prevent this flexion, special precaution must be taken by placing rolls or bolsters under the shoulders of the small child or infant. Alternatively, a specially made pediatric spine board designed to account for these differences may be used.

Radiologic Differences in the Cervical Spine Between Children and Adults

The cervical spine of the infant and child has distinct radiographic differences from that of the adult; many of these are directly attributed to multiple primary and secondary centers of ossification and synchondroses. It is important not to mistake these normal findings for fractures (Table 1). Normal findings in the pediatric spine include the persistence of a lucent zone in the anterior region of the atlas (called the neurocentral synchondrosis), which fuses by the seventh year. The odontoid synchondrosis is seen as a lucent area in the waist of the dens and fuses at 3 to 6 years of age. The atlantodental interval (ADI) is increased in children compared to adults, with up to 5 mm being considered normal. Vertebral bodies of children are more rounded and wedged anteriorly than those of the adult and can be mistaken for compression fractures. Notching of the anterior and posterior vertebral body is normal and results from nutrient vessels entering at these regions and the ring apophyses. In the child, the retropharyngeal space is up to 8 mm wide. The width of this space is increased if the child is crying. Pseudosubluxation up to 4 mm of C2 onto C3 is common and can be differentiated from true subluxation by obtaining extension radiographs. True subluxation may be present when reduction does not occur. The C2-C3 articulation is a normal fulcrum of pediatric cervical spine movement and accounts for this appearance. This is in contrast to the normal fulcrum of movement in the older child and adult, which occurs at the C5-C6 level. Furthermore, the facets of the upper cervical spine are more horizontal than those of the lower cervical vertebrae, particularly in the younger child, which contributes to pseudosubluxation. Absence of cervical lordosis is another common normal finding in the pediatric population.

Elasticity of the Pediatric Spine

One of the major differences in the spine of the infant or child compared to that of the adult is the increased elasticity of a child's spine. The bones and ligaments of the pediatric spine tolerate up to four times as much stretch as the spinal cord, which may be why pediatric cervical spine injuries may present with severe cord injury and normal radiographs, a pattern of injury called spinal cord injury without radiographic abnormality (SCIWORA). Multiple contiguous or near-contiguous fractures are also much more common in the pediatric population because of the elasticity of the spine. This elasticity allows for dissipation of energy from the injury over multiple segments.

Periosteal Tube Fracture

An apparent spinal dislocation in a child younger than 8 to 10 years of age often heals following closed reduction because there is an intact periosteal tube connected to an undisplaced cartilage apophysis or an unossified vertebral fracture is present (Fig. 1). Older children are unable to heal through this mechanism and, therefore, are more

Table 1. Table of pediatric cervical norms

Neurocentral synchondroses	Lucent zones in atlas fuse by seventh year
Odontoid synchondroses	Lucent zone at waist of dens fuses by sixth year
Atlantodental space	Up to 5 mm
Retropharyngeal space	Up to 8 mm
Pseudosubluxation C2 on C3	Up to 4 mm
Pseudosubluxation of C3 on C4	Up to 3 mm

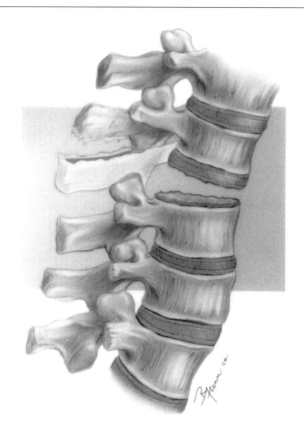

Fig. 1 A periosteal tube fracture (lumbar). (Reproduced with permission from Black BE, O'Brien E, Sponseller PD: Thoracic and lumbar spine injuries in children: Different than adults. *Contemp Orthop* 1994;29:253–260.)

adult-like in having less potential for spontaneous healing. In some cases, small children have undergone posterior fusion on apparent dislocations without an adequate trial of closed reduction. The inherent risks of these surgeries, which include potential growth into a hyperlordotic deformity, can be avoided if the injury heals well after closed reduction.

There are several other differences between young children and adults or older adolescents. Some reconstitution of the vertebral body may occur if the growth plates are not badly damaged. Long-term bracing may play a role in an attempt to improve deformities in these cases. Children tolerate immobilization better than adults. Bed rest and external immobilization, therefore, may be used for a prolonged period of time with very low risk of complications. The incidence of posttraumatic paralytic thoracolumbar spinal deformity is 100% in children younger than 10 years of age with quadriplegia and paraplegia. Typically, posttraumatic deformities eventually require surgical correction and stabilization.

Child abuse should always be considered in the differential diagnosis of pediatric spine injuries. The whiplash/shaken child syndrome is a strong indicator of child abuse. In these children, intracranial and intraocular hemorrhages, spinal cord injury, paralysis, and even death may be associated with significant spinal injury. Other signs of child abuse should be sought on physical examination and radiographic assessment.

Cervical Injuries

Atlanto-Occipital Dislocation
The atlanto-occipital articulation in children has little inherent bony stability and is reliant on ligamentous integrity. The true incidence of atlanto-occipital subluxation or dislocation in the pediatric trauma patient is unknown. Dislocation at this level is a rare finding that generally results in fatality. Many who survive are usually ventilator-dependent and remain quadriplegic. The injuries are very unstable. Initial stabilization with simple positioning to reduce the dislocation must be done with caution to avoid overdistraction of the occiput-C1 interval. In some cases, stability may develop after immobilization in a halo without fusion. Fusion should be performed in those who fail closed treatment.

Atlas Fractures
Atlas fractures are uncommon in the pediatric population. They may result in displacement of the lateral masses in a burst-type fracture pattern. Neurologic compromise is uncommon as the already capacious spinal canal is further enlarged by the spreading of bony fragments. Spinal cord damage, however, may occur with more significant amounts of force. Computed tomography (CT) offers the most precise imaging of these fractures. Proper gantry alignment is essential to avoid missing lesions that are not detected on plain radiographs. Conservative treatment is recommended for all atlas fractures. Most fractures heal well without incident, given proper immobilization in a halo vest. Serial CT scans may be used to assess fracture healing. Lateral radiographs of cervical flexion and extension should be obtained to assess for residual ligamentous instability after bony union is apparent.

Atlantoaxial (C1-C2) Disruptions
Several basic lesions involve the atlantoaxial articulation: traumatic ligamentous disruption, rotatory subluxation and/or dislocation, and odontoid epiphyseal separation or dens fractures. In the atlantoaxial region, Steel's rule of thirds is an important anatomic principle to remember. This principle states that the odontoid, spinal cord, and free space each occupy one third of the available space formed by the ring of C1. Therefore, atlantoaxial instability is more dangerous in the presence of an intact odontoid process because this diminishes the space available for the

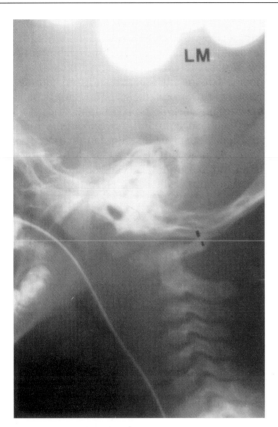

Fig. 2 A 2-year-old child sustained C1-C2 subluxation and transverse ligament rupture with an 8-mm atlantodental interval (ADI) in a motor vehicle accident. The child was neurologically intact. The patient was placed in halo cast for 2 months, but still had an atlantodental interval of 5 mm. A fusion of C1-C2 was performed with excellent results. (Reproduced with permission from Black BE, An H, Simpson G: Cervical spine injury in the skeletally immature patient, in *Surgery of the Cervical Spine.* London, England, Martin Dunitz, 1994, pp 293–305.)

Atlantoaxial Rotatory Subluxation and Dislocation

Atlantoaxial rotatory subluxation or dislocation may be caused by trauma or inflammatory processes, or may develop spontaneously without known etiology. Atlantoaxial subluxation secondary to inflammation is known as Grisel's syndrome. Fortunately, these conditions are usually mild, resolving spontaneously or with simple conservative measures. Most patients present with an acute onset of pain and torticollis. A few patients develop more gradual onset with little or no discomfort. Some patients may present with a fixed deformity of the C1-C2 subluxation, described as a "cock-Robin" appearance. Neurologic deficit and vertebral artery compromise are rare. Routine anteroposterior, lateral, and open-mouth odontoid radiographs are required in cases of suspected atlantoaxial rotatory subluxation.

The open-mouth odontoid radiograph will demonstrate asymmetry of the relationship between the lateral masses of C1 and the dens. On the lateral radiograph, the anterior atlas may appear to be wedge-shaped. Any increase in the atlanto-dens interval should be noted. Axial CT imaging is the definitive means of determining the extent of subluxation. Dynamic axial CT imaging of this interval can also be helpful in evaluating the rigidity of the deformity. In these patients, displacement should be reduced by traction, followed by placement into a halo vest for 8 weeks. General indications for surgical C1 to C2 arthrodesis include: neurologic involvement, failure to achieve and maintain correction (particularly common if the deformity is more than 6 weeks old at presentation), and recurrent deformity after 6 to 8 weeks of nonsurgical treatment.

Dens Fractures and Odontoid Epiphyseal Separations

Fracture of the dens is an uncommon injury in children. In most cases, there is a history of significant trauma. Most of these injuries can be readily diagnosed on plain radiographs but misinterpretation of the dentocentral synchondrosis as an odontoid fracture must be avoided. The conscious patient with an acute fracture will complain of pain and possibly a subjective sense of instability. Many of these children will hold the head with two hands to prevent motion.

In contrast to the high incidence of odontoid nonunion and potential for neurologic sequelae in adults, children typically experience a good result after conservative management. Pediatric odontoid fractures are treated by closed reduction and immobilization in a halo vest or Minerva cast for 12 weeks. Children are more tolerant of the prolonged immobilization than are adults.

Lateral cervical radiographs in flexion and extension are obtained at 12 weeks after injury. A collar is worn temporarily if no motion occurs at the fractured site (healed). If motion persists at the fracture site, posterior C1-C2 arthrodesis is recommended. Development of late atlantoaxial instability may complicate even a minimally dis-

cord. With acute disruptions of the ligaments, the atlantodens interval is increased as the atlas subluxates anteriorly from the odontoid (Fig. 2). Treatment consists of reduction in extension and then placement of the child in a halo cast or halo vest for 8 to 12 weeks, followed by awake, active, physician-supervised lateral radiographs of cervical flexion and extension to check for residual instability. If there is no instability, the child is placed into a cervical collar for several more weeks. To ensure that stability is maintained, it is important to obtain serial radiographs at 3-month intervals for 1 year. With persistent or recurrent instability, a posterior C1 to C2 arthrodesis is advised. A transverse incision at C1-C2 may be used in a small child so that dissection may be limited to the involved segments, reducing the possible complication of undesired extension of the fusion mass.

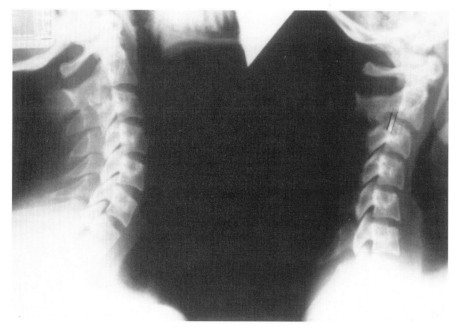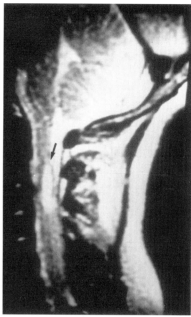

Fig. 3 Left, A 9-year-old sustained C2-C3 subluxation after a motor vehicle accident. Brown-Séquard syndrome was noted at presentation. **Right,** Magnetic resonance imaging shows cord edema. The patient was treated in a Philadelphia collar. Normal alignment returned with full resolution of neurologic deficits. (Reproduced with permission from Black BE, An H, Simpson G: Cervical spine injury in the skeletally immature patient, in *Surgery of the Cervical Spine.* London, England, Martin Dunitz, 1994, pp 293–305.)

placed odontoid fracture; therefore, follow-up must be performed at least until skeletal maturity.

In some cases, os odontoideum may be the result of a nonunion of a previously undiagnosed pediatric odontoid fracture. Posterior stabilization is recommended in cases of hypermobility accompanying an os odontoideum.

Pediatric Hangman's Fracture

Hangman's fractures, or pedicle fractures of C2, are uncommon in childhood. These injuries can result from either acute flexion or acute extension. Hangman's fractures typically are isolated lesions and usually are stable and heal well after closed reduction and maintenance in a halo vest for 8 weeks. Posterior C1 to C3 arthrodesis is indicated if nonunion occurs.

C2-C3 Subluxation and Dislocation

Pediatric C2-C3 subluxation and dislocation must be differentiated from pseudosubluxation (Fig. 3). True injury is usually associated with significant trauma and pain, with injuries to the head, face, neck, and chest. When true subluxation or dislocation is suspected, other associated fractures may be present and therefore a thorough examination is mandatory. Magnetic resonance imaging (MRI) is useful in assessing spinal cord injury, showing soft-tissue swelling and hemorrhage in this region. The spinal laminar line, the line formed by the anterior edges of the laminae

as viewed on the lateral cervical radiograph, is typically undisturbed in pseudosubluxation but is disrupted in true subluxation.

In children younger than 8 years of age, true C2-C3 subluxation or dislocation is likely to heal after closed reduction and immobilization in a halo vest. After the age of 8 years, the healing potential with closed management diminishes and fusion is generally required. A trial of immobilization for 8 weeks in a halo vest or two-poster brace should be done, followed by flexion and extension films.

Mid to Lower Cervical Spine Injuries

In older children and adolescents, upper cervical spine injuries become less frequent and lower cervical spine injuries become more prevalent. These injuries follow patterns similar to those seen in the adult. The age range in which the pediatric spine injury and healing potential becomes similar to the adult is 8 to 11 years. In younger children with subluxations or dislocations of the mid- to lower cervical spine, a trial of closed reduction and immobilization in a halo vest should be attempted because of the potential for healing (sometimes with autofusion). The neurologic status of the child with a lower cervical spine injury influences the treatment options. Postreduction MRI of the cervical spine is advised to rule out compression. With evidence of cord compression and an incomplete neurologic deficit, consideration should be given to surgical decom-

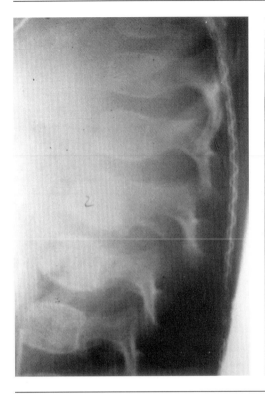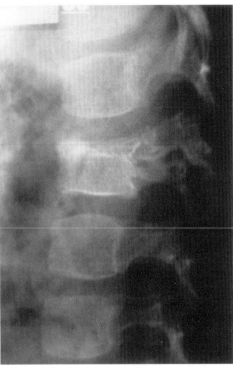

Fig. 4 Left, A 2-year-old child had a lap belt injury that resulted in apparent L2-L3 Chance dislocation. **Right,** At healing, double laminae are evidence of previous periosteal tube fracture mechanism.

pression and stabilization. Surgical intervention under these circumstances may allow for varied spinal cord recovery in incomplete injuries, or for nerve root recovery.

Thoracic and Lumbar Injuries

Healing of Apparent Dislocations in Small Children

Thoracic and lumbar dislocations in small children have excellent healing potential, but these same injuries in older children behave more as they do in adults and have less potential to heal with nonsurgical treatment. As mentioned earlier, the reason these injuries may have increased healing potential in the young child, without the need for surgery, is because they represent periosteal tube or physeal vertebral fractures rather than true dislocations (Fig. 4).

Multiple Levels of Fracture

In the pediatric age group, the increased flexibility of the thoracic and lumbar spine can dissipate the energy of injury, resulting in multiple contiguous or noncontiguous spinal fractures (Fig. 5). SCIWORA lesions may also occur because of the spine's flexibility.

Burst Fractures

Burst fractures are rare in children, usually occurring in adolescents in falls or vehicle accidents. Treatment follows

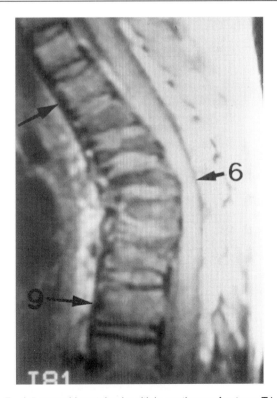

Fig. 5 A 5-year-old sustained multiple contiguous fractures T4 through T8, from a lap belt injury, resulting in paraplegia.

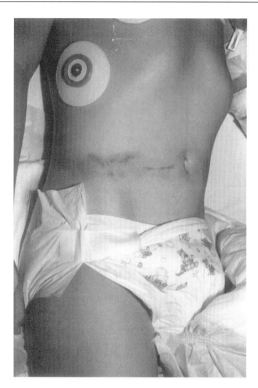

Fig. 6 Lap belt sign.

principles given for adults. The role of surgical fixation is debated in some cases. It may be considered where there is severe local kyphosis or a partial neurologic injury due to impingement by fragments from the middle column, which are displaced into the canal.

Lap Belt Injury

Lap belt injuries are a common cause of thoracic and lumbar fractures and dislocations in the pediatric population, particularly in children younger than 13 years of age. In this injury, the fulcrum of flexion is at the umbilicus. This flexion force at the umbilicus creates a larger and more destructive distraction force on the spine, leading to the Chance fracture or dislocation. The lap belt sign is a strip of ecchymosis at the level where the lap belt was secured (Fig. 6). Patients with the lap belt sign should have a complete workup for possible associated neurologic, spinal, and visceral injuries.

The orthopaedic management of lap belt injuries in children is influenced by the patient's neurologic status. For the pediatric Chance fracture or apparent dislocation in children up to 9 years of age who are neurologically intact, closed repositioning followed by spica cast (incorporating both legs) is recommended. If the patient has a complete neurologic deficit and imaging has shown that there is no surgically correctable lesion, closed reduction and spica casting including both legs under general anesthesia but without somatosensory-evoked potential (SSEP) is recom-

2 point restraint

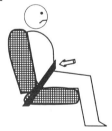

IMPROPER FIT

Lapbelt should not pull across stomach

Shoulder strap doesn't touch shoulder (young children are not tall enough)

3 point restraint

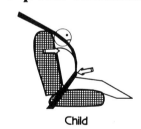

Child

2 point restraint

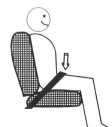

PROPER FIT

Lapbelt is pulled across thighs

Shoulder strap is touching shoulder (children should sit on a cushion)

3 point restraint

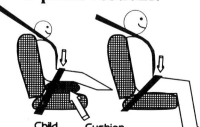

Child   Cushion

Fig. 7 Illustration demonstrating fitting of restraints. (Reproduced with permission from Black BE, O'Brien E, Sponseller PD: Thoracic and lumbar spine injuries in children: Different than adults. *Contemp Orthop* 1994;29:253–260.)

mended. If the patient has a partial neurologic deficit, the imaging should be studied after closed reduction.

If impingement on cord or nerve roots persists, open reduction with decompression and internal fixation should be considered. In general, children tolerate immobilization well. If the patient does not stabilize after appropriate closed reduction and immobilization of a Chance fracture or an apparent dislocation, then late open reduction and internal fixation with fusion is required. Posterior compression instrumentation achieves stable fixation. Some children younger than 9 years of age may have severe associated injuries that preclude prolonged cast immobilization or the hyperextension positioning required in a cast. Although young, these children need open reduction and internal fixation with posterior compression instrumentation.

Many children 4 through 8 years of age are too large for child restraints and too small for proper fitting of the lap belt or a 3-point restraint. Because of their small size, when these children are placed in a seat with a lap belt, the belt typically is placed over the umbilical region. If they are in a 3-point restraint, the shoulder restraint misses them and the lap belt portion is generally at the umbilicus, placing the child at risk for lap belt injuries. When properly fitted, the lap belt is placed over the proximal anterior thighs so that flexion occurs at the hips. Proper fitting should reduce the risk of spinal and visceral injuries. Dissemination of knowledge about proper fitting of the lap belt may reduce the frequency of lap belt injuries in both children and adults.

In addition, a properly fitted 3-point restraint (lap belt with shoulder harness) should reduce the risk of lap belt injuries (Fig. 7). With the use of a booster seat or bolster, the 3-point restraint or lap belt can fit the child properly. In addition, most automobiles have back seat lap belts instead of 3-point restraints, and children are the most common back seat passengers. Some car models have rear seat three point restraints, and in many automobiles rear seat lap belts can be converted to 3-point restraints. Despite the risk of severe injuries inherent in using 3-point restraints and lap belts, use of these restraints reduces morbidity or mortality compared with not using restraints.

Annotated Bibliography

Aufdermaur M: Spinal injuries in juveniles: Necropsy findings in twelve cases. *J Bone Joint Surg* 1974;56B: 513–519.

Necropsy study of spinal injuries in children shows radiographic and histologic evidence of injuries to vertebral cartilage end plates.

Birney TJ, Hanley EN Jr: Traumatic cervical spine injuries in childhood and adolescence. *Spine* 1989;14:1277–1282.

The authors reviewed 61 children and adolescents ranging in age from newborn to 17 years with traumatic cervical spine injuries treated over a 10-year period. Injury to upper cervical levels occurred more commonly in the younger patients. With increased age, lower cervical levels became predominant. Forty-four percent of patients incurred neurologic injury.

Black BE, O'Brien E, Sponseller PD: Thoracic and lumbar spine injuries in children: Different than in adults. *Contemp Orthop* 1994;29:253–260.

This is the largest review of children's thoracic and lumbar spine injuries in the orthopaedic literature. Thirty-eight children, birth through age 17, are reviewed in this, the first clinical description of periosteal sleeve fracture mimicking lumbar dislocations in small children. Appropriate use of motor vehicle restraints is reviewed. Distinct differences of thoracic and lumbar spine injuries in children and their treatments are elucidated.

Crawford AH: Operative treatment of spine fractures in children. *Orthop Clin North Am* 1990;21:325–339.

The author discusses cervical, thoracic, and lumbar injuries and their treatments in the pediatric population. Multiple cases and their treatments are shown, including seat belt injuries.

Flanders AE, Schaefer DM, Doan HT, et al: Acute cervical spine trauma: Correlation of MR imaging findings with degree of neurologic deficit. *Radiology* 1990;177:25–33.

The retrospective review of 78 patients with acute cervical spinal cord injuries correlates injuries and MRI findings.

Hadley MN, Zabramski JM, Browner CM, et al: Pediatric spinal trauma: Review of 122 cases of spinal cord and vertebral column injuries. *J Neurosurg* 1988;68:18–24.

The authors review 122 spine injuries in children. Anatomic and biomechanical features distinguish immature pediatric spine from mature adolescent spine. The frequencies of injury types, level of injury, and neurologic compromise varied with the age of the patient.

Herzenberg JE, Hensinger RN, Dedrick DK, et al: Emergency transport and positioning of young children who have an injury of the cervical spine: The standard backboard may be hazardous. *J Bone Joint Surg* 1989; 71A:15–22.

Ten children younger than 7 years of age with unstable cervical spine injuries were reviewed. The authors show how a young child positioned on standard back board has the neck passively forced into relative kyphosis. The authors recommend avoiding undesirable cervical flexion in young children during emergency transport and radiography by using a recess for the occiput to lower the head or using a pad to raise the chest while maintaining the neck extension and avoiding the dangerous passive kyphosis.

Mayfield JK, Erkkila JC, Winter RB: Spine deformity subsequent to acquired childhood spinal cord injury. *J Bone Joint Surg* 1981;63A:1401–1411.

Forty children who incurred spinal cord injury between birth and 18 years of age were reviewed 2 to 26.8 years after injury. All 25 patients who were injured before the adolescent growth spurt developed paralytic spinal deformity. Brace management was difficult. Most patients required fusion. Increased surgical complications were noted.

Pang D, Wilberger JE Jr: Spinal cord injury without radiographic abnormalities in children. *J Neurosurg* 1982;57:114–129.

Spinal cord injury without radiographic abnormality (SCIWORA) is described. Inherent elasticity of the vertebral column and other age-related anatomic peculiarities render the pediatric spine exceedingly vulnerable to deformity. The resultant neurologic lesions included a high incidence of complete and partial cord lesions.

Rathbone D, Johnson G, Letts M: Spinal cord concussion in pediatric athletes. *J Pediatr Orthop* 1992;12:616–620.

The authors reviewed 12 children with cord concussion. Predisposing factors in pediatric athletes were found to be spinal stenosis and hyperflexibility of the pediatric spine. It is strongly recommended that athletes with predisposition and history of cord concussion not be returned to contact sports until further epidemiologic data concerning long-term follow-up and predisposition to future cord injury have been established.

Rumball K, Jarvis J: Seat-belt injuries of the spine in young children. *J Bone Joint Surg* 1992;74B:571–574.

In this review of ten cases of seat belt injuries in skeletally immature patients at a tertiary referral center, seat belt sign correlated to high incidence of spinal and/or intra-abdominal injuries.

Torg JS, Pavlov H, Genuario SE, et al: Neurapraxia of the cervical spinal cord with transient quadriplegia. *J Bone Joint Surg* 1986;68A:1354–1370.

The authors studied neurapraxia of the spinal cord with transient quadriplegia in patients with negative cervical spine radiographs. Developmental spinal stenosis was noted in 17 patients, congenital fusion, in five patients; cervical instability, in four patients; and intervertebral disk disease, in six patients. The Torg ratio is described as the ratio of spinal canal width to the vertebral body width on a lateral radiograph. A ratio of less than 0.80 is indicative of significant cervical stenosis.

33

Polytrauma

Trauma is the leading cause of mortality in children older than 1 year of age. Polytrauma refers to injury to multiple organ systems, or multiple organs within a system. Skeletal injury is present in nearly one half of patients with polytrauma. Therefore, the orthopaedic surgeon must coordinate treatment plans with other medical specialists. Communication and diagnostic acumen are improved by knowledge of injury patterns. The following is a brief overview of polytrauma management for the orthopaedist who treats injured children.

Initial Evaluation

Children younger than 14 years of age who have suffered severe trauma are best cared for in centers specializing in pediatric care that have a predefined working hierarchy in place. The child's physiologic responses to stress, airway maintenance, physical examination, imaging studies, and needs for fluids and medications are different from those of the adult. Usually, the leader of the trauma team is a general pediatric surgeon or pediatric critical care specialist. All other specialists whose expertise may be required should be consulted early, so that they can be involved with subsequent studies and treatments. For instance,

computed tomography (CT) of the patient's acetabulum, head, and abdomen may be combined in one procedure; fracture stabilization may be combined with laparotomy.

Certain tests should be performed according to protocol. Radiographs of the skull, entire spine, chest, abdomen, and pelvis should be taken in the obtunded patient. In the alert patient, physical examination should determine any necessary radiographs. Radiographs of the skull should be taken in the conscious patient who has scalp tenderness, lacerations, or hematoma. Laboratory tests should include blood type and crossmatch, electrolytes, amylase, renal function studies, and blood count.

Head Injury

Head injury accounts for the most serious morbidity and mortality in children after trauma occurs. A Glasgow Coma Scale (GCS) determination should be performed immediately after trauma and periodically repeated. For younger children there is a modified GCS (Table 1). The physical examination should include a search for localizing neurologic signs, and serial examinations should be performed to assess neurologic status.

Despite the presence of open cranial sutures, the inci-

Table 1. Glasgow Coma Scale

Score	Older than 5 yrs	1 to 5 yrs	Younger than 1 yr
Best Motor Response (of 6)			**(of 5)**
6	Obeys commands	Obeys commands	
5	Localizes pain	Localizes pain	Localizes pain
4	Withdrawal	Withdrawal	Abnormal withdrawal
3	Flexion to pain	Abnormal flexion	Abnormal flexion
2	Extensor rigidity	Extensor rigidity	Abnormal extension
1	None	None	None
Best Verbal Response			
5	Oriented	Appropriate words	Smiles/cries appropriately
4	Confused	Inappropriate words	Cries
3	Inappropriate words	Cries/screams	Cries inappropriately
2	Incomprehensible speech	Grunts	Grunts
1	None	None	None
Eye Opening			
4	Spontaneous	Spontaneous	Spontaneous
3	To speech	To speech	To shout
2	To pain	To pain	To pain
1	None	None	None

dence of elevated intracranial pressure after head injury in children is about 60%. CT is the study of choice for imaging a head injury. Indications for CT include a GCS score of 8 or lower, depressed skull fracture, unconsciousness, focal neurologic signs, or cerebrospinal fluid leakage.

Indications for intracranial pressure (ICP) monitoring include a GCS score of 8 or lower, or CT showing a suggestion of swelling. ICP may be monitored via a catheter transducer device inserted into the epidural, subarachnoid, or ventricular spaces. The device placed in the ventricular space may be used for drainage, but it also carries a greater risk of causing infection.

Another important parameter to monitor is the cerebral perfusion pressure (CPP), the difference between mean arterial pressure and ICP. A normal measurement is at least 60 mm Hg. Serial measurements are mandatory.

Severe head injury may be accompanied by major skeletal injuries, such as open fracture, that require immediate surgery. The surgeon should be aware that different anesthetic agents affect cerebral perfusion in different ways. Inhalation agents tend to raise intracranial pressure and intravenous agents tend to lower it. Hyperventilation can reduce ICP by decreasing carbon dioxide and producing cerebral vasoconstriction. Mannitol administration and maintenance of a mean arterial pressure of more than 80 mm Hg are also helpful. The anesthesiologist should attempt to maintain perfusion pressure and oxygen saturation. No absolute contraindication to performing a necessary orthopaedic procedure exists, as long as any other, more urgent operable injuries are treated first, and intracranial and arterial pressures are adequately monitored. In rare cases only, such as complex skull fractures, is this not possible.

Head injury may be a cause of mortality and serious morbidity; however, the orthopaedic surgeon should not base treatment on a predicted outcome, and should provide treatment as though the patient will have optimum recovery. Most patients with a GCS score greater than 8, and many with a lower score, will have a very good outcome. Treatment should be geared toward eventual maximal function. In those few patients who have persistent problems and are eventually removed from life support, treatment of fractures generally should be continued until death occurs.

Children with head injuries benefit from rigid fixation of unstable fractures for two reasons. First, the physical encumbrance of traction interferes with frequent imaging scans, operations, and skin care. Second, patients with head injuries may go through a phase of agitation or spasticity a few weeks later that may complicate traction or cast treatment. There is no evidence, however, that rigid internal or external fixation improves management of increased ICP. Therefore, fixation may be performed at a time best suited for the patient's overall situation; on the day of injury or in the period after, sometimes combined with other surgeries.

Hospital admission is necessary for patients who have any neurologic deficit, seizure, fresh skull fracture, unconsciousness lasting longer than 5 minutes, or an unexplained mechanism of injury suggesting the possibility of child abuse. This guideline is useful to determine whether children with mild to moderate head injuries should be admitted to the hospital.

Abdominal Trauma

All children presenting with major trauma are evaluated for the possibility of abdominal injury. In the alert patient, evaluation takes the form of a physical examination and a search for telltale lap seat belt marks, lacerations, ecchymoses, or guarding. If any of these conditions are present or the patient is obtunded, a computed tomogram with intravenous contrast is obtained. CT of the abdomen may be combined with any other area of the body that requires imaging, such as the head or extremities. CT can demonstrate the anatomic locations of solid organ injury, such as spleen, liver, or kidney lacerations, as well as hollow organ injuries, as in the stomach, small intestine, and colon. Diagnostic peritoneal lavage is not performed routinely in children; that is, the presence of blood in the abdomen alone is not an indication for laparotomy. The need for laparotomy is determined instead by the specific organ injured and the clinical stability of the patient. If the patient is clinically unstable or is undergoing emergency surgery for cranial decompression, peritoneal lavage may be useful.

Injuries of the spleen previously were treated by splenectomy; however, this procedure often resulted in an increased risk of postoperative overwhelming sepsis. Currently, most splenic injuries are treated by observation only, provided that the patient's blood loss is less than half of the body's blood volume and the patient's vital signs are stable. Liver lacerations are treated according to the same principles. Intestinal injuries are treated by observation only or by segmental resection. Rupture of the diaphragm becomes apparent with an abnormal chest radiograph, such as the bowel located in the chest, or by respiratory embarrassment; surgical repair is mandatory. Gastric perforation is manifested by guarding, free air on the abdominal film, and coffee-ground aspirate on peritoneal lavage. Surgical repair for this condition is also mandatory.

Thoracic Injury

Thoracic injury occurs in approximately one quarter of children who sustain serious trauma. Rib fractures may serve as signs of thoracic trauma, but are less common in children than in adults because of increased elasticity of the chest wall. Rib fractures may also suggest child abuse. Pulmonary contusion is common and is treated by fluid restriction and, if needed, positive-pressure ventilation. Pneumothorax is usually treated with tube thoracostomy, although it may be managed by observation if it covers an area smaller than 15% of the pleural space and the patient's vital signs are stable. Hemothorax may occur because of bleeding from intercostal vessels or pulmonary parenchyma, and is also treated by tube thoracostomy. If bleeding exceeds about 2 ml/kg/hr from the chest tube, thoracotomy to control the source of bleeding should be performed. Pulmonary fat embolism may be seen in teens and young adults; however, it is rarely recognized in young children. Manifestations of pulmonary fat embolism are tachypnea, tachycardia, or increasing respiratory distress after a lucid interval in the first few days after trauma, accompanied by disorientation and petechiae. Pulmonary fat embolism is usually seen in association with long-bone fractures. Respiratory support and, in some cases, steroids are used for treatment.

Later Complications

Certain syndromes may occur as sequelae or complications of polytraumas. Deep venous thrombosis is seen in adults with pelvis and lower extremity injuries; however, it is rarely seen in children under the age of 16 years, so routine prophylaxis is not indicated. Multisystem organ failure also rarely occurs in children because of the greater resilience of the renal, hepatic, and pulmonary systems. The imperative for rigid fracture fixation that exists for adults to prevent multisystem organ failure does not exist for children.

If attention has been focused on obvious fractures or dislocations in the polytrauma patient, it is important that less obvious skeletal injuries do not go unrecognized. Unrecognized skeletal injuries may occur in as many as one third of polytrauma patients. Routine technetium bone scan imaging has been recommended as a means of detecting unrecognized fractures. In one study of 48 patients younger than 22 years old who sustained multiple trauma, bone scans were performed and unrecognized fractures were found in 40% (19 patients). However, only 13% (six patients) required treatment modifications, and none required surgery. Thus, the appropriate use of radionucleotide imaging has yet to be defined for this problem. A more practical approach is to perform a complete reexamination 24 hours and 48 hours after trauma in the patient who sustained a high-energy injury, employing radiography as needed. Bone scans may be used for those who are difficult to examine.

The need for a positive nitrogen balance in the traumatized patient is well-documented. Increased metabolic demands necessitate early and aggressive nutritional support. Enteral nutrition should be utilized when the patient's electrolytes have stabilized and it can meet all caloric requirements. If enteral means are not possible or cannot accomplish this goal, then the parenteral route should be used. In general, some form of nutritional support should be commenced within 24 hours after injury and should not be delayed more than 72 hours.

Injury Assessment

Injury severity scales are useful tools in the classification of multisystem injuries. The Modified Injury Severity Scale (MISS) reliably predicts both morbidity and mortality rates. The MISS score is obtained by adding the severity ratings of the three organ systems that are most severely injured. In one study, a MISS score of 25 or greater predicted those patients with an increased risk of morbidity and mortality. Eichelberger compared the trauma outcome in 1,009 children under 15 years of age with adult trauma victims. A combination of the Trauma Score (TS) and the Injury Severity Score (ISS) was used for assessment. No statistically significant difference existed between the pediatric patients and the adult patients. Injury severity scales provide a valuable method for assessing the prognoses of children who experience multisystem trauma. Long-term disability occurs in a minority of patients, generally because of head and spinal cord injuries.

Annotated Bibliography

Mechanisms of Injury

Beaver BL, Moore VL, Peclet M, et al: Characteristics of pediatric firearm fatalities. *J Pediatr Surg* 1990;25:97–100.

These authors reviewed the records of children younger than 16 years of age who were killed by firearms in the state of Maryland. They found that children were most likely to be killed in the home environment by a known assailant and to die from severe head injury.

National Safety Council: *Accident Facts: 1992.* Chicago, IL, National Safety Council, 1992.

Peclet MH, Newman KD, Eichelberger MR, et al: Patterns of injury in children. *J Pediatr Surg* 1990;25: 85–91.

This article discusses the patterns of injury in children who were admitted to Children's National Medical Center, Washington, DC, over a 34-month period. The authors found the greatest mortality rate was associated with child abuse, gunshots/stabbings, and drowning. The greatest number of accidental deaths were due to motor vehicle related accidents. The overall mortality rate was 2%.

Major causes of accident mortality among children: United States, 1988. *Stat Bull Metrop Insur Co* 1992; 73:2–8.

Acute Evaluation

Bruce DA (ed): *Rehabilitation of the Adult and Child With Traumatic Brain Injury,* ed 2. Philadelphia, PA, FA Davis, 1990, p 529.

Heinrich SD, Gallagher D, Harris M, et al: Undiagnosed fractures in severely injured children and young adults: Identification with technetium imaging. *J Bone Joint Surg* 1994;76A:561–572.

Forty-eight patients younger than 22 years of age with multiple injuries, head injury, or both, underwent technetium bone scanning to look for undiagnosed fractures. Ninety-four areas of increased activity were found in 30 patients. Subsequent radiographs revealed 19 fractures. Treatment was altered in six patients, with a cast applied in all cases. The authors conclude that technetium radionucleotide imaging is a useful adjuvant to the orthopaedic evaluation.

Newman KD, Eichelberger MR, Randolph JG: Abdominal injury, in Eichelberger MR, Pratsch GL (eds): *Pediatric Trauma Care.* Rockville, MD, Aspen, 1988, pp 101–104.

This is an excellent review of current management.

Nichols DG, Yaster M, Lappe DG, et al (eds): *The Golden Hour: The Handbook of Advanced Pediatric Life Support,* ed 2. St. Louis, MO, Mosby-Year Book, 1996, pp 289–359.

Injury Assessment

Eichelberger MR, Mangubat EA, Sacco WJ, et al: Outcome analysis of blunt injury in children. *J Trauma* 1988;28:1109–1117.

The TRISS was utilized to compare the efficacy of the Injury Severity Score and the Trauma Score in predicting outcome in trauma patients. In this study, 1,009 pediatric patients were compared with 16,764 adults from the Major Trauma Outcome Study. The TRISS proved accurate in predicting survival versus death in children. A Trauma score of 14 or fewer and an Injury Severity Score greater than 15 were found to define a severe injury in this group.

Marcus RE, Millis MF, Thompson GH: Multiple injury in children. *J Bone Joint Surg* 1983;65A:1290–1294.

The authors studied 34 children with severe injuries and correlated the Modified Injury Severity Scale (MISS) with their

morbidity. They found the MISS score correlated well with residual impairment and morbidity. A MISS score of 25 or fewer was associated with a 30% incidence of residual impairment; a score between 26 and 40, a 33% incidence; and a score of greater than 40 points, a 100% incidence of residual impairment.

Mayer T, Walker ML, Clark P: Further experience with the modified ISS. *J Trauma* 1984;24:31–34.

This prospective study of 250 pediatric patients with multiple trauma demonstrated the accuracy of the Modified Injury Severity Scale (MISS) in predicting morbidity and mortality. A MISS score of fewer than 25 was associated with no mortalities and only 1% morbidity, while a score of 25 or greater was associated with a 40% mortality and 30% morbidity rate. In addition, the neural MISS score was also found to be accurate in predicting mortality. A neural MISS score of 5 indicated a 73% mortality, while a score of 4 indicated an 8% mortality, and a score of 3, only a 2% mortality.

Wesson DE, Williams JI, Spence LJ, et al: Functional outcome in pediatric trauma. *J Trauma* 1989;29:589–592.

Two-hundred fifty pediatric trauma patients admitted over the study period were evaluated at time of hospital discharge and 6 months after discharge to determine functional outcome. A disability rate of 88% was noted at discharge; this had dropped to 54% at 6 months. These authors found that more than half the cases of disability were due to head or spinal trauma. Lower extremity injuries accounted for an additional 25% of disabilities.

Management

Loder RT: Pediatric polytrauma: Orthopaedic care and hospital course. *J Orthop Trauma* 1987;1:48–54.

Records and radiographs of 78 polytrauma patients younger than 16 years of age were reviewed. The results showed that children with a neural Modified Injury Severity Scale (MISS) score of 3 or 4, with a concomitant chest or abdominal injury with a MISS score of 3 or greater, who had a fracture requiring immobilization, were at greater risk for complications. The author recommends considering early fracture stabilization for these patients. For patients with a neural MISS score of 3 or 4, without a chest or abdominal injury scoring 3 or above, who do not awaken from a coma within 3 days, the author recommends delayed internal fixation.

Ziv I, Rang M: Treatment of femoral fracture in the child with head injury. *J Bone Joint Surg* 1983;65B:276–278.

The authors retrospectively studied 51 children with femoral fractures and head injury and recommended intramedullary fixation for children with head injury who were older than 5 years of age. They felt skin traction was appropriate for children with head injuries who were younger than 5 years of age.

34

Child Abuse

Introduction

The term child maltreatment includes both abuse and neglect by those responsible for a child's care. Maltreatment affects children from all economic and cultural groups. The National Center for Child Abuse and Neglect estimates that each year more than 1.5 million children are maltreated. All health care professionals are responsible for reporting cases of suspected abuse. Conversely, because of the psychological harm to families that can occur when children are removed from their homes unnecessarily, it is imperative that health care professionals perform an extensive interview with an examination of the patient, and exercise careful consideration before reporting such cases.

Denial, avoidance, and overreaction are pitfalls that should be avoided by the physician when attempting to recognize and treat children who are victims of child abuse. Studies have found that private practitioners and physicians in smaller towns are less likely to report child abuse. Overreaction to suspected child abuse, however, has created problems for innocent families of all types, particularly those whose children have osteogenesis imperfecta. As a result, the Osteogenesis Imperfecta Foundation has begun a publicity campaign about children with this condition who have been removed from their homes because of the suspicion of abuse. Not only does overreaction harm innocent families, but it also hampers organized efforts in the identification and prevention of child abuse. Criteria for removing the child from the home must be developed and evenly applied without bias related to culture, social, or economic status.

Abuse to children can be physical, sexual, or psychological. For this review, the term child abuse is defined as physical abuse in which the child is injured by a caregiver on one or more occasions. In 1962, Kemp introduced the term battered-child syndrome, which described the very young child who experienced repeated episodes of severe physical injury inflicted by a caregiver. Only a minority of child abuse cases are of this severity, yet any young child subjected to abuse is at risk of becoming a battered child.

Child neglect occurs when a caregiver fails to provide adequate supervision, protection, nutrition, or nurture for a dependent child. Most states consider a child younger than 12 years of age who is left alone and without supervision to be neglected. Orthopaedists may see children who have been injured in accidents when they were inadequately supervised; this scenario may represent neglect. Suspected child neglect should be reported.

There is an abundance of child abuse articles in the literature. Over the past 15 years, more than 5,600 citations and 400 review articles have been published. A journal devoted to this topic, *Child Abuse and Neglect*, has been in circulation since 1976.

Fractures in Child Abuse

The pattern of multiple fractures at various stages of healing is indicative of child abuse, provided there is no underlying bone disease (Fig.1). However, no single fracture pattern is considered diagnostic. Several studies have shown that fractures caused by child abuse are indistinguishable from those resulting from other mechanisms of injury. The most commonly fractured bones are the humerus, femur, and tibia, and the most common fracture pattern is transverse. Most children who are abused have a single fracture. Metaphyseal, or so-called "corner" fractures, occur in only 25% of child abuse cases. Only 2% of children aged 1 to 5 years with isolated, unwitnessed femur fractures are found to be victims of child abuse. A larger percentage of children (6%) sustain fractures while running or falling from low heights. Therefore, such mechanisms of injury should not be dismissed as impossible. Unwitnessed fractures in the preambulatory child, however, are much more likely to be caused by abuse.

Evaluation

If child abuse is suspected, early consultation with appropriate protective services is needed because orthopaedic surgeons are not experts in the social assessment. Physical signs should be carefully evaluated and documented during the physical examination. Multiple bruises, especially over the perineum or back, can be readily recognized. Soft-tissue injuries may outnumber fractures. Every major joint should be checked for effusion and stiffness. Failure to thrive may be indicative of neglect. Photographs are helpful in documenting the physical findings.

Imaging studies should be individualized, and lateral radiographs of the skull, anteroposterior views of all four extremities, and a chest radiograph should be obtained. Rib detail films may be helpful. A bone scan may be used to localize recent injuries.

Responsibilities of the Orthopaedist in Suspected Child Abuse

The orthopaedist must be thorough, competent, and objective when dealing with cases of suspected child abuse.

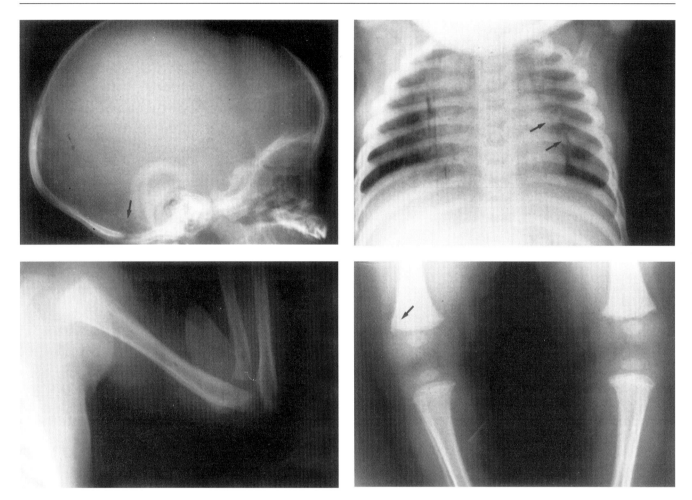

Fig. 1   Three-month-old infant with constellation of radiographic findings consistent with battered-child syndrome. **Top left,** Posterior occipital skull fracture (arrow). **Top right,** Rib fractures at various stages of healing (arrows). **Bottom left,** Humeral periosteal reaction. **Bottom right,** Physeal and corner metaphyseal fractures of distal femur and proximal tibia.

The eight principles outlined below provide guidance in the evaluation of suspected child abuse.

(1) *A history should be obtained regarding all injuries.* The physician should personally obtain a history from the parents or caregivers and the child, if possible, regarding all injuries. Discrepancies between history and physical examination are the most important findings triggering further investigation. The physician is a more credible expert in the courtroom or before a judge when direct testimony can be given about the history of injury provided by the parents or caregivers. This history should be compared with that obtained by other health care professionals.

(2) *The possibility of child abuse should be considered in the differential diagnosis of many injuries in children.* Child abuse should be considered wherever the history and examination are divergent, or whenever the injury does not fit the developmental age of the child (for example, fractures in a nonambulatory child). Considering child abuse

as a possibility is not the same as making the diagnosis. However, once child abuse is suspected, the physician is required by law to report it to authorities for further investigation.

(3) *The whole child must be examined.* The skin, head, back, and all extremities must be examined. An examination of genitalia and the rectum is indicated whenever the diagnosis of child abuse is deemed a strong possibility.

(4) *Other possibilities for injury should also be considered.* Tibia pseudarthrosis, osteogenesis imperfecta, fibrous dysplasia, rickets, or any disorder that affects bone density may lead to fracture. As experts in musculoskeletal care, orthopaedic surgeons possess the knowledge and experience to make the decisions that are sometimes needed in cases of suspected child abuse.

(5) *The examining physician should communicate personally with the social worker or case worker.* Physicians should characterize their suspicions: no suspicion; low suspicion;

high suspicion; conclusive evidence of child abuse; or cannot determine. Social service professionals typically rely on the physician for an index of suspicion, which will affect further investigation and disposition.

(6) *The examining physician should consult with other physicians for assistance in evaluating the child suspected to be abused.* Oral surgeons should be consulted to evaluate bite marks that could possibly have been inflicted by a human. Ophthalmologists should be asked to examine for retinal hemorrhage in younger children who may have been shaken. Gynecologists should be asked to perform pelvic examination whenever indicated.

(7) *Evaluation and treatment should be conducted with a nonjudgmental attitude.* If the physician believes that he or she cannot be impartial and nonjudgmental, another physician should assume treatment.

(8) *Findings should be documented in the medical record and a copy should be saved in personally held records.* Documentation is vital because subsequent investigations and court cases can be prolonged for months or years. Physicians should save a copy of the consultation in personal office files. Hospital records may be lost or incomplete and the physician may have difficulty remembering the details necessary for credible testimony.

By exercising skill and judgment, the pediatric orthopaedic surgeon can often be of great help in the process of evaluating and treating abused children.

Annotated Bibliography

Carty HM: Fractures caused by child abuse. *J Bone Joint Surg* 1993;75B:849–857.

Dr. Cary, a pediatric radiologist, reviews the radiologic features of child abuse, using the literature and her experience from Royal Liverpool Children's National Health Service Trust. She reports that in children younger than 1 year of age, fractures from accidental causes are less common than from child abuse. The following fractures were considered to have a high specificity for child abuse, most frequently under 3 years of age: metaphyseal fractures, rib fractures, scapular fractures, fractures of the outer end of the clavicle, vertebral fractures or subluxation, finger injuries in nonambulatory children, fractures of different ages, bilateral fractures, and complex skull fractures.

Dent JA, Paterson CR: Fractures in early childhood: Osteogenesis imperfecta or child abuse? *J Pediatr Orthop* 1991;11:184–186.

Radiographs of 194 fractures sustained by 39 children younger than 5 years of age with OI were studied and compared with radiographs of 84 fractures sustained by 69 normal children of the same age. The results of this study do not support the view that a particular fracture pattern renders the diagnosis of OI unlikely.

King J, Diefendorf D, Apthorp J, et al: Analysis of 429 fractures in 189 battered children. *J Pediatr Orthop* 1988;8:585–589.

This report remains the largest review of fractures in child abuse. Approximately 750 children seen at the Children's Hospital of Los Angeles between 1971 and 1981 were diagnosed by the courts or a Social Services team as victims of physical child abuse. Of these children, 189 had 429 fractures. Approximately half the children had a single fracture, usually transverse. The most commonly fractured bones were the humerus, femur, and tibia.

Kleinman PK, Belanger PL, Karellas A, et al: Normal metaphyseal radiologic variants not to be confused with findings of infant abuse. *Am J Roentgenol* 1991;156:781–783.

Postmortem high-detail skeletal radiography of 78 infants who died of the sudden infant syndrome was performed during a 3-year period. Review of the studies reveals a variety of distinct radiographic variants that should not be confused with the metaphyseal injuries caused by abuse of infants.

Kowal-Vern A, Paxton TP, Ros SP, et al: Fractures in the under–3-year-old age cohort. *Clin Pediatr* 1992;31:653–659.

Of 124 children younger than 3 years of age who were admitted with a fracture between 1984 and 1989 to Loyola University Medical Center, 29 were thought to be cases of child abuse. The determinations were based on inadequate explanation of injury, multiple injuries, presence of classic child abuse injuries, and physical findings inconsistent with history. Skull and rib fractures were the most common fractures in the defined child abuse cases.

Leventhal JM, Thomas SA, Rosenfield NS, et al: Fractures in young children: Distinguishing child abuse from unintentional injuries. *Am J Dis Child* 1993;147:87–92.

Each case was rated using predefined criteria assessed by two clinicians and two pediatric radiologists, who reached a consensus on a seven-point scale ranging from definite child abuse to definite unintentional injury. A total of 253 fractures were identified in 215 children, of which 24.2% were categorized as abuse, 8.4% as unknown, and 67.4% as unintentional injuries. Fractures that were considered likely due to abuse were (1) fractures in children whose caregivers reported either a change in the child's behavior, but noted no accidental event, or who reported only a minor fall, which elicited an injury that was more severe than might have been expected; (2) fractures of the radius/ulna, tibia/fibula, or femur in children younger than 1 year of age; or (3) midshaft or metaphyseal fractures of the humerus.

Loder RT, Bookout C: Fractures patterns in battered children. *J Orthop Trauma* 1991;5:428–433.

Cases of 75 battered children with fractures over a 2-year period were reviewed. The average age was 16 months; 57% were boys. There were 154 fractures (two per child); 77% were acute and 23% were old. The most common fracture occurred in the skull (32%), and the most common long bone fracture occurred in the tibia (16%). The most common long bone fracture pattern was transverse (41%); corner fractures accounted for 28% of long bone fractures. An isolated acute fracture was the orthopaedic injury in 65% of the children, whereas multiple fractures in various stages of healing were present in only 13% of children.

McMahon P, Grossman W, Gaffney M, et al: Soft-tissue injury as an indication of child abuse. *J Bone Joint Surg* 1995;77A:1179–1183.

Soft-tissue injuries were found in 92% of children suspected of being abused. Abuse should be especially suspected in children under 9 months with soft-tissue injury.

Thomas SA, Rosenfeld NS, Leventhal JM, et al: Long-bone fractures in young children: Distinguishing accidental injuries from child abuse. *Pediatrics* 1991;88: 471–476.

The medical records and radiographs of 215 children younger than 3 years of age with fractures during a 5-year period were retrospectively reviewed in an attempt to elucidate the mechanism of childhood fractures. Two clinicians (a pediatrician and senior medical student) and two pediatric radiologists rated the likelihood that the fracture was either accidental or due to child abuse. Long bone fractures were strongly associated with abuse. Fourteen children had fractures of the humerus. Eleven were considered to be the result of child abuse, and three, the result of accidents. The latter three were supracondylar elbow fractures in children who fell from a tricycle, a rocking horse, or down stairs. There were 25 femur fractures. Nine were found to be from abuse, 14 were found to be from accidents, and two could not be rated. Sixty percent of femur fractures in infants younger than 1 year of age were due to abuse. Although it is taught that femur fractures in young children are inflicted unless proven otherwise, in this study it was found that femur fractures often are accidental and that the femur can be fractured when the running child trips and falls.

Index

Page numbers in italics refer to figures or figure legends.